Cerebral Visual Impairment in Children

Josef Zihl • Gordon N. Dutton

Cerebral Visual Impairment in Children

Visuoperceptive and Visuocognitive Disorders

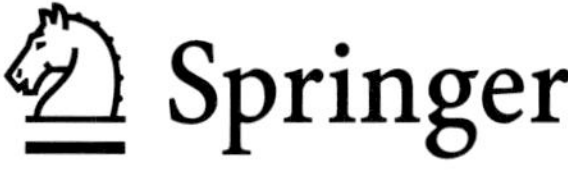

Josef Zihl
LMU Munich
Department of Psychology
München
Germany

Gordon N. Dutton
Department of Visual Science
Glasgow Caledonian University
Glasgow
UK

ISBN 978-3-7091-1924-2 ISBN 978-3-7091-1815-3 (eBook)
DOI 10.1007/978-3-7091-1815-3
Springer Wien Heidelberg New York Dordrecht London

Printed on acid-free paper

Springer is part of Springer Science+Business Media (www.springer.com)

Preface

Despite the heterogeneity of the umbrella term cerebral visual impairment (CVI) to denote visual dysfunction in early childhood that results from a wide range of developmental disorders and brain injuries, research on CVI and its translation into practice has undergone a remarkable transformation during the last 10 years. Not only are the differences between the developing and the developed brain and the patterns of visual dysfunction better understood, but the concepts concerning functional plasticity, particularly in the developmental phases of the brain, have also been empirically established. This remarkable progress has been possible due to the successful marriage between the so-called basic neuroscience disciplines and clinical neuroscience, including in particular (paediatric) neurology, neuro-ophthalmology and neuropsychology. Basic neuroscience has taken on board clinical knowledge, while clinical research has been guided by fundamental neuroscientific evidence. Consequently, both approaches have benefitted reciprocally and are now in a position to contribute significantly to assessment, diagnostic classification and intervention, founded upon a common evidence-based framework.

This book has primarily been written for all those who work with and for children with CVI: ophthalmologists, paediatric neurologists, psychologists, orthoptists, optometrists, occupational therapists, physiotherapists, speech therapists, teachers and many others. Thus, we have in essence chosen an interdisciplinary approach. This is salient because most children with CVI manifest additional functional impairments in the various domains of cognition, speech and language, motor activities, motivation and mood. Therefore, we deemed it appropriate to consider the accompanying nonvisual impairments, so as to ensure that diagnostic assessment is complete and that intervention procedures are tailor-made for the special combination of visual and nonvisual impairment patterns in each affected child. The use of a common professional language is a crucial prerequisite for successful and satisfactory co-operation between the different disciplines involved in the habilitation and education of children with CVI. We therefore have employed a language that is hopefully comprehensible to all professions (the glossary at the end of the book providing additional help).

We want to dedicate this book to all the children with CVI who have helped us to understand that their oft-times incomplete and sometimes confusing or even irritating visual worlds are nevertheless interesting and exciting ones that are worth identifying, characterising, explaining and acting upon.

Josef Zihl and Gordon N. Dutton thank the children and their parents for their agreed contributions in Chap. 6 (the anonymised report to parents) and Chap. 9 and Prof. Dr. Siegfried Priglinger for providing material for the latter chapter. Part of this book is based on the German monograph *Sehstörungen bei Kindern – visuoperzeptive und visuokognitive Störungen bei Kindern mit CVI* (*Visual disorders in children – Visuoperceptive und visuocognitive dysfunction in children with CVI*) by J. Zihl, K. Mendius, S. Schuett and S. Priglinger (Wien and New York, Springer, 2012), while GD wishes to thank Helen Krushave and Nicola McDowell for their major contributions to cases 7 and 8, respectively, in Chap. 9. JZ thanks Katharina Mendius and Susanne Schuett for their help with the literature used in the German monograph. Furthermore, JZ expresses his thanks to Walter Untermarzoner and his family in Villanders (South Tyrol, Italy), for their hospitality and for providing their wonderful alpine hut as a kind of writing office for this book, and to Sepp and Pia, for their generous care with excellent food and wine during his stay in this special retreat.

Both authors appreciate the care and support of Katrin Lenhart and Wilma McHugh from Springer in realising the publication of the book.

Munich, Germany — Josef Zihl
Glasgow, UK — Gordon N. Dutton

Contents

Introduction

1

Perception provides the means to access and engage with our physical and social environment and to learn through this process. It is essential for the acquisition of knowledge through short- and long-term experiences and for the guidance and control of our behaviour and movements. Perception comprises all activities involved in the recording, processing and coding of information, including cognitive (e.g. attention, memory, planning and supervision), motor (e.g. eye, hand, limb and body movements) and emotional components (e.g. affective evaluation). The neurobiological foundation of the range of perceptual functions and capacities comprises the peripheral (sense organs) and central nervous system components that are specialised to process, code and evaluate the information recorded and to make it accessible for further mental and behavioural activities. The integration of this myriad data set within respective brain structures constitutes a crucial prerequisite for temporally and spatially coherent perception, action and experience (Mather 2006; Goldstein 2010).

The different perceptual systems (vision, audition, taste, smell, the somatosensory system and sense of balance) possess similar neurobiological principles of construction. Stimuli are registered in the sensory organs, are translated into reliable neuronal codes and are transmitted to the central structures serving the respective sensory systems. Information processing and coding predominantly occurs in networked elements of the cerebral cortex. This guarantees detection, localisation and discrimination as well as the more complex capacities of identification, recognition and association, as well as storage of visual stimuli. Functional neuronal units in sensory cortical areas are specialised in processing and coding for specific pieces of sensory information. For example, the visual cortex possesses different areas for the analysis of colour, form, movement and spatial information (e.g. position, distance, direction) and for objects, faces, places and text material (letters, words and syntax). The auditory cortex contains areas specialised in processing and coding of sounds, pitch, music and speech. In the somatosensory cortex, various qualities of tactile, proprioceptive and kinaesthetic stimuli are processed and coded in separate areas (for comprehensive reviews, see Goldstein 2010; Yantis 2013). This so-called

J. Zihl, G.N. Dutton, *Cerebral Visual Impairment in Children: Visuoperceptive and Visuocognitive Disorders*, DOI 10.1007/978-3-7091-1815-3_1

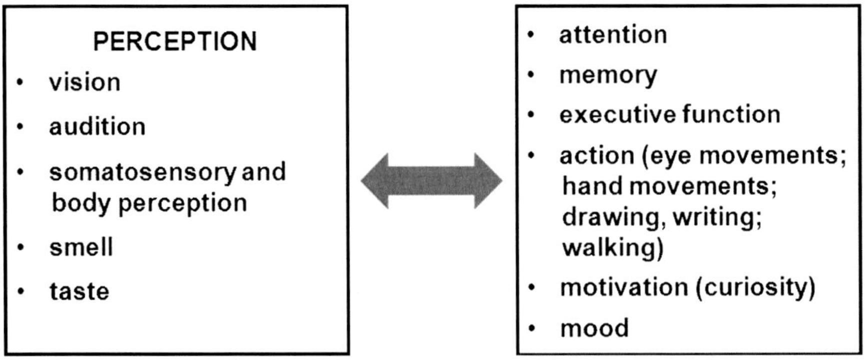

Fig. 1.1 A framework of mental functioning, where visual perception is embedded and interacting reciprocally

functional specialisation of the cerebral cortex enables the brain to process information (e.g. object features) in parallel and serial modes in one or in several sensory modalities, which are then integrated in consecutive steps to a uni- or multimodal percept. The final goal of visual development is to establish 'primary' visual perception, which integrates the active observer with subjective visual experience, i.e. perception is linked to a first-person perspective that mediates between conflicting visual information, on the one hand, and expectation and experience, on the other (Pollen 2011).

Perception does not operate in isolation, but is embedded in a network of mental functions. Figure 1.1 shows the various components of and interactions between the various components of this network. Attention, memory, executive function, motivation, mood and emotions as well as language and action have an impact on perception but are also reciprocally influenced by perception. These mutual interactions mean that disorders of perception are not only caused by direct disturbance of a specific perceptual system (so-called primary perceptual disorders) but can also result as a consequence of dysfunction of the other functional systems, because processes of stimulus registration, processing and encoding may be indirectly affected (so-called secondary disorders) and thereby impair perceptual ability and capacity. This concept applies particularly to the development of perceptual functions and capacities in early childhood. The normal development of perception relies crucially upon cognitive, motor, motivational and emotional components reaching the requisite milestones. A child will not explore the environment in the absence of adequate curiosity, nor will the child focus interest on and fixate a stimulus for detailed processing, identification and storage, without adequate attention. The child cannot gain experience with guidance and control of motor response and behaviour, nor develop and acquire action routines without perceptual learning and the requisite memory capacity. Moreover, perception is fundamental for the development of attention, memory, executive function, sensorimotor activities, language, motivation and emotion (see also Chaps. 3 and 5).

The brain is built of complex and highly developed networks, comprising many functional systems (see Table 1.1). Learning to interact with the physical and social world is mediated by experience, progressive optimisation of these systems/subsystems and their interactions and underpins successful development. Any disorder of brain development, either due to unfavourable congenital factors or to acquired impairment of normally developing or developed brain, can affect capacities in the various functional domains, either selectively or in combination, and disrupt or delay their further development.

The development of the central nervous system (CNS) takes place through generation of neurons (neurogenesis) to differentiation of the cerebral cortex, in relatively regulated steps (Sanes et al. 2006). In early childhood, the capacity of the CNS to adapt to changes of internal (i.e. processes and alterations in the brain) or external conditions (i.e. stimuli in the environment) is maximal; this facility is referred to as developmental (neuro)plasticity (Johnson 2001). Selection, optimisation and compensation, and their intermediary processes, have been considered to be fundamental components of the 'architecture' of human ontogeny, which is incomplete and thus allows flexible adaptation to internal and external changes to achieve and maintain a 'positive balance between gains and losses' throughout the life span (Baltes 1997, p. 366). To some extent, the child's brain possesses the potential of self-regulation and autonomy as it builds its intrinsic structure (Ryan et al. 1997) on which functional systems are based, in particular those concerned with coding and storing information, i.e. with gaining and learning from perceptual experience. As Black (1998, p. 168) has emphasised, many regions of the brain are 'responsive to experience' but differ with respect to their functional specialisation and the timing of their development. In addition, plasticity is 'typically embedded in a developmental programme' and requires appropriate timing and quality of sensory input. Experience-dependent plasticity in the visual cortex is at the same time also practice-dependent plasticity, which manifests particularly in so-called sensitive periods. During these periods, neural circuitries are formed, which at the physiological level are associated with receptor activation and inhibition. Transmitters (e.g. NMDA and GABA) play a crucial role in determining onset and closure of the time window of the sensitive period (Murphy et al. 2005). As a consequence, early visual deprivation, for example, arising from early bilateral congenital cataracts, can limit plasticity for 'recovery' of visual acuity and contrast sensitivity, and the age of treatment plays an important role, with early surgery affording the best outcome (Gelbart et al. 1982; Maurer et al. 2006).

An enriched, age-appropriate complex environment triggers and accelerates the morphological and functional maturation of the visual system, with maternal behaviour (or that of the first person of reference) representing and acting as a fundamental 'mediator' (van Praag et al. 2000; Baroncelli et al. 2010). Visual experience is also necessary for the maturation of multisensory neurons and the integration of multimodal spatial information, as well as the development of spatial cognition (Pasqualotto and Proulx 2012). Systematic and repeated perceptual learning results in specific and lasting improvements in lower (pattern orientation; Jehee et al. 2012) and higher (face and texture processing; Hussain et al. 2011)

Table 1.1 Functional systems and associated functions/capacities (A) and associated brain structures (B): a simplified overview

A. Functional systems

Perceptual systems

Vision: visual field, acuity and contras vision, form and shape perception, colour vision and visual space perception, including stereopsis, movement vision, visual recognition (objects, faces, letters, paths and places, etc.)

Audition: perception of sounds, voice, music and speech; spatial audition

Somatosensory perception: touch, proprioception, kinaesthesis; body perception

Olfactory perception: detection, discrimination and identification/recognition of smell stimuli

Gustatory perception: detection, discrimination and identification/recognition of gustatory stimuli

Social perception: identification/recognition of social stimuli in the various perceptual domains, particularly in vision and audition

Cognitive systems

Attention

Intensity: level and duration of maintenance of alertness; mental processing speed

Selectivity: focused attention (concentration), divided attention, attentional flexibility (attention regulation)

Spatial attention: shifts of attention in space; field of attention

Memory

Time dimension: short-term memory, working memory, long-term memory; prospective memory

Content dimension: episodic, semantic and procedural memory

Executive function

Cognition: planning, problem solving, flexibility, (self-)monitoring, multitasking

Behaviour: response inhibition, flexibility and control of (internally and externally triggered/guided) behaviour

Speech and language

Understanding and producing verbal language; reading and writing

Emotional and motivational systems

Emotions: feelings and mood and appropriate regulation

Motivation: activation and modulation of mental processes and behaviour and appropriate regulation

Sensorimotor or motor systems

Gross motor functions: body posture and control of body movements, including movements of legs (e.g. walking) and arm movements

Fine motor functions: hand movements (grasping and manipulating of objects)

Articulation: production of speech

Oculomotor functions: vergence, accommodation; saccades, pursuit movements, fixation

B. Brain structures	
Occipital lobe	Vision
Temporal lobe	Vision (visual identification and visual memory); language perception; verbal memory

(continued)

Table 1.1 (continued)

Parietal lobe	Space (visual and multimodal); visuomotor guidance (gaze, hand movements); somatosensory perception, body representation
Frontal lobe	Motor activities (planning, execution and control; praxis) Executive cognitive functions Regulation of motivation and emotional responses/mood adaptation processes (e.g. environment-intention)
Limbic system	Motivation, mood, emotional behaviour Memory Emotional evaluation of internal and external stimuli
Midbrain, brainstem	Alertness, attention (intensity)
Cerebellum	Motor activities (including cognitive adaption processes of motor responses)

visual as well as cognitive capacities (e.g. working memory; Jolles et al. 2012) not only in the adult but also in the young child. However, changes in neural circuitry can also occur after sensitive periods have ended and can, to a lesser degree, influence spatial and temporal integration modes in the visual cortex and contribute to further maturation of visual functions (Murphy et al. 2005). The final outcome of developmental regulation of associative learning in perception and cognition may be understood as a 'balance of plasticity and stability that is optimal for information processing and storage' (Dumas 2005, p. 189). Interestingly, periods of maximal learning capacity in brain development correspond to the behavioural development during the first year of life and are also paralleled with the degree of glucose metabolism within salient functional units. In the newborn, primary sensory and motor cortical structures, cingulate cortex, thalamus, brainstem, cerebellum (vermis) and hippocampi show the highest degree of glucose utilisation. At 2–3 months of age, glucose metabolism increases in the primary visual cortex, parietal and temporal cortex, basal ganglia and cerebellar hemispheres. In the first 4 years, the child's brain shows more than twice the glucose consumption of the adult brain; this high rate is maintained until about 10 years of age. At the age of 16–18 years, brain glucose metabolism gradually declines and eventually corresponds to adult values (Chugani 1998). Therefore, 'sensitive' periods in terms of brain maturation exist not only for perceptual systems but also for cognitive development in general (e.g. Gale et al. 2004), whereby 'biocultural' factors influence plasticity within different time scales (e.g. moment to moment and throughout the life span) and multiple neurobiological, cognitive, behavioural and sociocultural levels (Li 2003).

The elevated developmental sensitivity to internal and external changes can result in both positive and negative outcomes. Every disruption of the developmental process, either because of brain dysfunction disturbing self-regulation and autonomy or due to unfavourable environmental conditions, has morphological and/or physiological consequences, because plasticity, as an intrinsic property of the CNS, is always operating as internal and external factors change (Ryan et al. 1997; Nava and Roder 2011). Consequences of dynamic 'maladaptation' manifest themselves in delays or disruptions of functional development. It is important to note that ‘young is not always better’ in terms of neuroplasticity, as a factor in overcoming consequences of unfavourable conditions, but that the developing brain may also be more vulnerable than the adult brain in some respects (Giza and Prins 2006). Thus, brain plasticity and vulnerability may rather represent ‘extremes along a continuum’ of morphological and functional change (Anderson et al. 2011). This is an important fact, because it signifies that neuroplasticity continues to operate life-long. Although the window of critical periods for the development of particular brain functions may be almost closed, the larger door of brain plasticity may still remain (sufficiently wide) open and thus offer the opportunity to improve impaired brain functions in older childhood and even in adulthood (e.g. Baltes 1997; Li et al. 2006; Kolb et al. 2011; Kolb and Teskey 2012; Zihl et al. 2014). Thus, despite age-related decline of maximal learning capacity, residual plasticity can enhance functional efficiency by systematic practice beyond the sensitive period (Ostrovsky et al. 2006; Astle et al. 2011). Measures aimed at improving functional outcome levels after acquired brain injury in adults are contingent upon prior life experience (May 2011). However, developmental plasticity, and thus functional outcome of brain dysfunction, is set by the risk associated with the degree and extent of brain injury (severity, dimensions and topography of brain injury), the maturational state of the brain system involved, the integrity of brain structures belonging to the affected intra- and interhemispheric network(s) and associated medical conditions (e.g. epilepsy, medication). In addition, the outcome may be moderated by age at and time since the onset of brain dysfunction as well as the functional resources (‘reserve’) available within the child’s brain and by social environment (family, school and community) (Chugani et al. 1996; Dennis 2000).

In the following, some principles of development are presented in more detail, to aid understanding of the origin and classification of developmental disorders:

(a) *The child’s brain develops in close reciprocal interaction with the environment.* Brain development depends on the presence of adequate (specific) stimuli within both physical and social environments (Evans 2006). During sensitive periods, the brain is particularly ‘plastic’; the absence of an adequately stimulating environment can impair or disrupt development. The various functions and capacities of the visual system develop mainly in the first 2 years, while normal development of basic social functions develops during the first 3 years. For the development of language, the sensitive period seems to end after the fourth year, but further important developmental steps take place as far as the end of the 14th year (Cole and Cole 2001; see also Chaps. 2 and 3), while fundamental executive functions are not fully developed before the end of puberty (Jurado and Rosselli 2007). Of course, environmental stimuli are not only effective in the sensitive periods, as both favourable and unfavourable environmental factors influence development throughout the entire life span.

(b) *The developing brain possesses its maximum plasticity in early childhood.* Brain plasticity, understood as the capacity to adapt to normal and pathological conditions either in the environment or within the organism, or in both, seems to be maximal in early childhood, although it is preserved and is therefore available throughout life (Baltes 1997; Li et al. 2006; Zihl et al. 2014). Congenital and acquired brain dysfunction can cause transient but also persistent, chronic effects. In addition, a child with persistent dysfunction not only has to cope with the consequences of congenital or early-acquired brain dysfunction but has also to manage the effects upon development of the spared (intact) functions and capacities. According to Grafman (2000), several possibilities exist for the reorganisation of an injured brain. (1) The function in question is relocated to a homologous cortical area, which can, however, be associated with so-called crowding effects in the same area. For example, after injury to left hemisphere structures that are crucial for language, language development may take place in homologous right hemisphere structures. This relocation can impair or even disrupt the development of the function/capacity originally destined for this structure, i.e. spatial capacities, while verbal capacities show good recovery (Chiricozzi et al. 2005). (2) In the case of missing visual input, respective cortical areas can instead process information from another (e.g. auditory or tactile) sensory modality. It is, for example, known that subjects with congenital blindness process Braille letter information in the visual cortex using a retinotopically specific reorganisation of visual cortical areas (Cheung et al. 2009), which is associated with higher activation in early- than in late-onset blindness (Sadato et al. 1998; Wittenberg et al 2004). In addition, in children with congenital blindness, visual cortical areas can also participate in 'high-level' cognitive functions, including processing of language by 'finger reading' (Gizewski et al. 2003; Bedny and Saxe 2012). (3) Cortical areas can be expanded in size by systematic practice. Representational plasticity has particularly been demonstrated in the auditory (Pantev et al. 2003) and the somatosensory systems (Xerri et al. 1999). (4) Injured cortical areas can be supported by intact areas serving the same or a similar function or capacity or by bypassing of information through alternative afferent pathways. In early injury to the striate cortex, expansion of visual association areas may be larger than in adulthood, or visual input can reach extrastriate visual areas via thalamo-cortical afferents that bypass striate cortex (Guzzetta et al. 2010). However, processes of plasticity available in the (very) young brain may not operate with the same efficacy as in later stages of development with respect to reorganisation of the visual, sensorimotor and language systems (Cioni et al. 2011). Another possibility is enhancement of processing efficacy and thus improvement of perceptual performance in another modality; e.g. early (but not late) blindness can enhance auditory perception (Wan et al. 2010). There is cogent fMRI evidence that the facility of echolocation that develops or can be trained as a substitute for visual perception and navigation is served in the occipital lobes (Thaler et al. 2011) and middle temporal lobes with analogous anatomical and functional specialisation (Arnott et al. 2013). Finally, under certain conditions, limited neurogenesis seems possible (Quadrato and Di Giovanni 2013) although the significance of this phenomenon is far from clear in humans.

(c) *The development of the brain and also of mental functions is dynamic in nature and proceeds in phases at intra- and interindividually differing rates.*

The development of the brain and thus of mental functions does not proceed in a linear fashion. The complex interaction between genes, maturation and environmental stimulation becomes manifest in gradual, discrete and discontinuous courses, which differ between functional systems and individuals. This lack of homogeneity poses a great challenge for the diagnostics of functional profiles and their courses. Furthermore, specific developmental stages of interaction and integration are required in each period of development because the individual steps are, at least in part, subsequently built upon one another. Every functional system, i.e. perception, attention, memory, executive function, language, action, motivation and emotion, which is unable to supply its particular contribution to the development in its respective period, and each internal and external factor that diminishes this contribution can delay or disrupt the normal course of development. Depending on the extent of the CNS dysfunction, a global delay or impairment in specific development can result, occurring either in isolation or in combination with other functional brain disorders.

(d) *An age-specific interplay exists between cognitive, emotional and social functions, with the networked character of information exchange being the relevant feature.*
Progress in all phases of development is intrinsically tied to motivation to gain information (curiosity), motor activities (intentional actions) and their repetition and responses to the diversity of environmental stimuli. The network character of processing and coding of information is therefore of special significance. Behaviour mirrors the cooperation of diverse cognitive, motivational, emotional and social functions and represents the interplay of different functional systems in terms of a final common pathway product. Whether or not any of these processes in any of the involved networks manifest alongside this common pathway can dictate the final outcome and lead to the display of behavioural abnormalities. The diagnostic classification of such behavioural abnormalities sometimes poses a major challenge, especially on account of the reciprocal cross-linking of mental functions. The resulting impairments are to be expected in more than one domain (see Chap. 5).

Developmental plasticity can be understood in terms of specific *and* universal learning capacity; this capacity does not seem, however, to be unlimited. One major reason for such limitation is the association of dysfunctions caused by congenital and acquired conditions of the CNS. As a rule, several functional systems are affected in their development, among them, motivation and curiosity, respectively, as well as attention and executive functions, i.e. systems that are crucial for flexible adaptation to the consequences of CNS dysfunction. For visual disorders, particularly those acquired in early childhood, comprehensive assessment of dysfunction in other domains is therefore necessary. A complete diagnostic evaluation is required to characterise both negative and positive functional patterns relating to the developmental stage of the child. On the basis of the patterns elicited, appropriate tailor-made intervention measures can be applied and delivered. These measures should help to reduce the degree of specific (and non-specific) dysfunction and thus the severity of disability, so that the child has a better chance to use all resources and means available to enhance development. As a final outcome, the aspiration is for the child to ultimately attain maximal independence in a fruitful and fulfilling adult life.

When specific functions are impaired, the combination of specific interventions with non-specific more holistic measures is required for optimal habilitation. Customised specific measures are framed within global intervention measures to enhance attention, curiosity, motivation and intent. This approach consisting of an ingenious combination of functional specialisation and integration and of differentiation and interaction of processes and activities fulfils the principles of construction and functional organisation of the CNS. Knowledge, understanding and implementation of these principles should constitute the guiding headline for all measures and activities of intervention and facilitation of the child's development.

Habilitative and therapeutic action should thus always be guided by systematic and critical analysis and self-reflection of our personal experiences in the framework of valid expert knowledge and empirical evidence; this attitude is also helpful in coping with the responsibility for our therapeutic actions and procedures. In the case of children with cerebral visual disorders, our diagnostic and therapeutic actions and procedures should be based on and guided by the neurobiological and neuropsychological concepts of vision and visual perception, which consider the modes of operation of the peripheral and central visual systems, as well as their development and interaction with other functional domains. Because many children with cerebral visual disorders suffer from additional cognitive, motor and motivational difficulties (see Chap. 5), the planned integration of the various interventional measures, particularly in very young children, is a crucial prerequisite for their optimal efficacy. Therefore, only shared, coordinated concepts and procedures contributed by the range of experts and professions in the field, with well-informed parental engagement, will eventually guarantee success in the complex and often complicated interventions required for the visually impaired child, for whom a critical issue is to ensure that all elements of every approach used, fall well within each of the predetermined day-to-day perceptual limitations (see Chap. 5).

Measures of intervention are, in general, ideally aimed at interacting directly with functional impairments to achieve an effective reduction of each and every disability. Such measures imply specific and systematic intervention procedures. However, if such measures cannot be applied because of the severity of the functional impairments, or if they are no longer effective, resulting in the aim of intervention not being achieved, then pragmatically orientated measures are sensible and appropriate. Such conditions include very low vision with low curiosity and interest in the visual world, or the perceptual world in general, or very low levels of attention in terms of alertness to maintain a critical minimum of attention over time, in order to process and store visual information and experience (see Chaps. 7 and 8).

2 Development and Neurobiological Foundations of Visual Perception

2.1 Visual and Oculomotor Functions and Their Significance for Visual Perception

The main foundations of the various perceptual capacities are built on peripheral (sense organs) and central components of the sensory systems, particularly in the cerebral cortex, which are specialised in the analysis and coding of sensory information, translating the outcome into experience, and making it accessible for use. Figure 2.1 shows a schematic sketch of the brain with the cortical structures relevant for vision, audition, body perception, language, and motor action. The integration of processed information and synthesis of the segregated outputs are essential prerequisites for coherent perception, experience and action (Goldstein 2010; Yantis 2013). A great deal of information about the environment is of a visual nature, i.e. the world within our brains is a predominantly visual one. The prominent role of the visual modality is, however, not only limited to perception. Major elements of experiences, memories and conceptions concerning the external world are based on vision, as are language (e.g. object labels), emotional experiences, and gross (e.g. walking) and fine motor actions (e.g. hand and finger movements). Finally, human curiosity, particularly in more distant space, i.e. beyond the space of grasp and touch, is mainly directed toward visual aspects of the surroundings. Children with cerebral visual disorders are therefore confronted with the very special condition of coping with a world that they can encompass only in part and with great effort, often without access to detailed prior visual experience and knowledge.

According to the level of complexity, perceptual capacities can be classified as "lower" and "higher" visual capacities; another principle of classification refers to the type of visual information and material, which is processed. "Lower" or elementary visual capacities comprise the visual field, visual light and dark adaptation, visual acuity and spatial contrast sensitivity, colour vision, and spatial vision (localisation, distance and direction perception, monocular and binocular depth perception, including stereopsis). "Higher" or more complex visual capacities include visual identification and recognition, topological and geographical orientation, and text and number

J. Zihl, G.N. Dutton, *Cerebral Visual Impairment in Children: Visuoperceptive and Visuocognitive Disorders*, DOI 10.1007/978-3-7091-1815-3_2

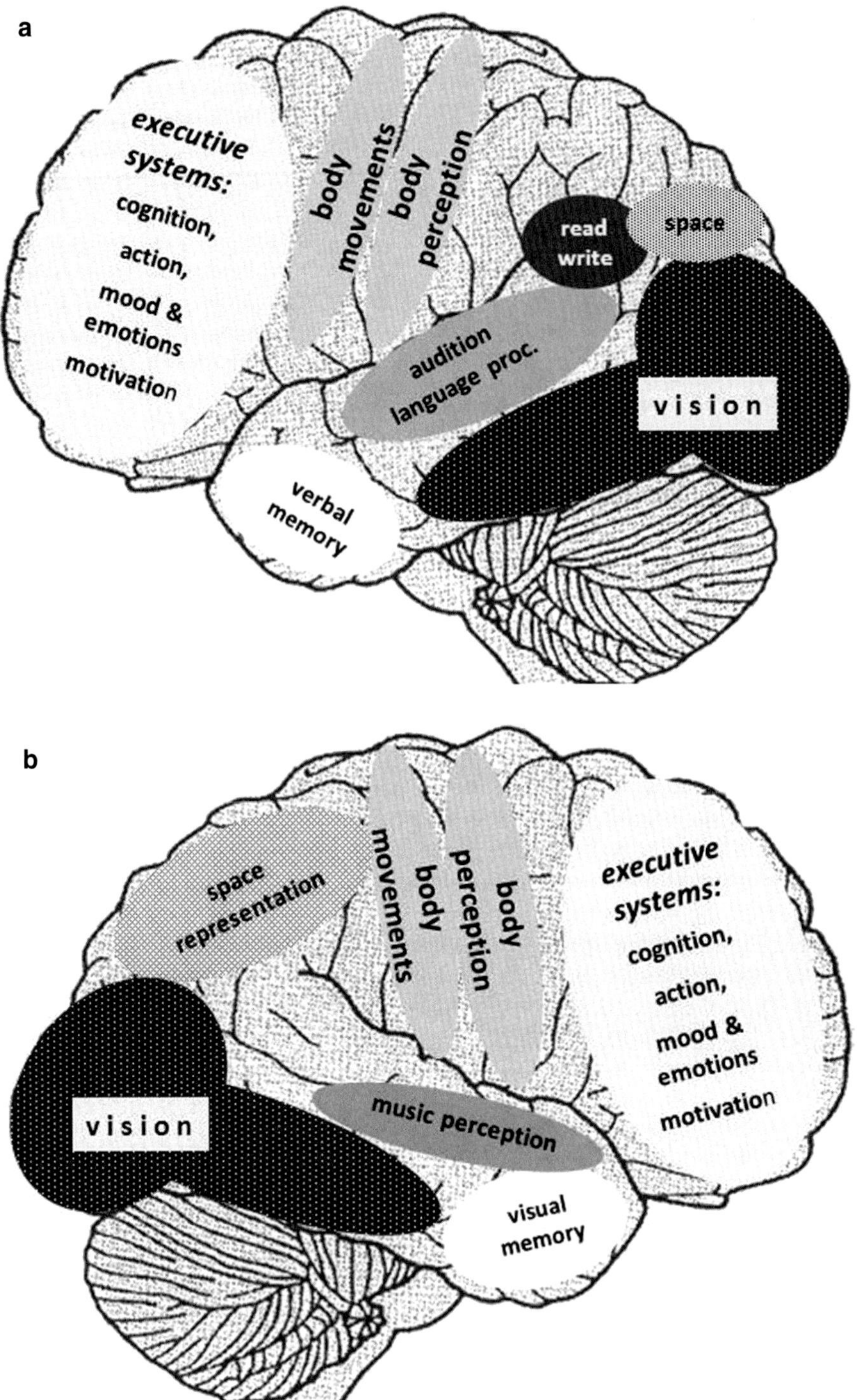

Fig. 2.1 Schematic sketches of the brain showing the regions specialised for various mental functions. (**a**) the left side of the brain. (**b**) the right side of the brain

processing. Moment-to-moment visual mapping of the surrounding environment provides both the substrate for visual search and the principal means of bringing about guidance of movement through our surroundings (Goodale 2011). The various visual capacities are built on the availability and interplay of several visual functions, with varying degrees of involvement of cognition, which make them visual-cognitive abilities, but nevertheless represent genuine visual functions at different levels of organisation.

The visual system can be characterised as a sequence of structures and functions, which transform physical light stimuli into neuronal signals and process them at successively higher levels of organisation. At the most basic level, the visual system operates as an optical measuring system, comprising components that focus optical stimuli as images onto the retina of the left and right eyes with the help of the adaptation system, for mapping the image on corresponding retinal locations so that the two monocular images meld into one image with the help of the vergence system. Accommodation and vergence are coupled: in far vision, both lines of sight are in parallel, i.e. vergence is close to zero, while in near vision vergence increases as well as accommodation. The two retinal images are finally fused in the visual cortex to a coherent percept; the small disparity between the two retinal images is in addition used for finely graduated stereoscopic acuity and stereopsis.

The mobility of the eyes allows a more accurate inspection of objects and their details, respectively, by precise and accurate fixation. Mechanisms in the brain stem, the mid brain and the thalamus and in the cortex are involved in the guidance and control of eye movements, so that we can fixate stationary and moving visual stimuli (Fig. 2.2). Disorders of eye movements can therefore impair visual information processing and thus visual perception, either because oculomotor scanning and fixation shifts in space are impaired or because precise fixation of stimuli for further fine analysis becomes difficult if not impossible. The visual system and the oculomotor systems are intimately connected with each other, and have to co-operate closely to enable fast and reliable visual information processing.

Cognition, in particular, attention and executive functions, and motivation are also involved in visual perception and contribute to the reliability and efficiency of the visual system (see Chap. 3). The close temporal and spatial interplay of the visual system with cognitive, and eye and head movement systems, guarantee high speed, reliable visual information processing and coding even in complex visual task conditions in daily living activities. Table 2.1 shows essential prerequisites for the reliable representation of the visual world in the brain.

In summary, the various functions and capacities of visual perception can hardly be reliably separated from each other, either because they are based on each other (e.g. visual acuity on accommodation; detection and spatial localisation of stimuli on visual field extent; visual identification and recognition, on colour, form, size and shape processing), or they depend on each other (e.g. fixation of stimuli and spatial localisation; visual acuity and fixation accuracy, and vice versa). Any classification of visual functions and capacities is, therefore somehow artificial, but is helpful to denote and define the particular functions and capacities described, and to better explain and understand the interplay between them. Table 2.2 contains a compilation of the visual and oculomotor functions and capacities and their

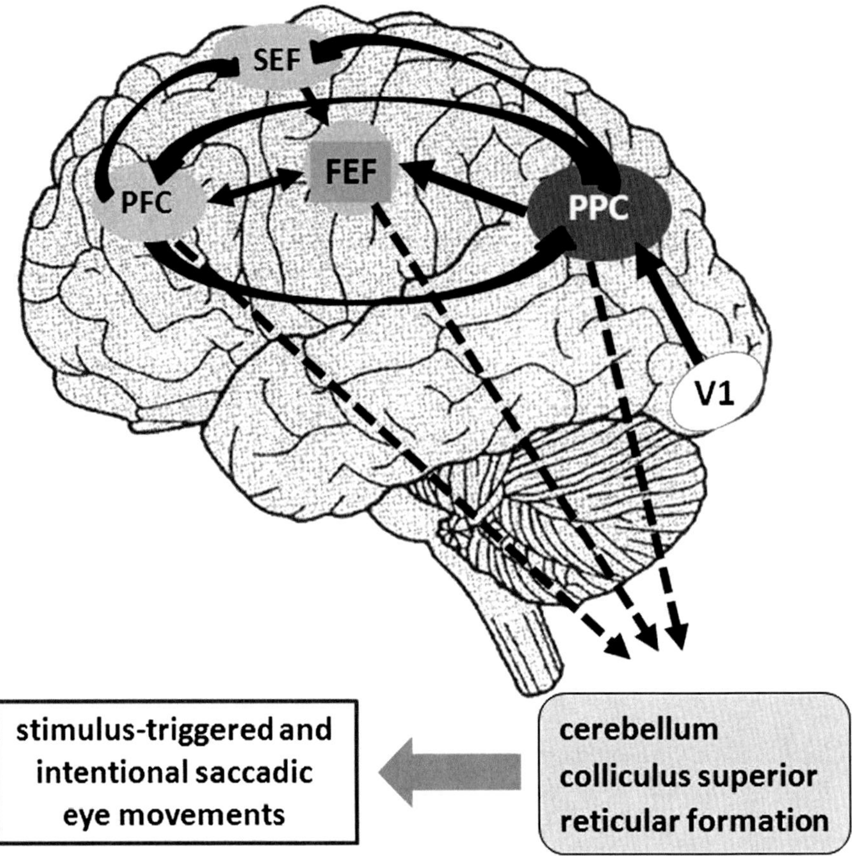

Fig. 2.2 Schematic sketch of CNS structures involved in the guidance of saccadic eye movements. *PFC* pre-frontal cortex, *FEF* frontal eye fields, *SEF* supplementary eye field, *PC* posterior parietal cortex, *V1* the visual cortex (Modified after Pierrot-Deseilligny et al. 1995)

Table 2.1 Prerequisites for an accurate and reliable representation of the visual world in the brain

Adequate differential sensitivity for visual stimulus dimensions and characteristics (resolution, brightness, shades of grey, colour, hue, size, form, orientation, position, depth, direction, etc.);
Selection of features for discrimination and identification (recognition) of complex stimuli (objects, faces, scenes, text information), including parallel and serial synthesis of single features to a whole;
Coding and storing of visual stimuli and their characteristic features in visual memory that are relevant for further identification and recognition;
Identification/recognition of complex visual stimuli despite differing conditions ´(visual constancy capacities)
Association with additional important information (use, denomination, episodic context, past experience)
Temporary storage of processed visual information until discrimination, identification, recognition and associations are complete (visual working memory)
Long term storage of processed visual information (visual long-term memory)

Table 2.2 Summary of visual sensory and oculomotor functions and capacities and their significance in the context of visual perception

Visual field	Overview; detection and localisation of stimuli; parallel processing of spatially distributed stimuli ("simultaneous perception"); hazard detection; guidance of movement
Spatial contrast sensitivity	Spatial resolution of contours and form elements; visual acuity, stereoacuity
Visual acuity	Form vision, stereoacuity, text processing
Colour vision	Object identification and recognition
Form vision	Object, face, and scene perception; text processing
Space perception	Localisation, distance and direction perception, monocular and binocular (stereopsis) depth perception; topographical orientation
Object perception	Identification and recognition of objects of different categories
Face perception	Identification and recognition of (familiar) faces, including age, gender and facial expression
Accommodation	Contrast sensitivity, visual acuity, stereoacuity, form vision
Vergence	Binocular vision, visual acuity, stereopsis
Saccades	Transport of the fovea to targets; scanning of objects, scenes, and text material
Smooth pursuit eye movements	Fixation of a moving target
OKN	Stabilisation of visual perception by resetting the eyes during prolonged movement of the surrounding and Direct gaze toward oncoming visual stimuli
VOR	Stabilisation of visual perception during body motion

OKN optokinetic nystagmus, *VOR* vestibulo-ocular reflex

respective functional significance. "Function" refers to basic components of vision. They subserve but do not represent genuine visual-perceptual capacities. Such functions include, for example, oculomotor components, visual adaptation, and contrast sensitivity. "Visual capacities" refer to components of visual perception that support more complex visual abilities, (e.g. visual acuity for form vision, form vision for object and face perception).

2.2 Neurobiological Foundations of Vision

The neurobiological foundation of visual perception is mainly in the retina and geniculo-striate pathway (optic tract, optic radiation), and the striate cortex, which is located in the posterior brain (occipital cortex). The visual cortex consists of the primary visual cortical area (striate cortex, Brodmann area [BA] 17, V1) and the so-called extrastriate or visual association cortex, which consists of more than 30 areas that differ with respect to the processing and coding properties of their neurons, and their connections with other visual and non-visual areas. These 'higher-order' visual areas process and code the various dimensions of visual information, e.g. brightness, contour, orientation, form, colour, motion, spatial attributes (position, distance, direction, etc.), and complex visual stimuli, e.g. objects, faces, and places and routes (landmarks) (Goldstein 2010; Yantis 2013; Zihl 2014). The central visual system – like other central sensory systems – shows parallel organisation with hierarchical components. This organisation principle is known as "functional segregation" or "functional specialisation" (e.g. Zeki 1993; Cowey 1994; Rainer and Logothetis 2003; Grill-Spector and Malach 2004), which increases over the course of development (Dobkins 2009). This model implies parallel and serial processing and coding in terms of division of labour, i.e. each area is more or less specialised for the processing and coding of a particular visual stimulus dimension; the aggregated organisation is based on parallel and serial processing modes. The various visual areas are reciprocally interconnected; exchange of information and thus interaction is possible in bottom-up (stimulus-driven) and top-down (intention-driven) directions. Within the extrastriate visual cortex, prominent processing pathways have been identified, which are either specialised in processing and coding spatial information (the occipital-parietal or WHERE-pathway) or object properties (the ventral, occipito-temporal, or WHAT pathway) (Desimone and Ungerleider 1989). This two-route model of visual spatial and visual object information processing has been converted into a two-route model of visual action (dorsal route) and visual perception (ventral route) (Goodale and Westwood 2004; Milner and Goodale 2006, 2008; Goodale and Milner 2010). Although there is some neuropsychological evidence for dissociation of either visual- spatial/visual object processing and visual-action/visual-perceptual deficits after injury to the ventral and dorsal route, respectively, both models may be too simplistic to explain visual perception as a coherent, integrated outcome of processing and coding (Schenk 2006; Schenk and McIntosh 2010; De Haan and Cowey 2011). In particular, the interplay between visual areas and both global and local integration of the various pieces of information into a coherent percept as a whole, and the various parallel and serial convergent and divergent processes within and between the two routes, which allow the processing of a large amount of information within a given time window and in the actual context of perception, intention and action, cannot be fully explained by either model. Co-operation and interaction between the two streams and other components of a distributed network involving also posterior and inferior parietal and prefrontal structures guarantee spatial and temporal coherence of processing of visual information via attention and working memory, also subserving visually guided action and spatial navigation (Goodale and Westwood 2004; Konen and Kastner 2008; Singh-Curry and Husain 2009; Kravits et al. 2011). The dual route model of cortical visual processing in terms of WHERE (dorsal route) and WHAT (ventral route) is still used in the literature and there is evidence, that in the context of focal brain pathology affecting these brain areas this model offers some sense and utility (e.g. Dutton and Jacobson 2001; Dutton 2009; Klaver et al. 2011). For the sake of simplicity, we too refer to this model in the context of describing behavioural manifestations of damage to the visual brain without implying that it exhaustively explains visual perceptual disorders.

Interestingly, early clinical and pathological anatomy observations are in support of the functional specialisation model of the visual brain because of selective loss of single visual capacities, for example, colour vision, visual space perception, and visual recognition (Zeki 1993; Kanwisher 2010; Barton 2011; Zihl 2011). In addition, the visual brain is able to identify and recognise visual stimuli despite changes in their appearance, and thus in the images produced on the retina, concerning, for example, brightness, colour, shape, orientation, location, and perspective of the observer. This capacity is called visual perceptual constancy, and is part of visual concept learning, which requires perceptual organisation and is based on bottom-up and top-down processes (Quinn and Bhatt 2001, 2009). It plays an important role in the adjustment of the visual system to the perception of an object or object property as constant even though our sensation changes (Goldstein 2010; Yantis 2013), and depends on occipito-temporal (ventral) structures (Turnbull et al. 1997; Goldstein 2010; Yantis 2013). For the sake of simplicity, we refer also to this model without implying that it too exhaustively explains visual perception.

Visual information is transmitted from the retina via the optic nerves, lateral geniculate bodies, optic tracts and optic radiations to the primary visual cortices (V1), from where it is distributed to areas in the visual association cortices (extrastriate visual areas) for further processing (Fig. 2.3). As already mentioned, these visual areas are specialised for the processing and coding of visual stimulus dimensions, for example, colour, form and shape, motion, and spatial aspects (location, distance, direction, and depth). Brain imaging studies in healthy subjects have confirmed the model of functional specialisation of the visual cortex, and have also added additional empirical evidence for the dual-route processing model, showing that processing of spatial information is associated with more dorsal activation, while processing of object properties, objects and faces, etc. is associated with more ventral activation (Corbetta et al. 1991, 1993; Tootell et al. 1996; Kravits et al. 2011; Sewards 2011). Disturbance of one of these areas causes selective loss of the respective visual capacity; thereby visual spatial impairments are typically associated with dorsal injury, while impairments in the perception of colour, shape, objects and faces are associated with ventral injury (Kanwisher 2010; Zihl 2011; see also Sect. 4.3).

The striate cortex, and extrastriate visual areas are topographically organised, i.e. they possess a representation of the visual field. This topography is very precise in V1, where the central 15° of visual field cover around 37 % of the striate cortex (Wong and Sharpe 1999), and is characterised by high topographical precision, such that a definite retinal position (central visual field) or area (peripheral visual field) corresponds to a definite cortical position or area in V1, that correlates with the diameter of the receptive fields of neurons (Daniel and Whitteridge 1961; Wandell et al. 2007; Benson et al. 2012). The fovea comprises 0.5° on either side of the centre of the visual field (total diameter: 1°), while the macula extends to a radius of 4.5° (total diameter: 9°). There is still no accepted definition on the diameter of the fovea, which according to various authors varies between 0.8 and 2° of visual angle. There is convincing evidence that the central 0.5° of the visual field is represented in both striate cortices; this explains foveal sparing even after total destruction of one striate cortex (Huber 1962; Bunt et al. 1977; Sharpe et al. 1979; Horton and Hoyd 1991). The topographical representations of the visual field in extrastriate visual areas become more and more imprecise, i.e. receptive fields become larger and larger, and eventually cover one quadrant or one hemifield, and may even extend

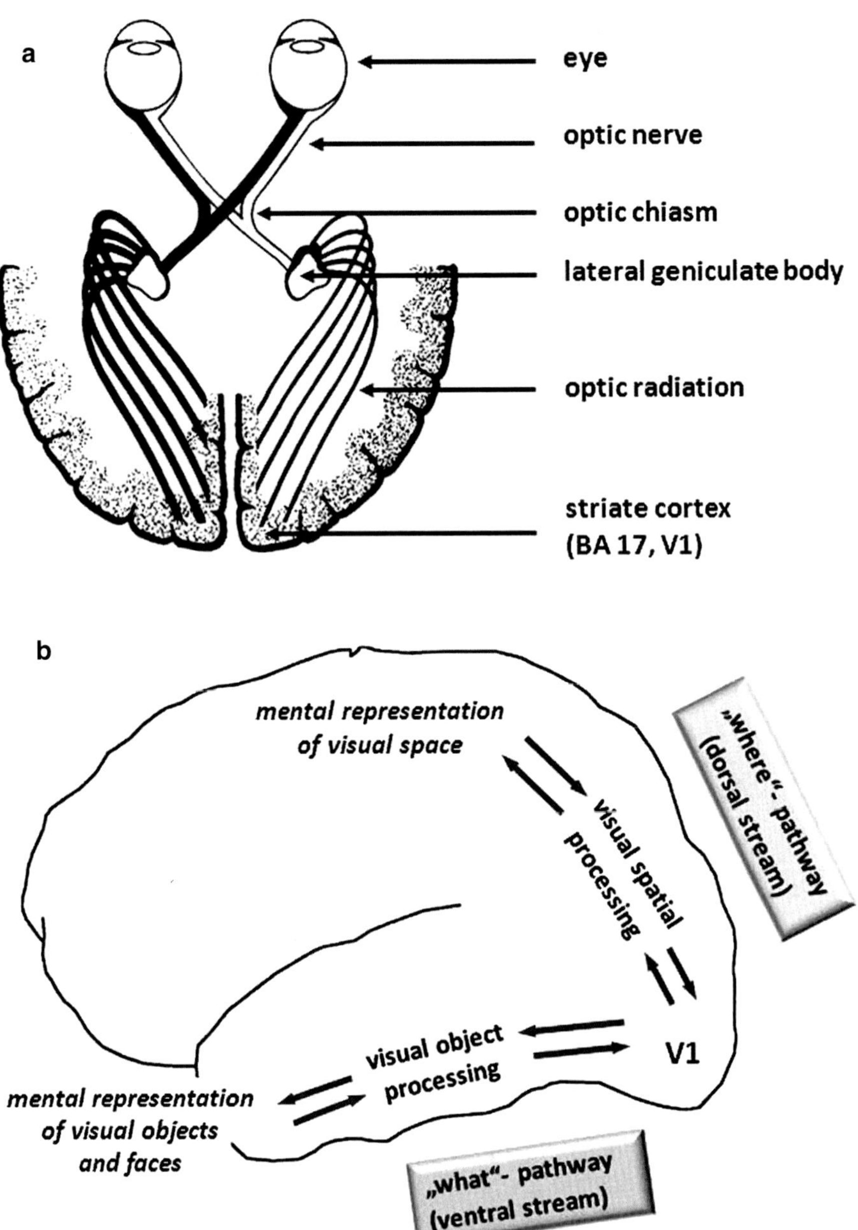

Fig. 2.3 (**a**) The visual afferent system from the eye to the striate cortex and (**b**) Routes of visual processing (After Ungerleider and Mishkin 1982, and Milner and Goodale 2006; modified after Zihl 2011). BA 17: Brodmann area 17 (striate cortex, V1)

into the other visual hemifield, whereby the magnification factor decreases with eccentricity but remains constant in extrastriate visual areas when related to striate cortex conditions (Dumoulin and Wandell 2008; Harvey and Dumoulin 2011). Top-down (executive, attentional, motivational and emotional) influences modulate selection of particular inputs to visual cortical neurons and enable them to "assume different functional states according to the task being executed", in an adaptive way by means of feedback pathways (Gilbert and Li 2013, p. 350).

2.3 Development of Vision and of Its Neurobiological Foundations

To a major extent, vision is a skill that depends on learning and use, just as other skills such as walking or talking. The development of vision is characterised by a more or less regular sequence. Periods of morphological development are paralleled or followed by functional development, mostly influenced and guided by environmental factors, i.e. the disposition and nature of visual stimuli. While the auditory system already shows an advanced functional developmental stage at birth, the visual system primarily commences its functional development after birth. In the first months, a baby shows rapid development in nearly all visual functions and capacities, although visual acuity and visual contrast sensitivity at distance still need months and even years to fully develop (Granrud 1993; Slater 1998a, b; Atkinson 2000; Braddick and Atkinson 2011). Table 2.3 summarises the normal development of visual and oculomotor functions and capacities in the first year.

The development of the visual system also depends on the stage of maturation of the eye, and takes place in serial steps (Banks and Shannon 1993; Candy 2006; Iliescu and Dannemiller 2008). The critical period of development of the eye and particularly the retina occurs between the second and fourth month of pregnancy. The differentiation of the cellular retinal elements starts in the central retina, the fovea; the ganglion cells develop before the receptors. In the sixth month the eye lids open for the first time and the macula, the inner part of the retina (diameter: 10°) begins to differentiate; this process is completed several months after birth. At the time of birth particularly the receptors in the fovea are wide, have not reached their final density, and need visual stimuli for their functional refinement (Tian and Copenhagen 2003). This fact explains the poor visual acuity in this period of early childhood, which is about 10–30 times lower than that of an adult. At the end of the first year the development of the retina is nearly complete; however, smaller morphological changes can still be observed till the end of the fourth year. It is important to note that the development of visual spatial (and temporal) resolution of the visual system is tightly coupled with the development of the oculomotor system, in particular pupil movement, accommodation, and vergence (Schor 1985; Charman and Voisin 1993; Charman 2004).

The brain structures involved in visual information processing begin their development by weeks 13–15 of gestation (Chi et al. 1977; Table 2.4). The visual midbrain (lateral geniculate body, LGB) and the primary visual cortex (striate cortex, V1) develop rapidly; the thickness of the striate cortex and the number of interneurons and fibre connections within and between areas in the visual cortex, and between these areas and other structures of the brain increase. Visual modularity also increases over the course of development (Dobkins 2009), but development

Table 2.3 Development of visual and oculomotor functions and capacities

Age	Functions/capacities
Birth	Blinks (rapid closing and opening of the eye lids)
	Slow pupil responses to day light
	Very limited accommodation
	Visual acuity ~ 20/150
	Responses to light, motion, and colour
	Oculomotor scanning of the visual environment in ~ 5–10 % of waking time
	Oculomotor scanning and searching movements for e.g. Light stimuli or contours within a radius of about 45°
M 1–2	Threshold for light detection decreases, visual acuity increases
	Oculomotor scanning and searching eye movements within a radius of 60–90°
	Increase in precision of smooth pursuit eye movements
	Incipient binocular vision starting at about 6 weeks
M 2–4	Increase in accommodation power
	Conjugate eye movements in all directions
	Eyelids close when stimuli (e.g. hand movements) appear suddenly before the eyes
	Oculomotor scanning of the visual environment in ~ 30–40 % of waking time
	Oculomotor scanning and searching eye movements within a radius of 180°
	Baby observes his own hand(s) when manipulating objects
	Baby shows defense reactions for objects approaching in collision course
M 4–6	Visual acuity increases further
	Binocular vision is established
	Visual identification/recognition of particular objects and faces/persons possible
M 6–12	Visual acuity is 20/100
	Baby avoids visual depth

Modified after Reinis and Goldman (1980)
M month of life

Tables 2.4 Temporal development of regional brain structures

Lobe	Gestational age (weeks)	Sulci/fissures	Gyri
Occipital	10–27	Calcarine fissure; parieto-occipital and lateral; occipital sulci	Superior and inferior occipital gyri; lingual gyrus cuneus; occipito-temporal gyrus
Parietal	10–26	Parieto-occipital fissure; interparietal sulcus; interhemispheric fissure; Rolandic and postrolandic sulci	Superior, middle, inferior parietal lobules; angular and supramarginal gyrus; cingulate and postrolandic gyri
Temporal	14–30	Sylvian fissure; superior, middle and inferior temporal sulci	Superior, middle, inferior temporal gyrus; fusiform gyrus; parahippocampal gyrus
Frontal	10–28	Superior and inferior frontal sulcus; cingulate sulcus; olfactory sulcus	Superior, middle, anterior gyri; insula; cingulate gyrus

Modified after Chi et al. (1977)

of visual cortical areas depends on stimulus-specific visual experience (Quin et al. 2013). The two main visual information processing pathways in the brain show different developmental timing. The ventral (i.e. occipito-temporal) visual pathway shows prolonged development and appear less "plastic" compared to the dorsal (i.e. occipito-parietal) visual pathway; in contrast, fibre connections within the ventral pathway mature earlier (Klaver et al. 2011; Dormal et al. 2012). The morphological development of the visual brain is the crucial basis for the functional development of the various substructures, and their co-operativity, as well as their connectivity with other functional systems, for example the attention, memory, executive and motivation and reward systems. Learning by selection is a fundamental principle in visual development; it depends on an efficient attentional mechanism for information processing (Amso and Johnson 2006). Attention also plays an important role in recognition memory development during early childhood (Rose et al. 2001); it modulates active vision in (spatial) selection and processing, but also in coding and representation of visual information (Berman and Colby 2009). Emotional evaluation of visual stimuli supports vision by enhancing selection of stimuli, based on the affective impact of past visual sensation and experience (Barrett and Bar 2009). 'Affective learning', i.e. repeated systematic experience with task-relevant affective information, for example, colours or faces, not only modulates visual association cortical areas and connected prefrontal structures, but also enhances response activity and functional connectivity within the primary visual cortex (Damaraju et al. 2009) indicating that stimulus-emotion associations are powerful learning conditions even at low-level visual processing stages. Interestingly, facial expression ("emotional faces") in particular captures attention, i.e. children preferentially direct spatial attention in the direction of such faces (Elam et al. 2010).

It appears that the prenatal development of the visual system occurs at a basic level without visual stimulation and associated experience. In contrast, the postnatal development of the visual system is both, environment- and practice-dependent; it is environment and action – "anticipatory". Early visual experience is required for further development of the structures and functions of the visual system to make use of the visual information provided by the environment, and to develop the necessary adjustments to this visual environment (Berardi et al. 2000; Maurer et al. 2008; Lewis and Maurer 2009). This principle applies also to the development of the so-called receptive fields, i.e. the region of the visual field that is covered by a neuron, in which a stimulus can elicit the best response of this neuron, regarding its size as well as its specialisation of processing, and coding properties, and its interactions. Monocular visual deprivation, for example, caused by improper alignment of the eyes (known as strabismus, squint, or heterotropia), or anisometropia (a greater refractive error developing in one eye), causing amblyopia is associated with underdevelopment of the corresponding visual cortex: the number of functionally intact neurons decreases, the receptive fields do not fully develop or can shrink, and neurons do not arrive at the normally occurring high degree of specialisation in processing and coding of the finer details of visual patterns (Bi et al. 2011). Similarly, bilateral amblyopia can compound untreated bilateral refractive error (Abrahamsson et al. 1990) and developmental disorders affecting the peripheral part of the visual system, where the associated sensory deprivation can cause amblyopia, therefore lead to delayed or even impaired morphological and functional development of the central components of the visual system (Kiorpes and McKee, 1999; Sireteanu 2000; Maurer et al. 2005, 2008; Lewis and Maurer 2009). This delay or impairment may affect both the differentiation of the visual system as well as the specialisation of the neurons with regard to their processing and coding properties. Consequently, incoming sensory information may be processed only incompletely, imprecisely or incorrectly, and integration of information may be impaired, despite the central structures of the visual system being intact. This condition of additional bilateral amblyopia may thus induce or compound difficulties with the development of a sufficiently valid and reliable representation of the visual world in terms of fine differentiation within visual categories, the identification and recognition of visual stimuli, the guidance and control of motor activities and of complex actions, and the development and optimisation by perceptual learning.

2.3.1 Visual Field

Definition. The *visual field* is the extent of visual space over which vision is possible with the eyes held in a particular position, typically straight ahead. In the adult, the measurable binocular visual field extends over 70° of visual angle to the left and right side from the fovea, the upper visual field over 50°, and the lower visual field over 60°. Therefore, the total binocular visual field size is at least 140° in the horizontal and 110° in the vertical dimension (Zihl 2011). On confrontation testing the visual field can extend up to 100° temporally for each eye for detection of movement, and movement of one's own foot can be perceived within a normal stride while looking straight ahead.

Newborn babies only respond to large, high-contrast stimuli that appear in their line of sight or close by, i.e. in the central portion of their visual field. Thus newborn babies are not blind for stimuli appearing in the visual field periphery, but do not respond because the extent of their visual field does not exceed ~30° (Maurer et al. 2008). However, even within the first month the diameter of the visual field extends markedly; at the age of 4–8 weeks the minimum size of the visual field is about 30° in both hemifields (Schwartz et al. 1987; Werth 2007, 2008). The quantitative assessment of the visual field classically requires accurate and stable fixation of a central stimulus and a valid response to the appearance of a peripheral stimulus as indicator for its detection (see Chap. 6). Both requisites do not reliably exist in the first months. However, searching eye movements can be observed within a radius of 60–90° by the end of the second month (the so-called field of search). At the end of month 4, the field of search expands to a radius of about 180°, i.e. 90° to either side. This observation may be taken as evidence that at the end of the fourth month the visual field allows a sufficient view over the visual surroundings, provided that the stimuli are large, of high-contrast, and/or are moving. An essential prerequisite for detecting peripheral stimuli and being responsive in terms of orienting responses (eye and head movements, grasping) is an adequate level of alertness and attention, and of visual curiosity for the visual world. These prerequisites are not always sufficiently available in the first months (Richards and Hunter 1998). At the beginning of the second year, children show a visual field extent similar to that of

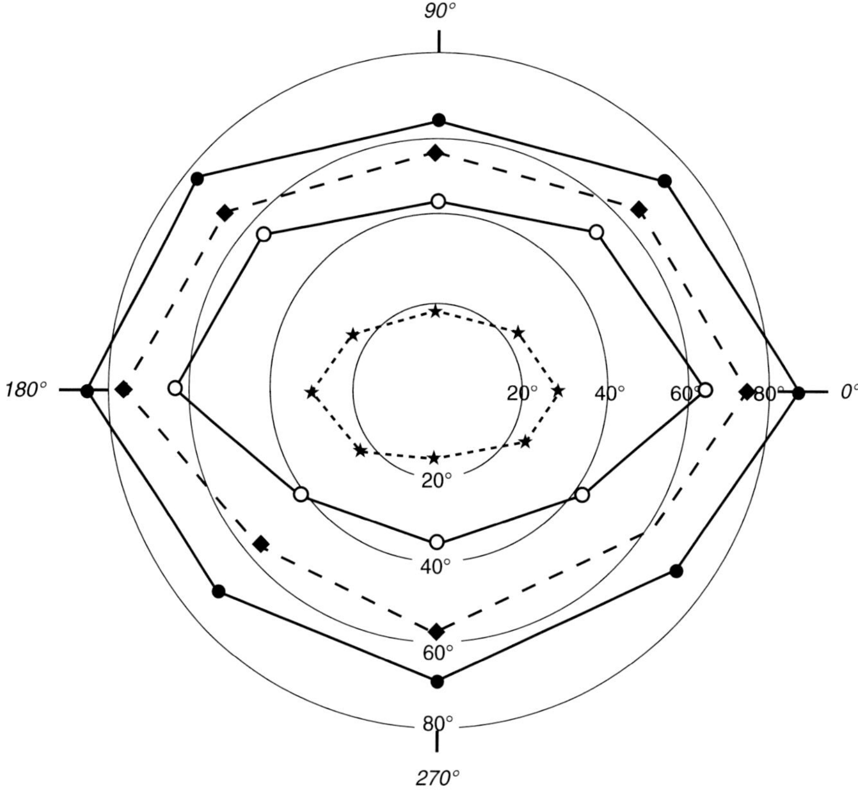

Fig. 2.4 Development of visual field (Adapted from Schwartz et al. 1987, Dobson et al. 1998, and Hargadon et al. 2010). ★- -★: 2 months of age, o—o: 9 months of age, ◆ - - ◆: 6 years, ●-●: adult

older children and even adults when kinetic perimetry is used (Dobson et al. 1998; Delaney et al. 2005; Werth 2008). From the age of 2 years on, kinetic perimetry can be used for the assessment of the visual field (Cummings et al. 1988; see Fig. 2.4), while automated eye movement detection methods now can be used to objectively test attentional visual fields in young children (Murray et al. 2013). It has to be considered, however, that at this age the field of attention has still not fully developed, and young children may, therefore, ignore peripheral stimuli, particularly when they appear simultaneously in both hemifields.

2.3.2 Visual Adaptation

Definition. Visual adaptation allows the flexible adjustment of vision to changing light intensities in the mesopic (daylight conditions), photopic (higher illumination levels), and scotopic conditions (night conditions). Thus, visual adaptation is the ability of the visual system to adjust to higher levels (*light adaptation*) or to lower levels of light (*dark adaptation*), in order to restore visual sensitivity (acuity, contrast sensitivity). Light adaptation takes a few minutes, while complete dark adaptation takes up to 30 min (Rushton 1972).

Thresholds for detection of light stimuli are increased for all three conditions in the first weeks, but decline to about the adult levels at the end of the third month (Brown 1990). Thus in the first 3 months infants are only minimally protected, particularly from intense light levels, and are therefore very sensitive to bright light, which causes discomfort from glare. In contrast, time for dark adaptation in children may be similar to adults (Hansen and Fulton 1986; Fulton and Hansen 1987).

2.3.3 Visual Contrast Sensitivity and Visual Acuity

Definition. Visual contrast sensitivity (*spatial contrast vision*) refers to visual spatial resolution, and defines an individual's capacity to detect subtle differences in light and dark shading in a pattern, an object, or a scene. In the adult, visual contrast sensitivity is highest for gratings of intermediate spatial frequencies (4–8 cycles/degree) and lower for both coarser and finer gratings. *Visual acuity* is the individual's capacity to detect small spatial gaps in a figure (e.g. circle or square) of maximum contrast (black and white), or between two parts of a figure (minimum separabile), to discriminate and identify single forms, letters, or numbers, or to process text material (reading acuity) (Zihl 2011). Formal measures specify the lighting conditions.

The capacity to discriminate visual stimuli with high accuracy and reliability depends crucially on the spatial resolution power of the visual system. Visual spatial resolution is the basis of visual spatial contrast sensitivity, and represents also an essential prerequisite for visual acuity and stereopsis. In comparison with adults, spatial contrast sensitivity in neonates is lower by a factor of 50, while visual acuity is lower by a factor of 40 (Banks and Shannon 1993; Maurer and Lewis 2001a, b; Cioni et al. 2006). In children, visual spatial contrast sensitivity is assessed behaviourally using preferential looking paradigms (PL) and registration of orienting eye movement responses. Both methods make use of the fact that children show preferred orienting responses to gratings that they can see as patterns, i.e., they can discriminate gratings differing in spatial separation (width of bars) and contrast (contrast between bars). Another method is to record pattern-evoked visual potentials; the amplitude of P1 can be taken as an indicator for contrast sensitivity (for details, see Chap. 6). Figure 2.5 shows the results of oculomotor orienting responses, preferential looking, and visual evoked potentials to gratings differing in spatial frequency and contrast sensitivity for months 1, 2, 3 and 4 (Hainline 1998). There is a striking increase in sensitivity in this developmental period, with respect to both spatial frequency and contrast; in addition, the peak of sensitivity moves towards higher frequencies. While the development of sensitivity for lower spatial frequencies appears more or less complete at the end of year 4, sensitivity for higher spatial frequencies (>10 cycles/degree, c/deg) appears complete by the age of about 8 years (Gwiazda et al. 1997; Ellemberg et al. 1999; Maurer and Lewis 2001a, b; Adams and Courage 2002; Cioni et al. 2006; Daw 2006). The gradual increase in spatial contrast

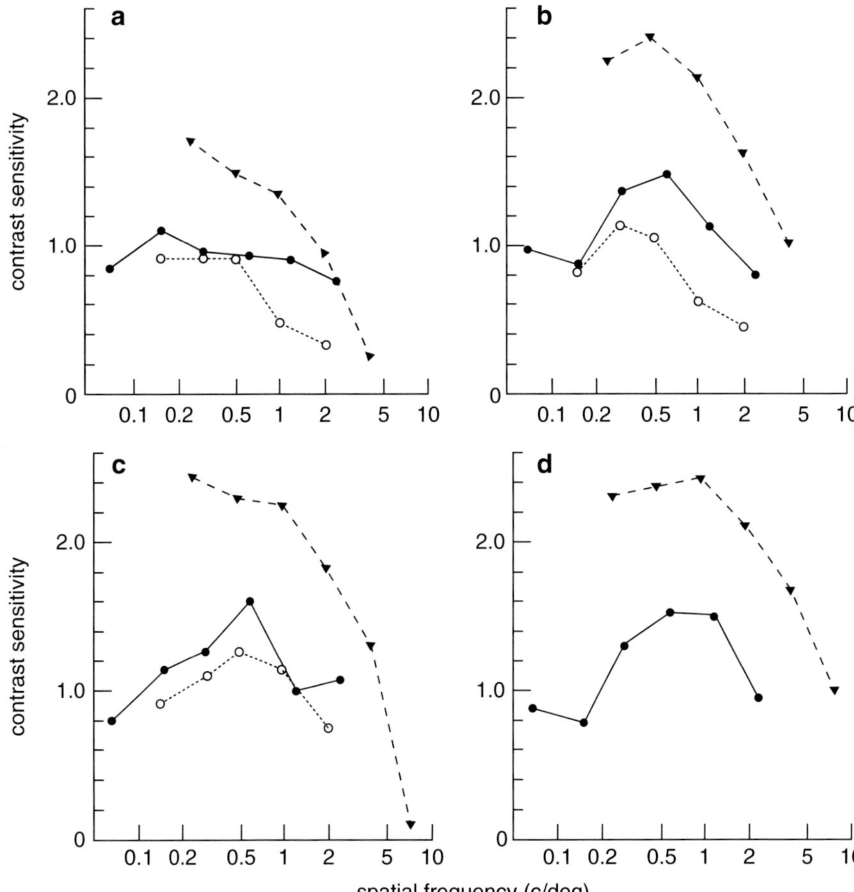

Fig. 2.5 Development of contrast sensitivity between the 1st (**a**) and the 4th month (**d**) of life depending on the method of assessment (Adapted from Hainline 1998. © Psychology Press reprinted with permission). ●–●: saccadic orienting responses; ○···○: forced preferential looking; ▼- -▼: visual evoked responses (VEP). Note that for VEP-responses higher contrast sensitivity values were obtained compared with behavioural responses

sensitivity (and also of visual acuity) can be explained by the concomitant morphological development of the fovea (Cioni et al. 2006; Daw 2006).

Concerning near vision in young children, contrast sensitivity may be sufficiently developed for adequate discrimination and recognition of complex visual stimuli (objects, faces) and stimulus details by the end of the first year. Valid and reliable assessment of visual acuity is possible during infancy (Mash and Dobson 2005), but is more accurate by about the second year (Lithander 1997). Table 2.5 shows visual acuity values for form, assessed in 89 children aged 2–4 years (Lithander 1997) Spatial resolution for form (so-called minimum separable) increases considerably in this period from 2.10 to 1.30 min of arc, while Snellen

Table 2.5 Minimum separable (MS; in min of arc) and Snellen-values for 89 children between 2 and 4 years of age

Age (months)	MS (SD)	Snellen
24–29	2.10 (0.60)	0.48
30–35	1.81 (0.41)	0.55
36–41	1.49 (0.26)	0.67
42–48	1.30 (0.24)	0.77

Modified after Lithander (1997)
Note decrease in SD with increasing age
SD 1 standard deviation

Table 2.6 Development of colour discrimination under isoluminant conditions

Age (weeks)	Discriminable colour hues
4	Red-green
8	Red-green, red-blue, red-purple, red-yellow, green-yellow
12	Red-green, red-yellow

Modified after Banks and Shannon (1993)
Colour discrimination capacity depends on stimulus size; at 4 and 8 weeks, minimal diameter of stimuli is 8°, at 12 weeks it is 4°

acuity increases from 6/12 (0.48 decimal; 0.3 logMAR) to 6/8 (0.77 decimal; 0.1 logMAR). Thus visual acuity increases by about fivefold in the first 6 months, and by the age of 6–7 years visual acuity appears more or less fully developed (Maurer and Lewis 2001a, b; Duckman 2006).

2.3.4 Colour Vision

Definition. Colour vision is the capacity to distinguish visual stimuli on the basis of the wavelengths of light they emit. The discrimination of colour hues depends on the functional capacity of the cones, which has developed incompletely by the end of the first year (Banks and Shannon 1993). However, even newborns show evidence of a kind of rudimentary colour vision (Abramov and Gordon 2006); by the age of 4 weeks children can discriminate green and red (Adams and Courage 1995). The rapid development of light and contrast sensitivity in the first 2 months is followed by the development of sensitivity to colours, provided that the colour stimuli are large and of high contrast (Brown 1990; Abramov and Gordon 2006). Table 2.6 shows the development of colour discrimination for primary colours; discrimination of red, green and blue may be detectable even earlier, if coloured OKN stimuli are used (Zemach and Teller 2007; Zemach et al. 2007). Coloured stimuli possibly appear less intense during the first months, because children at this age require a higher colour contrast for accurate discrimination (Morrone et al. 1990; Allen et al. 1993; Teller and Lindsey 1993). However, children may be able to use colour as a feature to discriminate, identify and recognise objects. If they are confronted with coloured and colourless objects, they prefer the coloured ones; thus colour represents an already prominent visual attribute in early childhood (Catherwood et al. 1996). At the age of 6 months, the capacity for colour discrimination appears similar to adults (Franklin and Davies 2004; Abramov and Gordon 2006).

2.3.5 Visual Space Perception

Definition. Visual spatial functions comprise the processing of spatial properties of optical stimuli and include position, distance, depth, and direction (horizontal, vertical and straight ahead) as well as of spatial relations of stimuli (objects) in a scene, of both a three- and a two-dimensional nature (Zihl 2011).

Even during the first days after birth, babies can locate a visual stimulus within a radius covering 45°, but localisation accuracy is low (Roucoux et al. 1983). At the age of 5 months babies can execute accurate saccadic eye shifts to stimuli (Hainline 1998), while saccadic accuracy corresponds to that of adults by the age of 4 years (Fukushima et al. 2000). In early childhood, the perception of distance in the straight-ahead direction is better in the binocular than in the monocular viewing condition. By the age of 5 months babies can reach correctly for visual objects under monocular conditions in 65 % of stimulus presentations, but in 89 % of trials under binocular conditions (Granrud et al. 1984). Before this age, babies do not show systematically guided reaching actions, although distance perception may be present even earlier (Daw 2006; Stiles et al. 2008). More complex visual-spatial capacities, including representation and translation of visual spatial information into visually guided control when copying or drawing, require many years of experience and practice and are not sufficiently developed before the age of 9 years, whereby perceptual abilities precede space representation and graphomotor abilities (Del Guidice et al. 2000).

Stereopsis develops rapidly between months 3 and 6; stereoacuity improves within a few weeks from very low levels of acuity to disparities of ~1 min of arc (Held 1993). At the end of the first year stereoacuity increases further to 30–40 s of arc, provided that contrast sensitivity and vergence are appropriately developed. Stereoacuity is eventually fully developed at the age of 6 years, with girls showing significantly better stereoacuity values between 4 and 6 years (Hainline 1998; Daw 2006; Duckman and Du 2006; Pola 2006).

2.3.6 Form and Object Perception

Definition. Form and pattern perception comprises the discrimination, identification and recognition of forms and Gestalten on the basis of their spatial features, e.g. length and orientation of lines, and spatial pattern properties. *Object perception* refers to the same visual capacities concerning real objects, which are characterised by global (e.g. size, shape) and local (e.g. form, figural and colour details) properties, and by special (shared only by a single object or object class), and generic features (shared by all objects of a category, but also other objects, not belonging to that category).

Table 2.7 Some fundamental associations between context conditions and early visual perceptual activities

If the baby is awake and alert and light is not too bright, eyes are open
If light conditions are appropriate, but no forms/patterns are in the line of sight, the baby begins to search for contours with the help of gaze shifts
After a contour has been found, search stops, and fixation remains at the contour or close to this for a longer time

Modified after Haith (1980)

Table 2.8 Preferred (italics) and less attractive visual stimuli for infants

High contrast vs. low contrast stimuli
Larger vs. smaller forms and objects
Moving vs. stationary objects
Patterned vs. plain stimuli
Horizontal vs. vertical and oblique lines
Curvilinear vs. rectilinear patterns
3-dimensional vs. 2-dimensional objects
Objects in direct line of sight vs. peripheral
Faces and face-like stimuli vs. other forms

Modified after Slater (1998a, b)

Both, simple and complex visual stimuli are available for the newborn baby in its "new" world, but at this time the visual system is hardly able to process and code such information. Alertness and curiosity are two fundamental prerequisites for early visual activities of the baby (Table 2.7). Despite the limited stage of development of the peripheral and central visual systems at this age, babies show remarkable preferences for more complex visual stimuli (see Table 2.8). This incongruity between the physiological stages of development and the perceptual preferences exhibited has been interpreted in favour of inherent visual capacities (Maurer et al. 2008; McKone et al. 2009; Hunnius and Bekkering 2010). In particular, faces attract attention, and are fixated for longer than other complex visual stimuli (Elam et al. 2010; see below). The combination of visual curiosity, indicating motivation for information supply, focusing and maintenance of attention and fixation upon faces, and repeated processing of faces, appears particularly attractive for the rapidly developing visual brain, suggestive of specific stimulus preference and prior expectation, respectively. Face processing requires close coordination of and cooperation between engaged visual cortical areas, but also cognitive and motivation/reward systems, and thus facilitates and promotes the bottom-up and top-down interplay of the functional systems involved.

As mentioned above, newborns do not find all kinds of visual stimuli equally attractive and interesting, as indicated by oculomotor orienting responses and fixation times. At the age of 6 weeks babies can discriminate orientations of contours. Given the developmental state of contrast vision and visual acuity, it is not surprising that they prefer objects with coarse contours and lines in contrast to fine form or figural details. At the age of 3 months children can discriminate angles built from contours. At 4 months of age they can use form and object features for identification and recognition; the integration of features to a whole ('Gestalt') is, however, not possible before month 10. The development of form and pattern perception is characterised by an early tendency for the construction of Gestalten. Consequently, children show a stronger bias in terms of faster responses towards global processing of complex forms, at least up to the age of 10 years (Mondloch et al. 2003). With increasing visual development, and thus an increase in visual perceptual experiences, in cognitive capacities (attention, memory, executive functions) in general, and specific capacities involved in visual perception, young children prefer increasingly complex visual stimuli (Aslin and Smith 1988; Johnson 2003; Sireteanu et al. 2003; Maurer et al. 2008). Visual selection processes (Amso and Johnson 2006) and memory for complex visual stimuli (Rose et al. 2001) play an important role in the development of object perception in the first year of life. Viewing preference during visual and manual exploration grows rapidly during the first 3 years of age; in this period children prefer planar views and views of objects in an upright position in preference to other viewing directions and spatial axes (Pereira et al. 2010). Development of visual object recognition shows fast progress between 6 and 11 years of life, indicating that this complex 'higher-order' visual capacity requires intensive visual experience, with integration of the various processes involved, including figure-ground separation, form and figure completion, segregation of overlapping figures, and object constancy (Bova et al. 2007).

2.3.7 Visual Categorisation, Concept Formation and Constancy

The visual world offers ecological structures and spatial stimulus organisation, which facilitate and support the coherent perception of objects, scenes, humans and events (Gibson 1979). It appears that infants possess, at an early stage, various perceptual organisation principles that serve as a means of arranging the visual world into perceptual categories. Concept formation allows the child to identify and recognise figures, forms and objects, independent of external factors, e.g. lighting, shadows and occlusion of parts, visual context etc., as well as of internal factors related to the observer, e.g. perspective, distance, and episodic context. Concept formation is the basis for visual constancy, i.e. an object keeps its identity despite changes in internal or external factors. Constancy guarantees increasing independence of (concretistic) visual perception from the actual appearance of a visual stimulus, and thus enhances autonomy for action. The final product of concept formation is the 'prototypical' Gestalt, without losing the progressively developing capacity for fine discrimination and differentiation of stimuli and stimulus features within a given category. Elementary form and object constancy can be observed soon after birth indicating that constancy is most likely an innate capacity. Size constancy can be demonstrated around month 7 (Aslin and Smith 1988; Slater et al. 1990; Johnson 2003; Rakinson and Oakes 2003; Sireteanu et al. 2003; Maurer et al. 2008). Table 2.9 shows the typical sequence of Gestalt constancy principles in development. Gestalt principles facilitate the discriminability and classification

Table 2.9 Temporal sequence of the appearance of Gestalt principles in visual development

Principle of similarity: as of M 3
Principle of closure of forms and figures: as of M 3–4
Principle of coherence of objects and parts of objects: as of M 3–5
Principle of object segregation and object abstraction (figure-ground, continuity, effective Gestalt): as of M 8–10

Modified after Slater (1998a, b)
M month of life

of visual objects, and promote thereby the further development of object constancy, but top-down influences guiding perceptual learning in terms of organisation and categorisation of visual information and visual concept formation, and their interactions with bottom-up processes are crucial for gaining valid and reliable constructs about the various aspects of the visual world (Quinn and Bhatt 2009).

The combination of the faculty of discrimination of complex visual stimuli on the one hand, and the accuracy and reliability of their classification and categorisation, respectively, on the other, is a good example of the close matching of apparently opposite developmental principles of the visual brain. The marked increase in visual information processing capacity does not develop without concomitant development of rules concerning how visual information has to be allocated and classified for saving of processed and classified information in visual memory. Part of this process is the definitely challenging ability to assign specific stimulus features, e.g. colour, form and size, to different objects, i.e. to be able to discover that different objects, e.g. ball, apple, bowl, share common features (form, colour, size), irrespective of the fact that they belong to different object classes. Repeated systematic practice with the identification and recognition of different objects sharing common features or properties, results in reliable and fast coding and representation of objects in visual memory. This representation also comprises knowledge about variations in appearance, semantic and pragmatic significance, use, and eventually categorisation and denomination. This object information constitutes the basis for the formation of modality-specific, i.e. visual, and supra-modal concepts of the objects in question (Quinn 1998, 2003; Quinn and Bhatt 2001; Rakinson and Oakes 2003). Although infants as young as 3 months are able to use various visual Gestalt cues to organise visual patterns, e.g. common motion, connectedness, continuity, proximity (Quinn and Bhatt 2009), it is not surprising, that top-down visual organisation processes in scene and object recognition, and the underlying processes in the brain, need several years of development, because intensive and repeated perceptual and concept learning is required, which is probably not complete until the age of 11 years (Bova et al. 2007).

Categorisation requires concept formation. Even very young children can recognise an object or face seen under different conditions, especially when these conditions possess high ecological relevance for the child. The ability to form concepts can be understood as an essential prerequisite to attain increasing familiarity with perceptual effects, and thus progressive certainty and safety in manipulating objects. Elementary visual memory capacities can be observed by a few weeks after birth, with rapid improvement over the first 12 months (see Sect. 2.3.8). The development of visual memory is possibly enhanced by the innate visual stimulus preferences (see Sect. 2.3.6). A special case of visual stimulus preference is faces.

2.3.8 Face Perception

Face perception represents a special case of object perception, which refers only to facial properties and attributes, both within and between facial categories. Visual face perception plays a particular role within visual development. Babies already prefer faces shortly after birth, i.e. without prior perceptual experience; this observation has led to the assumption of an innate perceptual mechanism underlying the preference of faces and facial expressions (Pascalis and Slater 2003; de Haan 2008; McKone et al. 2009). In the first weeks after birth, fast perceptual learning takes place, which is mainly devoted to faces, particularly the face of the mother or of another relevant person. This face, which is seen and thus processed with high daily frequency in different contexts, is favoured over other faces and "serves" probably also as a tool for the optimisation of visual social perception and acquisition of knowledge concerning the significance of facial expressions (see Sect. 2.3.10). This systematic and regular experience with one face, or a few familiar faces, is the basis for perceptual "tuning" in terms of progressive specialisation of the face-processing system (Simion et al. 2007) and the recognition and interpretation of facial expressions of other persons later in life (Mondloch et al. 2003; Bushnell 2011). Of course, the voice of the mother or of another relevant person also plays an important role (Sai 2005). At the age of 4 months children can recognise familiar faces even when typical, for example by a haircut (Turati et al. 2008). This implies that children at this age features are removed, can use characteristic individual facial features to identify a person. At the age of 6 months children prefer natural ('real') faces to photographs or line drawings of faces, independently of age, gender and skin colour of the faces (Rubinstein et al. 1999). As for objects, the development of the faculty of face discrimination is paralleled by an improvement in concept formation and consequently in face categorisation including face class (girls vs. boys, younger vs. older persons) and identity (father, siblings, grandparents, aunts, uncles, etc.). At the age of about 10 years, children's representation of identity becomes expression-independent like in adults (Mian and Mondloch 2012).

Faces possibly also exhibit a high natural preference bias and accelerate visual learning, because their discrimination, identification and recognition, respectively, play a crucial role in social perception (see Sect. 2.3.10). Already in the first month children prefer faces to objects; at month 3 children fixate faces longer than objects, particularly the eye and mouth regions (Table 2.10). The identification and interpretation, (understanding) of facial expression probably develop in the second year; faces that do not mimic movements stop a child from smiling or trigger looking the other way. At the age of 3 months, children respond differentially to facial expressions: "happy" faces trigger positive responses; "sad" faces trigger negative responses (Table 2.11). This period is followed by a phase of imitation of facial

Table 2.10 Inspection times (in % of total observation times) and smiling times (in % of inspection times) of 3–6 month old children for different face variations and for an object with similar figural complexity

Face variation	Inspection time (%)	Smiling (%)
Static neutral face	42	03
Moving neutral face	80	18
Happy face	76	30
Sad face	74	10
Eyes looking at child	78	14
Eyes looking away from child	70	07
Object	38	02

Modified after Ellsworth et al. (1993)

Table 2.11 Development of visual discrimination capacity for facial expressions in the first year

Pair of expressions	Age
Happy – surprised	Birth
Happy – sad	Birth
Happy – angry	M 3
Happy – anxious	M 7
Sad – surprised	Birth
Sad – anxious	M 5
Angry – sad	M 5
Angry – anxious	M 5
Angry – surprised	M 5
Anxious – surprised	M 6

Modified after de Haan and Nelson (1998)
M month of life, *age* time of first appearance of this capacity

expressions made by the mother (or relevant person). Eye contact plays a particular role in the perception and interpretation of facial expression. At the age of 2 months children show a vivid interest in eyes; at the age of 4 months they can discriminate between different directions of gaze of the other party. Reciprocal looking activates increasingly more selective attention ("joint attention") and social responses in both communicating partners (De Haan and Nelson 1998; Pascalis and Slater 2003; de Haan 2008; McKone et al. 2009; Elam et al. 2010; see Sect. 2.3.10).

2.3.9 Text Processing and Reading

Reading includes processing of text stimuli and understanding their meaning at the semantic level. Reading requires various functional prerequisites including visual, oculomotor, and cognitive functions that facilitate reception, processing, and understanding of spatially distributed visual-verbal information (Findlay and Gilchrist

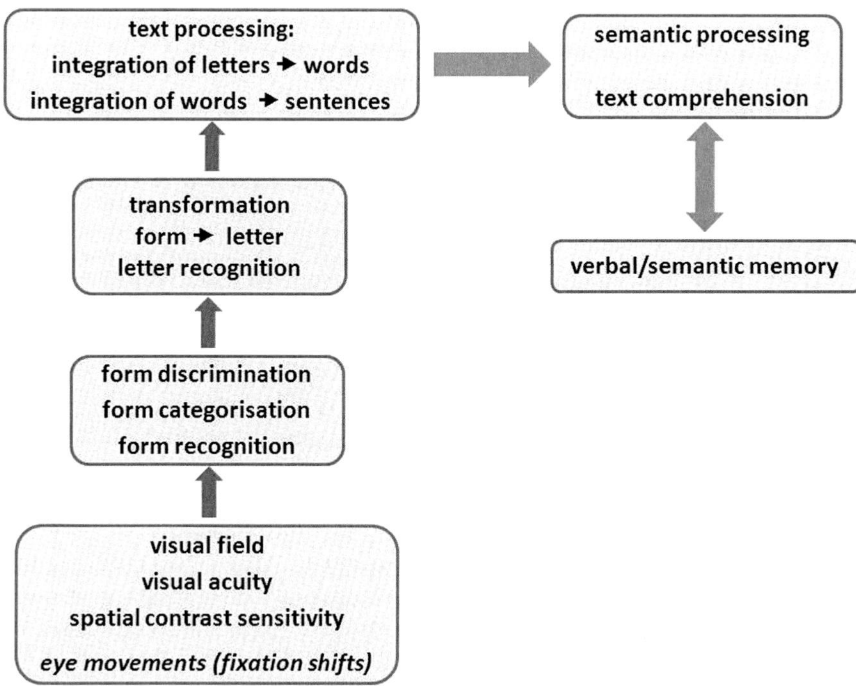

Fig. 2.6 The hierarchical process of text processing to reading: the visual capacities and processes involved in lower and higher level analysis

2003). Thus reading is based on a complex coordination of processes involved in processing and understanding of text material. A sufficient central visual field, acuity, contrast sensitivity, form and letter discrimination, integration of letters into words, and appropriate guidance of fixation shifts, bring about efficient text processing (Fig. 2.6). Letter identification efficiency depends on perceivability, bias, and similarity of letters (Mueller and Weidemann 2012), and on consistency of letter font (Sanocki and Dyson 2012). At the semantic level, the translation of visual letter and word information into verbal information is essential for speech comprehension; processed linguistic information is stored in verbal memory. Occipito-temporal structures in the left hemisphere, which are specialised for text processing and reading, in particular the so-called visual word form area (VWFA), are involved in reading (Dehaene and Cohen 2011; Wandell 2011). The VWFA is also "the likely substrate for the interaction of the top-down processing of symbolic meanings with the analysis of bottom-up properties of sensory inputs making the VWFA the location where the symbolic meaning of both words and non-word objects is represented" (Song et al. 2012). VWFA activation is highly selective for individual real words (Glezer et al. 2009), although words are processed at multiple levels in the visual brain (Szwed et al. 2011). The VWFA also possesses sensitivity for letters and words in terms of visual field position invariance (Braet et al. 2012; Rauschecker et al. 2012), and shows the best activation for high word visibility (Rauschecker et al. 2011). Consequently, processing of case-and letter-deviant forms is associated with increased demands in the VWFA (Kronbichler et al. 2009), which is in agreement with observations on longer fixation durations when text material is faint (White and Staub 2012). The activity patterns in these cortical regions develop to mature levels with increased proficiency at both the morphological and functional level (Schlaggar and McCandliss 2007; Schlaggar and Church 2009).

Reading eye movements parallel word and text processing, including reading span (span of parallel processing of text stimuli, equivalent to fixation duration), preview benefit (processing of text stimuli right from the actual fixation position), and spatio-temporal sequence of saccadic shifts and fixations (Rayner 2009). Children at the age of 7–11 years show similar fixation durations in reading as adults, indicating that differences in reading speed are indicative of the level of difficulty in semantic processing rather than in text processing (Blythe et al. 2009). The various visual, oculomotor and cognitive functions involved in reading develop only after systematic and specific practice with visual text material. The development of an efficient text processing capacity is the biggest obstacle for children in acquiring the skill of reading (Rayner et al. 2001). Only after text processing has become a routine does reading in terms of understanding text material become a skill. In the first 4–5 years, language development is mainly based on processing of auditory verbal information and producing spoken language. After the first year children possess on average 100 words; at the age of 6 years the passive vocabulary comprises around 14,000 words. Sensitivity to word visibility increases between 7 and 12 years of age, which is associated with developmental changes in activation in left occipito-temporal regions (Ben-Schachar et al. 2011). The acquisition of reading skills requires systematic practice over several years, which typically begins with school entrance. At the age of 10 years children normally can read at a good level, and development of at least the routine processes of reading is complete (Ashby and Rayner 2006; Goswami 2008). This does not imply that reading cannot be improved and optimised later on, but the training process may be much more laborious and eventually less efficient with respect to the acquisition of skilled reading.

2.3.10 Social Perception and Social Behaviour

The human brain is intrinsically organised to develop in a social context and thus to develop social behaviour for communication in a general and specific sense with other individuals, particularly through face and eye gaze processing, perception of biological motion and of the actions of others (Grossmann and Johnson 2007). "Social behaviour" includes a variety of functions, capacities and abilities, for example, independence, giving due regard to social rules in social interactions, social adaptation, taking on the perspective of others ("theory of mind"), social cooperation and social competition. Humans develop a similar capacity to identify emotional signals of diverse facial expressions and translate them into social signals independent of culture (Leppanen and Nelson 2009). The ability to attend to negative emotional information develops earlier in the vocal than in the facial domain, but by the age of 7 months infants can reliably match emotion information and identify emotions across face and voice (Grossmann 2010). At the age of 4 months children can detect changes in face-voice pairings indicating that they are able to establish specific face-voice associations (Bahrick et al. 2005). Adequate facial expression perception and evaluation is also essential to prevent development of abnormal biases resulting from abnormal affect processing, which may represent a risk for the future development of depressive states (Bistricky et al. 2011). To gain skill in identification of social signals, humans pay particular attention to other humans, in particular members of their groups, so as to acquire valuable social information about their identity, emotions, and likely intent. Relevant social stimuli are processed by two distinct but integrated pathways and translated into 'social' signals: a subcortical route mediating crude but fast orienting responses, and a subcortical-cortical 'social system' that mediates and controls adaptive and flexible context- and experience-dependent responses and complex social behaviour (Klein et al. 2009). For the development of social functions, the parents' style of education, the social framework of the family, and the quality of social binding between the child and the relevant individuals, play an essential role (Wijnroks 1998; Fei-Ying Ng et al. 2004; Grossmann and Johnson 2007). On the other hand, learning individual responsive behaviour from parents facilitates development of social responsiveness and competence, as well as cognition and communication (Landry et al. 2006; Barrett and Fleming 2011).

An important aspect in this context is the child's capacity to focus attention and gaze at targets, which are also being attended to by another (e.g. the acting) person. The shifting to, and maintenance of attention upon such targets, i.e. the "capacity to coordinate one's own visual attention with that of another person" is called *joint attention* (Mundy and Jarrold 2010, p. 985). Joint attention is the process that allows two or more individuals to search for the same visual stimulus and shift attention and gaze to it. Joint attention cannot be observed before 10 months of age but from about 8 months on, a gaze-following response exists (Corkum and Moore 1998). At the age of 14 months children use the direction of gaze and the facial expression of an acting individual to conclude what the action goal might be (Liszkowski et al. 2004). At the end of the first year children can shift to and maintain attention in social situations for a sufficiently long time. Responding to joint attentional stimuli is significantly related to the development and use of executive self-regulatory processes at the age of 12 months (Van Hecke Vaughan et al. 2012). Eye gaze processing plays a crucial role in social perception and social development. It modulates processing of the accompanying stimulus and context information, under an executive network that regulates the infant's capacity to direct attention and respond to social signals of others, so as to share (social) experiences (Hoehl et al. 2009; Senju and Johnson 2009; Mundy and Jarrold 2010). Based on the gaze direction of another person, children can conclude that a stimulus is at a definite position in space (Elam et al. 2010) and which stimulus it might be. On the other hand, children can also "guide" the gaze and attention of another person to a particular location in space. This correspondence in visual behaviour enhances the development of other capacities, for example, shifting attention in space, regulation of the field of attention, visual recognition, and also visual naming (Grossmann and Johnson 2007; Tasker and Schmidt 2008). In addition, the infants' capacity to watch social interaction is not only an important developmental step from more passive to more active engagement, but it also plays a role in progressing from crawling to walking towards other people (Clearfield et al. 2008). Observational learning in social contexts continues in later childhood, and allows children and young adults to learn interpersonal interaction e.g. with teachers (Grossberg and Vladusich 2010).

Low vision, with low contrast sensitivity and acuity, diminishes the capacity to discriminate faces and facial expressions. This has the potential to interfere with the development of recognition, social engagement, shared attention and understanding of the emotional language conveyed by facial expression, unless faces are close enough, or sufficiently enhanced both on people, and on toys and pictures, so as to be rendered visible by falling within the constraints of functional vision from an early stage of development.

2.4 Attention in Vision

Visual perception and attention are closely interrelated; visual perception without visual attention is nearly impossible (and vice versa). Particularly illustrative examples of this close relationship are some fundamental relationships between the "functional" or "attentional" states, respectively, for the infant and its early visual activities (see Table 2.7), and the combination of visual field and attention. The distribution of attention in the sector of environment, which is covered by the visual field, allows global and fast processing of large parts of the visual environment (overview, vision at a glance), while narrowing attention to just a part of the scene or one object, or a small detail of an object, allows accurate processing of this information at a more local level. It is the precise temporal and spatial interplay of global and local processing that guarantees that the visual field becomes the field of attention and thus of perception. The diameter of the field of attention determines how much of our surrounding can be processed and how detailed and accurate this processing can be performed and used for visual perception. We are able to set our field of attention to a panorama view, with a very wide field of processing and coarse spatial resolution, but also to attain a detailed view, with a much smaller field of processing and fine spatial resolution, while covert attention is still operating, although probably not at the same level of efficiency. Thus, the field of visual attention may be as large as the visual field (global view), but may also be much smaller (local view). Global view allows complete perception of a scene; for processing of detail, local processing is required. Typically global perception precedes local analysis (so-called global precedence effect; Mondloch et al. 2003); global processing guarantees spatial orientation within a scene and thus can guide detailed analysis at different locations in the scene without losing the spatial context (Hochstein and Ahissar 2002). Attention influences visual information processing directly at lower and higher levels of cortical organisation by creating so-called saliency maps, which serve as "topographic representations of relative stimulus strength and behavioural relevance across visual space" (Treue 2003, p. 428). Saliency maps are closely linked to brain structures involved in oculomotor orienting responses to particular parts of a scene. Furthermore, transient storage of the scene along with locations of stimulus processing (fixation positions) in visual-spatial memory within the scene enables the subject to integrate scene information independent of fixation positions, and prevents the observer from carrying out unnecessary fixations and processing repetitions. Only in the case of uncertainty, i.e. inaccurate or incomplete updating of fixation positions, loss of spatial coherence of scene details, or missing significance of what has been already perceived, are parts of the scene or even the entire scene processed again. Efficient and accurate processing of a scene thus requires a flexible field of attention, which allows shifts of attention and thus of fixation, in an optimal spatio-temporal order, without losing coherence.

Children possess attentional capacities in the visual modality soon after birth. Newborns pay selective attention to stimuli in their visual environment, as demonstrated by stimulus preferences. Orienting responses triggered by external visual stimuli can be observed in the first month. The ability to shift visual attention intentionally within visual space is evident after the 4th month. At the age of 6 months children show similar attention and gaze shifting behaviours as adults; at this age children can also shift attention covertly, i.e. without concomitant orienting responses. Furthermore, their ability to intentionally explore their visual surroundings, as well as single objects, begins to grow. The distribution of attention in space also plays an important role in the development of guiding eye, head, and grasping movements (Hunnius et al. 2006; Hunnius 2007; Atkinson and Nardini 2008; Richards 2008; Sinclair and Taylor 2008). Spatial selective visual attention implies selection of important and relevant stimuli while ignoring less important and less relevant stimuli. This visual-attentional capacity develops rapidly within the first 4 months (Johnson et al. 1994; Johnson and Tucker 1996). Shifts of attention in space are typically associated with orienting eye, head and body responses, but can also occur covertly, i.e. without orienting responses. The control and regulation of attention in vision occurs either via external stimuli, or by intention, but the two factors can hardly be separated in typical everyday life activities (Hunnius 2007). The development of attention in vision appears completed by school age (~6 years) (Goldberg et al. 2001; Hunnius 2007; Atkinson and Nardini 2008; Richards 2008; Sinclair and Taylor 2008).

Low visual acuity, and contrast sensitivity, limited visual fields, the incomplete mapping typical of dorsal stream pathology, and the disordered recognition typical of ventral stream dysfunction, can all interfere with the ability to develop, engage and employ attentional skills, and early measures need to be taken to deal with these issues.

2.5 Visual Memory

Two different sources of information play a prominent role for the vision-based mental representation of objects: information about the spatial position (WHERE), and about the type of object, including object features (WHAT; see also Sect. 2.2).

The capacity to code spatial information appears to precede the capacity to code object features (Distler et al. 1996; Atkinson and Nardini 2008). The functional significance of this temporal order may be that object localisation also precedes object identification, which in turn requires the direction of attention and fixation to the position of the object in question, for detailed processing of the object features.

Even by the age of 3 months children possess knowledge about spatial relations, for example "above" and "below" (Gava et al. 2009). However, this knowledge is still very concrete, i.e. bound by the actual viewpoint of the child. At the age of 6–7 months children can code the positions of objects independent of the own point of view. Thus, the development of visual space perception and visual spatial memory can be understood as transition from an egocentric to an allocentric type of coding, which becomes progressively independent of the actual position of the observing child (Atkinson and Nardini 2008).

Concerning types of object, children at the age of 4 months are able to classify forms, figures and objects as "familiar", i.e. can build prototypes and categories of object stimuli. Duration of retention (recognition) increases monotonically between 2 and 18 months of age (Hartshorn et al. 1998). After 6 months of age visual memory performance is task-independent, i.e. no longer bound by the specific stimulus and/or task condition in which learning has occurred (Hartshorn and Rovee-Collier 1997). At 18 months of age children are able to reproduce visually observed actions with objects, despite changes in context relative to the original demonstration (Hayne et al. 2000), which is an essential prerequisite for observational learning (see Sect. 3.2). A very interesting observation concerns the perception and (pre-semantic) classification of animal "forms". At the age of 4 months children use different visual categories e.g. for dog, cat and bird; classification is mainly based on global visual features, which belong to a given category or distinguish between categories. Repeated visual experience with animals enhances concept formation and classification, so that discrimination of different types of dog, in contrast to cats or birds, improves progressively (Quinn 1998, 2003; Rakinson and Oakes 2003). Remembering stimuli and stimulus events entails encoding the experience; this determines which brain regions are reactivated during subsequent retrieval, e.g. in recognition, such that the same specific regions in the temporal lobe are activated during encoding and retrieval (Danker and Anderson 2010; Khan et al. 2011).

Low vision in all its forms limits what can be seen, and commensurately constrains the development of visual memory, which necessitates early implementation of sets of approaches matched to the specific disabilities and needs of the child.

2.6 Visual-Motor Functions

The development of visually guided motor activities not only depend on the current state of development of visual functioning, but the repeated execution of motor activities under visual guidance also impacts upon the development of visual functioning, in particular, visual-spatial perceptual capacities. Such motor activities comprise body movements (body control, sitting, walking), movements of hands and fingers (pointing, grasping, manipulating), and eye movements (saccadic eye movements, fixation, smooth pursuit eye movements; see Sect. 2.7) in such a way that they correspond with the developing internal mental three-dimensional representation of the external surroundings as this becomes progressively refined to reflect external 'reality'. In addition, the development of posture control requires vestibular function, whereby visual-vestibular interactions are of particular importance (Hainline 1998; Daw 2006; Pola 2006; Atkinson and Nardini 2008; Karatekin 2008). The capacity to accurately visually perceive and know what is vertical and what horizontal is in part contingent upon these interactions. The interplay of the various brain structures involved in motor (motor and pre-motor cortex, supplementary motor cortex, basal ganglia, brainstem and cerebellum) and visual functions (posterior parietal cortex, occipital cortex, temporal cortex) is essential for the development of visually guided motor activities. However, while motor activities are insufficiently developed, vision cannot or can only in part be used for the visual guidance of such activities (Del Guidice et al. 2000). It is currently popular to attribute all types of visual observation learning to the miraculous all-rounder called the mirror neuron system (Rizzolatti and Sinigaglia 2010). Although the universal role of the mirror neurons has been questioned, there is no doubt that this system is involved in understanding and emulating the actions of another, thus supporting learning of actions through visual observation. However, in determining the reasons why an agent performs a particular action, many other brain structures are involved (Sinigaglia 2013).

As examples, lack of visual clarity, of lower visual field, or specific optic ataxia can each interfere with visual guidance of movement of the upper and lower limbs, requiring early appropriate measures, such as tactile supplementation of visual guidance, to be facilitated and encouraged.

2.7 Ocular Motor Functions

2.7.1 Accommodation and Convergence

Accommodation is the process of adapting the refractive power of the lens of the eye to match changing distances of a visual stimulus, so that the image is and remains best focused. *Vergence* denotes the simultaneous movements of both eyes to maintain single binocular vision. Convergence is the simultaneous inward movement of both eyes to view objects in near space, while divergence is the simultaneous outward movement of the eyes to subsequently view objects in more distant positions; in both instances, the movement directions are opposite to one another. The near point for accommodation and convergence is about 10 cm during childhood; beyond 150 cm the contribution to single binocular vision decreases markedly. Under normal viewing conditions, changing fixation at different stimulus distances automatically triggers matched vergence and accommodation, also known as the *accommodation-convergence reflex*. Both vergence and accommodation are understood as calibration and recalibration processes to varying fixation distances, which are controlled by neural structures in the brainstem, cerebellum and cerebral cortex, and are in addition influenced by attention and the intention of visual information processing (see Leigh and Zee 2006, for a comprehensive review on eye movements).

Accommodation and convergence improve from about the second month on, and enable better focussing of visual stimuli (Currie and Manny 1997), but steady state accommodation may still be unstable (Candy and Bharadwaj 2007). By the age of 3–4 months the range of accommodation becomes similar to that of young adults (Hainline 1998; Daw 2006; Rosenfield 2006). The common development of accommodation coupled to convergence, allows the extension of spatial contrast sensitivity and visual acuity to greater observation distances, and enhances the fusion of monocular retinal images to combined binocular images. Accommodation and vergence latencies in infants between 7 and 23 weeks of age, tend to range between 1 and 2 s, but can also be in the adult range (<0.5 s; Tondel and Candy 2008). Male infants show earlier maturity of accommodative responses, which is possibly related to differences in refractive error (Horwood and Riddell 2008).

2.7.2 Fixation

Fixation marks the endpoint of a saccadic jump, i.e. when eyes have hit the target, and provides the basis for detailed processing of the stimulus by holding the image of the stimulus on the fovea. At the age of 1 month children can fixate visual stimuli for a short time (Roucoux et al. 1983). Until the age of about 5 months fixation duration is considerably shorter than adulthood, but depends, of course, also on the curiosity of the child as well as the attractiveness of the visual stimulus in question. Children's interests manifest in the resulting span of attention, which also limits the duration of fixation. Fixation stability at this age is low, and fixation is characterised by many small corrective saccades. The window of fixation, i.e. the area within which fixation is kept, has a diameter of ~0.8°; for comparison, the fixation window of an adult has a diameter of ~0.5° (Hainline 1998; Daw 2006; Pola 2006; Leigh and Zee 2006; Karatekin 2008).

2.7.3 Saccadic Eye Movements

Saccadic eye movements are very fast moves of the eyes that enable the observer to transport the fovea, i.e. the central part of the visual field with the highest acuity and contrast sensitivity capacities, to a position in space for fixation and further (local) processing of a visual stimulus. Saccadic eye movements are 'reflexive', i.e. generated to and triggered by novel stimuli in the visual, auditory or tactile environments that unexpectedly appear, or are volitional, for example intentionally triggered or generated to command. The latency for triggered saccades is about 200 ms; saccadic velocity is about 140°/s for small amplitudes (up to 5°), but can reach up to 500°/s for larger saccades (>40°), whereby saccadic velocity increases with increasing amplitude (the so-called main sequence). The saccadic accuracy is in the range

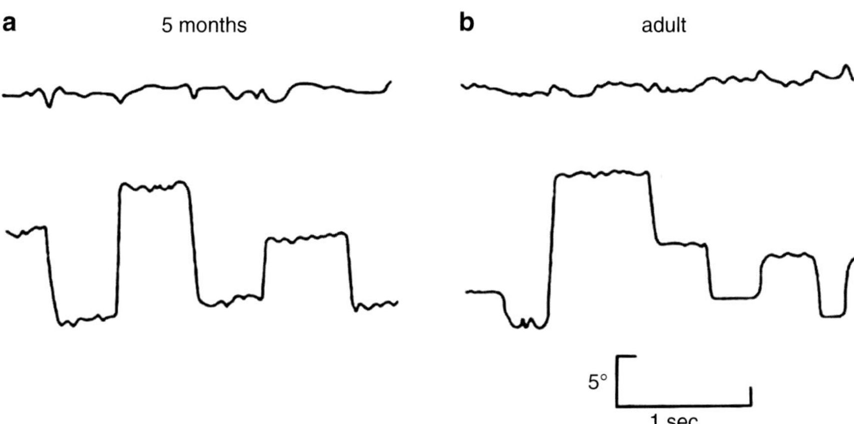

Fig. 2.7 Fixation stability (*upper image*: EOG-recordings) and saccadic eye movements (*lower image*: EOG-recordings) in a 5 month-old child (**a**) and in an adult (**b**). (Hainline 1998. © Psychology Press reprinted with permission)

of ±2°, whereby accurate fixation is attained by corrective saccades. Spontaneous saccades are seemingly random saccades occurring without engagement in a particular visual task (Leigh and Zee 2006).

Newborns already show saccadic eye movements with nearly normal main sequence characteristics. Saccadic speed is, however, reduced and saccades to more distant stimuli are fragmented until the end of the third month (so-called saccadic hypometria; Roucoux et al. 1983; see Fig. 2.7). This hypometria may be explained by the developmental stage of the saccadic system, but may also partly be due to the fact that the visual capacities available do not allow a more accurate visual spatial localisation and thus visual guidance of saccades (Hainline 1998; Daw 2006; Pola 2006; Karatekin 2008). Saccadic latencies are also prolonged in the first months. At the age of 3 months latencies are in the range of 600 ms for targets at a horizontal distance of 10° from the actual eye position, and about 900 ms for targets at a distance of 30°. At the age of 5 months the corresponding latencies decline to about 280 and 490 ms, respectively, implying that infants at the age of 3 months require about half a second to shift their gaze to and fixate a target at a distance of 10°, and about 1 s to shift their gaze to and fixate a target at distance of 30° (Regal et al. 1983).

2.7.4 Smooth Pursuit Eye Movements

Maintenance of fixation on a moving stimulus enables it to be accurately tracked, and at least in part, visually processed. There exists an upper physiological speed limit for pursuing a moving stimulus, which also depends on stimulus characteristics, in particular, size and contrast. This limit is at about 30–40°/s; above this speed small saccadic jumps appear to catch the moving stimulus, and the pursuit eye movement is no longer smooth. At much higher speeds the stimulus can only be pursued for very short distances, and large saccades are required to catch the stimulus and refixate upon it (Daw 2006; Pola 2006; Atkinson and Nardini 2008). Children can pursue moving visual stimuli already by the age of 4 weeks, provided that the stimulus speed does not exceed 20°/s. The main explanations for this limit are low visual acuity and movement vision capacity, but also low attention control (Rutsche et al. 2006). Interestingly children at this age can detect moving (and flickering) stimuli more reliably than stationary ones, and show more reliable orienting responses to moving stimuli (Wattam-Bell 1992, 1996a). This is explained by a preference for moving stimuli because they possess higher salience. The low capacity of movement vision in early childhood is also shown by the lack of ability to discriminate movement direction (Wattam-Bell 1996b) and the still marked inability to pursue moving stimuli with higher speed (Aslin and Smith 1988). Between 2 and 4 months of age, children improve considerably in their smooth pursuit ability (Gronqvist et al. 2011), whereby executive functions are already involved in predictive control (Rosander 2007). At the age of 4 months children can reliably differentiate between stimulus movement and self-movement (Dannemiller and Friedland 1989). It is likely that by this stage very young children use mainly binocular vision for movement perception, because this capacity has not been found under monocular conditions (Kellman 1993), but accurate binocular pursuit eye movements have been reported for stimulus speeds up to 40°/s (Roucoux et al. 1983; Hainline 1998; Daw 2006; Pola 2006; see Fig. 2.8).

Figure-ground discrimination based on movement vision is possible at the age of 3 months; at the age of 5 months, children use movement information to perceive the figure itself (Arteberry et al. 1993). At this age children prefer viewing biological movements, for example, hand movements, movements of walking and running, etc. Interestingly, binding of movement to an object or a person is not required, but a moving pattern consisting of illuminated dots can by this stage be integrated into a Gestalt (Fox and McDaniel 1982). The early appearance of this stimulus preference for biological movement indicates that this capacity is innate because the time since birth would be insufficient for the development of such a complex ability.

Spatial and temporal, visual and attentional deficits limit access to the moving image, potentially interfering with social interaction (e.g. by not seeing more rapid facial movements), access to information and mobility. Such limitations need to be sought, identified and acted upon in children with CVI.

2.7.5 Binocular Eye Movements and Binocular Vision

Binocular eye movements comprise saccades, smooth pursuit eye movements, vergence eye movements, optokinetic nystagmus (OKN) and the vestibular ocular reflex (VOR). In early infancy, eye movements already show high similarity with adulthood. However, control of eye movements at this time is still underdeveloped, although single oculomotor components already exist (Daw 2006; Pola 2006; Hunnius 2007; Atkinson and Nardini 2008; Karatekin 2008). The development of binocular vision particularly requires accommodation and convergence. Children

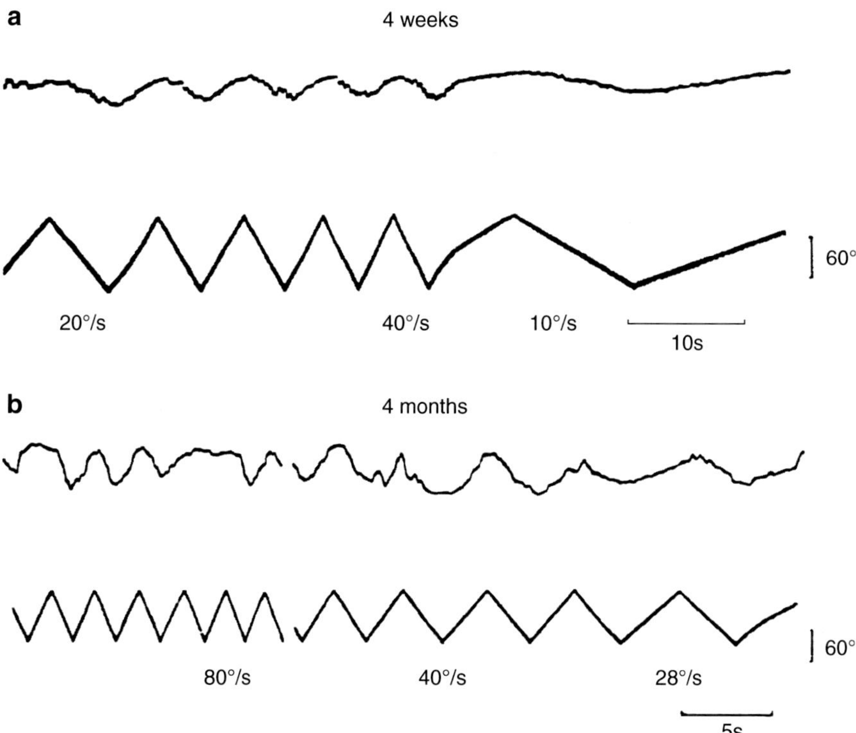

Fig. 2.8 Smooth pursuit movements recorded by EOG (*upper traces*), at 4 weeks (**a**) and 4 months of age (**b**) for different stimulus speed (deg/s) (*lower traces*). Note pronounced improvement in pursuit accuracy for higher speeds at 4 months. (Adapted from Roucoux et al. 1983. © Elsevier reprinted with permission)

possess elementary binocular vision at the age of 3 months; at this age stereopsis develops rapidly (see Sect. 2.3.5).

2.7.6 Visual Exploration and Visual Search

Visual exploration is the free intentional inspection of the surroundings, a scene or a large object without (fixed) instruction. In contrast, visual search is the ability to find a single defined target among distractors, which either pops out in the field of non-targets, or distractors (parallel search mode), or can only be found after carefully scanning the entire stimulus field (serial search mode; see Fig. 2.9) (Zihl 2011).

Visual exploration of the visual environment in general and of a scene or complex object in particular, while using search for defined particular stimuli in this environment or scene, is essential for gaining a global coarse representation of the spatial properties and directing attention and fixation to specific locations for local processing (Treue 2003). Both components subserve visual information processing and build

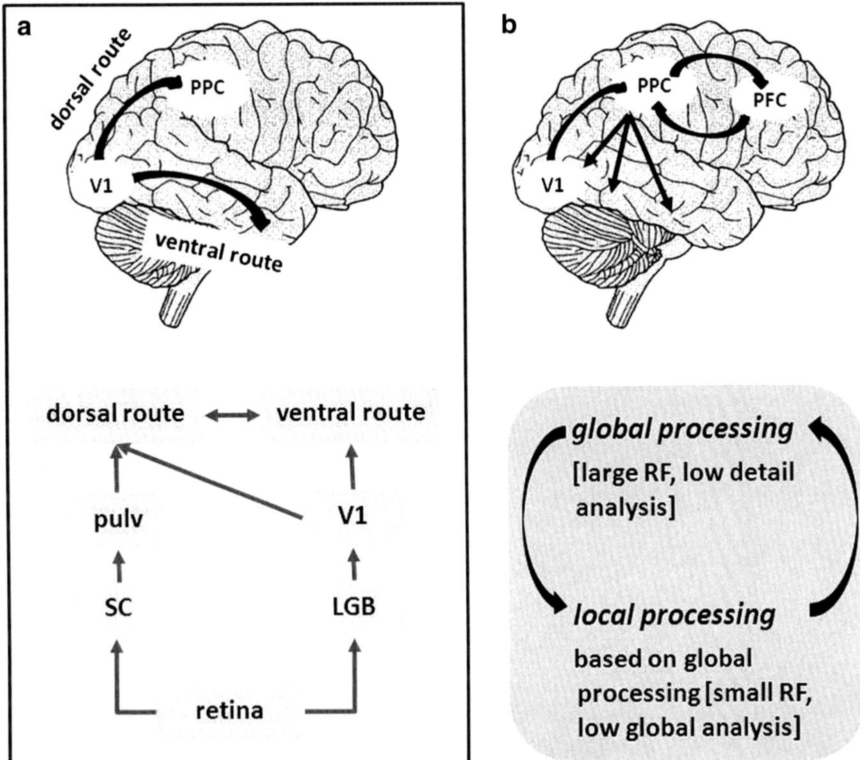

Fig. 2.9 Brain pathways for global–local visual processing. (**a**) Normal hierarchy bottom-up pathways from the eye to the dorsal and ventral visual processing streams. *SC* superior colliculus (midbrain), *pulv* the pulvinar (posterior thalamus), *LGB* (lateral geniculate body), *V1* visual area 1 (striate cortex). *PPC* posterior parietal cortex. (**b**) Reversed hierarchy pathways reaching first PPC for global processing (based on large receptive fields (RF) of neurons for coarse analysis), which guides subsequently local processing in the ventral route (based on smaller receptive fields of neurons for fine analysis) (Modified after Hochstein and Ahissar 2002)

the basis for mental representation of stimuli in space, and their quality in terms of object properties; and both operate by interaction with selective attention (Martinez-Conde et al. 2004; Himmelbach et al. 2006). Already in 3-month-old infants' visual selective attention enhances visual search and object perception (Amso and Johnson 2006). Thus, basic visual search operates bottom-up and top-down early in development (Taylor and Khan 2000), whereby object and face scanning may precede development of gaze shifting to peripheral stimuli (Hunnius et al. 2006). Spatially and temporally coherent oculomotor scan patterns develop gradually, because they require global vision and sufficiently reliable visual spatial orientation, as well as the capacity to accurately localise objects in space to maintain fixation upon them for a sufficient period. Face identity recognition performance in children strongly depends on accurate, detailed scanning of faces (Wilson et al. 2012). It is interesting to note that after birth, spontaneous gaze shifts are preceded by rapid changes in general body movement; this sequence changes after a few weeks (Robertson et al. 2001). Explorative abilities are well developed by about the age of 3 years (Del Guidice et al. 2000), but show progressive optimisation until 15 years of age (Keating et al. 1980). Visual search performance strongly depends on developmental processing capacity for stimulus dimensions, whereby colour and orientation can be more easily detected than size; conjunction (of two stimulus dimensions) and odd-one-out search performance (one stimulus differing from all the others, which are identical) continue to develop until 10 years of age (Donnelly et al. 2007). Of course, the developmental stage of visual spatial memory plays an essential role, in that lower memory span is associated with lower search speed (Smith et al. 2005).

Low vision in all its forms limits visual exploration, and acquisition of information, necessitating early institution of measures to render salient visual information accessible, as well as facilitating alternative strategies of safe and rewarding exploration founded on use of the other senses, to help optimise learning.

2.7.7 Optokinetic Nystagmus (OKN), the Vestibulo-Ocular Reflex (VOR) and Cerebellar Input

OKN and the VOR are closely associated with the vestibular system. They help to compensate for retinal image shifts during self-movement and thus support visual stabilisation of perception of the visual surroundings (Ackerley and Barnes 2011). OKN can be elicited soon after birth, but definitely by the age of 6 weeks (Banton and Bertenthal 1996). As a rule, at this age the OKN is asymmetrical, i.e. easier to elicit for centripetal (towards the nose) than for centrifugal movement direction of the optokinetic stimulus. At about the 4th–5th month of age, this asymmetry disappears under both binocular and monocular viewing conditions. The coordination between the visual and vestibular systems and associated motor responses, and the adjustment of interactions between these functional systems is not complete before the age of 6 years (Hainline 1998; Daw 2006; Pola 2006; Atkinson and Nardini 2008). External factors, for example when the child is carried, elicit head movements, and cause altered or instable fixations. However, appropriate eye movements, for example, a pursuit eye movement in the direction of the head movements, followed by a saccadic movement in the opposite direction, can efficiently compensate for these changes. This type of compensation is known as the VOR, which can already be observed from the first month of life (Regal et al. 1983). There is evidence that the cerebellar vermis plays a role in the discrimination of motion (Cattaneo et al. 2014).

2.7.8 Head Movements and Vision

Gaze shift typically also includes head shifts; under natural conditions, head shifts follow eye shifts, when eye shifts exceed ~15° (Leigh and Zee 2006). Head movements are thus integral components of both orienting responses to visual stimuli, and the child's intentional responses in the context of visual exploration and visual search. Already in the first month of life, infants use eye and head movements to shift their gaze in space; eye shifts follow head shifts, which reverses in late childhood (Netelenbos and Savelsbergh 2003; Murray et al. 2007). The interval between eye and head movements decreases rapidly, i.e. head movements follow saccadic eye shifts more frequently and more promptly (Bloch and Carchon 1992). Head movements are – as are saccadic eye movements – still very much fragmentary; interestingly, however, motor parameters, e.g. velocity and amplitude, are already similar to values of older children and of adults (Regal et al. 1983; Atkinson and Nardini 2008). The frequency and variability of head movements decreases between 4 and 15 years of age (Murray et al. 2007).

2.7.9 Grasping

Visually guided grasping movements are essential for children because they allow catching and manipulation of objects using arm, hand and fine finger movements. In addition, body movement and control are essential prerequisites for grasping. Some of the most relevant and interesting developmental steps of these motor actions and activities are summarised in Tables 2.12 and 2.13. Of course, visual capacities as well as cognitive and motivational factors (curiosity and pleasure in movement) determine the development and optimisation of all visually guided movements. Improvement in object manipulation begins at the age of 2–3 months, after the grasp reflex has disappeared and intentional grasping movements begin to develop. From the 4th month on, grasping movements become more and more guided by vision, particularly with respect to stimulus localisation, identification and evaluation, and whether the stimulus in question is an attractive and appropriate goal for a grasping movement (Atkinson and Nardini 2008). It is important to note, that children actively practice visually guided exploration to advance their reaching behaviour; passive observation is not sufficient (Libertus and Needham 2010).

2.8 Comments

As outlined in the previous sections, newborns can already perceive the visual world as a 'near' world, although acuity, contrast sensitivity, accommodation and vergence are still in their early developmental phase. The perceptual development reflects the morphological and physiological development of the brain in general, and the visual brain in particular. However, innate visual perceptual preferences allow children to perceive complex visual stimuli like faces, which may enhance

Table 2.12 Development of motor actions and skills

Age	Motor actions/skills
Birth	Primitive reflexes (e.g. oculo-cephalic reflex, tonic neck reflex, grasp reflex) Low muscle tonus; low motor coordination
M 1–2	Arms slightly stretched; begins to lift the chin
M 3–4	Hands are opened Beginning of visually guided grasping Increase of oral activities (sucking) Disappearance of primitive reflexes
M 5–6	Stretching of hands and grasping for objects Sitting in a tripod position
M 7–8	Can hold an object (for example, a cube) in each hand Can deliver an object from one hand to the other Improvement in holding objects Independent sitting, standing with help
M 9–10	Can hold bottle and drink out of it Can, unassisted, hold and eat a piece of biscuit Can put fingers into holes Can sit for a longer time without help Crawls and drags on the floor Tries to stand up without help
M 11–12	Uses a spoon; can hold a cup and drink out of it Opens and closes boxes Can walk and stand up with help

Modified after Reinis and Goldman (1980)
M month of life

visual and also cognitive and motor development. Nevertheless, an intimate interplay appears to exist between the neurobiological and the functional trajectories of visual development; they are interdependent and mutually enhance or impair each other. If one or other element does not develop adequately, and within certain time windows, whatever the reason may be, then the development of all the wonderful visual perceptual capacities and abilities will suffer, and in addition, all brain functions that depend on visual development may be affected directly or indirectly. Not much is known about the time windows that are crucial for particular visual developmental stages. Table 2.14 comprises a summary of visual behaviours in the first year of childhood.

Table 2.13 Stages of normal development in infancy and early childhood (time ranges in months, M, with 3 and 97 % confidence interval)

Activity	M (3–97 %)
Motor activities	
Turns to the side	3–7
Turns prone	4–8
Crawls prone	7–13
Semi-sitting position	8–14
Sits up	9–16
Plays in sitting position	10–17
Scrambles on hands and knees	8–16
Stands up without assistance	12–21
First free steps	13–21
Eating activities	
Opens the mouth when touched with the spoon	2–5
Opens the mouth when seeing the spoon	3–7
Eats with the spoon without assistance	15–24
Holds a cup and can tilt it	5–19
Drinks from the cup without help	6–17
Eye- hand coordination and playing	
Pursues a moving object	1–3
Observes own hand	1–5
Plays with own hands	3–5
Tries to reach objects	4–6
Grasps accurately	4–7
Manipulates an object in a variable way	6–9
Puts two objects together	8–14
Manages two or more objects	9–17
Builds with objects	10–27

Modified after Straßburg et al. (1997)

Table 2.14 Development of visual behaviour within the first 12 months

0–1 month
Looks at sources of light, turns eyes (using saccades) and head
Eye blinks (lid closures) as avoidance behaviour
Makes contact with eyes
Slow and jerky horizontal pursuit eye movements
2–3 months
Intensive eye contact
Interest in 'lip reading'
Interest in mobiles
Vertical pursuit eye movements
4–6 months
Observes own hands
Grasps for moving objects
Observes falling and rolling away of objects
Shift of fixation across midline
Gradual extension of the field of visual search
Beginning of uncoupling of eye from head movements
Smooth pursuit eye movements
7–10 months
Becomes aware of and detects smaller objects
Touches, and later grasps, stationary objects
Interested in scenes and pictures
Can identify partially occluded objects
Maintains eye contact over a distance of several meters
11–12 months
Good visual orientation in familiar surroundings
Looks through window and recognises familiar individuals
Visual recognition of pictures; plays hide and seek
Observes and examines objects in detail
Efficient visual communication (understands and uses facial expressions and gestures)

Modified after Hyvarinen (2000)

Development of Non-visual Mental Functions and Capacities

3

Visual perception does not act independently, but is orchestrated together with other mental functions and capacities. What happens when a child has lost his favourite toy and tries to find it? First, the child has to have sufficient interest to search for the toy (motivation). Then the child has to remember what the toy looks like to recognise it visually (visual memory). The process of visual searching then starts, with shifting the field of vision and transport of the fovea to places where the toy might be, using eye and head movements (attention, motor activities, and monitoring of the search process). It is important that the child maintains attention throughout the search process and avoids distraction by other toys (sustained attention and concentration; control of attention; response inhibition). In addition, the child needs to remember the areas already searched (visual working memory). Once the child has eventually found the toy and has recognised it as his favourite one (visual recognition and visual memory), the child may well be happy that search was successful (emotion, reward). This simple example shows that visual perception without motivation, attention, memory, executive function and action would not work successfully. The content and activity of visual perception are embedded in cognition, motivation, emotion, language and action. The respective functional brain systems interact in a reciprocal way with the visual system, and support visually guided activities. Without reference to these systems, neither normal nor impaired visual perception can be understood and explained. In the following sections, development of attention, learning and memory, executive functions, language, emotions, motivation and social behaviour are briefly described. For more detailed presentations, see Granrud (1993), Cole and Cole (2001), Johnson and de Haan (2010). There is evidence for some gender-specific differences in the development of cognition, which are mainly interpreted in the context of sex hormone differences (Berenbaum et al. 2003). Spatial abilities and working memory appear enhanced by androgens at several stages in development; boys may therefore show higher performance than girls in both domains. In contrast, verbal capacities (verbal memory, verbal fluency) are enhanced by oestrogens, which may explain why girls outperform boys in this domain.

J. Zihl, G.N. Dutton, *Cerebral Visual Impairment in Children: Visuoperceptive and Visuocognitive Disorders*, DOI 10.1007/978-3-7091-1815-3_3

3.1 Attention

Attention represents an essential and crucial basic resource of the brain for all activities, particularly in the domain of vision and cognition (e.g. Berman and Colby 2009). Van Zomeren and Brouwer (1994) have found it useful to distinguish between two dimensions of attention: *intensity* and *selectivity*, which are both regulated and controlled by a superordinate (executive) function that monitors and adapts attentional resources to the actual task demands. In both dimensions, several components can be identified, which are, however, closely interconnected within a common network. The dimension *intensity* comprises alertness (activation of global attentional resources), sustained attention (maintenance of a given level of attention over time), information processing and mental speed. The dimension *selectivity* includes the ability to focus on just one stimulus or stimulus configuration without being distracted by other stimuli or tasks (concentration), the ability to divide attention between two or more stimuli or stimulus configurations (divided attention), and the ability to shift attention between stimuli (attentional flexibility). In their taxonomy of attention, Chun et al. (2011) rely on targets, i.e. the types of information that attention is operating over. *External attention* refers to the selection and modulation of spatial and temporal properties and modality of sensory input, while *internal attention* refers to the selection, modulation, and maintenance of internally generated 'information', i.e. responses, task rules, working and long-term memory. Posner and Peterson (1990) have proposed a model of attentional brain systems comprising three components: *alerting* (brain stem) subserving alertness, *orienting* (thalamus and posterior parietal cortex) for attention in space, and *executive control* (pre-frontal cortex) for selective and divided attention, including multi-tasking, and the control of alertness and spatial attention. The original model has been extended to include *self-regulation* (prefrontal cortex; cingulate cortex), i.e. self-control of attentional responses (Petersen and Posner 2012). Spatial attention comprises the global distribution of attention over a wide or narrower part of the surroundings or a scene (field of attention) and the shift of attention to particular regions/locations in space (spatial attentional shifts).

In early child development, the various attentional functions show different trajectories. Components of intensity and simple functions of selectivity develop earlier, while components with higher sharing of executive function develop later and are not available before the age of 3 years (Colombo 2001; Jones et al. 2003; Kannass et al. 2006). Attention plays an important role in the development of vision, in particular visual search and object processing (Amso and Johnson 2006) and recognition memory (Rose et al. 2001), but also social interaction (Elam et al. 2010).

These developmental trajectories are briefly described and summarised below (after Anderson et al. 2001b; Colombo 2001; Klenberg et al. 2001; Anderson 2002; Ruff and Cappozoli 2003).

1st year. Wakefulness changes more and more into alertness with guided attention to external stimuli. In the first year, periods of wakefulness, and thus of alertness, increase in both frequency and duration; during such periods attention to visual stimuli can systematically be elicited and thereby improved. At the end of the third year, longer periods of alertness are well established within the circadian rhythm of the child. At the age of 10 months, children show less concentration when more than one stimulus (toy) is present in their field of attention. At the end of their first year, children show faster habituation to novel stimuli; consequently stimulus salience has to be increased in order to elicit a reliable response. This manifests a kind of a milestone in the development of attention: a change takes place, from predominantly externally (bottom-up) guided attention, to an increasingly stronger internal (intentional, top-down) guidance of attention that allows more independence from external events and thus more personal autonomy.

2nd–4th year. All attentional functions improve, in particular sustained attention and attentional capacities involving higher executive components. Multi-tasking however, still remains limited.

5th–16th year. Information processing and mental speed, sustained attention, concentration, attentional control and flexible adaptation to changing stimulus and task conditions increase further. Multi-tasking performance also improves, but complex multi-tasking is not fully developed until early adulthood.

3.2 Learning and Memory

Learning is the fundamental basis for recalling visual (and other) facts and experiences from memory. There exist various forms of learning, which differ with respect to the degree of 'conscious' control involved (implicit vs. explicit) and the more declarative or non-declarative character (Gabrieli 1998; Squire and Wixted 2011). *Classical conditioning* refers to the association of a neutral stimulus with a particular significance (the baby learns to associate the view of the little white bottle with 'food'). *Operant conditioning* denotes a form of learning through the outcomes of particular behaviours, whether they are pleasant and rewarding, or otherwise. *Learning by imitation (so-called model learning or observational learning)* denotes the type of learning when children acquire a behavioural response or even a complex type of behaviour by observing this behaviour as shown by another person. *Trial and error learning* may be taken literally and typically takes place in a new or very unfamiliar task condition, when subjects just try and test again and again until the outcome eventually fits. Of course, the processes of planning, problem solving and monitoring, as well as knowledge gained from experience are also involved in this type of learning. *Learning by insight* means that the outcome is gained by systematic consideration and testing of ideas based on previous experiences and inductive and deductive reasoning.

Once processed, information is stored and has to be recalled for use, in forming experiences and in guiding and regulating behaviour. Information in *short-term memory* can be kept for only a few seconds without further processing, while in *working memory*, information can be maintained and processed over minutes. Information important for the individual is then transmitted to *long-term memory*, from where it can be recalled even decades later. Long-term memory is organised as a store-house with separate compartments for events (episodic memory), facts and knowledge (semantic memory), and procedures (procedural memory). *Episodic memory* comprises autobiographical and public events of one's life, including details about who, what, where, when, and why and how. *Semantic memory* contains facts and knowledge. In *procedural memory* procedures are stored, i.e. how things are done. Most of these procedures are actions and complex motor activities, for example, walking, swimming, and skiing, but also waving a hand for a good bye, writing and drawing. In a more general sense, there also exist procedures in the domains of perception and cognition, for example, how to scan a scene for fast and complete comprehension, how to regulate attention when performing a task, how to learn a language, or how to monitor a complex action to avoid errors. After considerable practice such procedures usually become routine, and less cognitive (and sometimes also physical) effort is needed to carry out the activity in question. Interestingly, learning 'by looking' plays an important role in the infants' transition from crawling to walking (Clearfield et al. 2008). Episodes and facts can be easily put into words and communicated through language; in contrast, procedures and skills are very difficult to declare. Thus, episodic and semantic memory is also called *declarative memory*, while procedural memory is known as *non-declarative memory* (Squire and Wixted 2011). Episodes from the first 2–3 years can only imprecisely be recalled in childhood, and most cannot be remembered into adulthood, which is not explained by the time elapsed between event and time of recall but relates to the very young age of the brain at the time of storage (Eacott and Crawley 1999; Hayne 2004; Picard et al. 2009). Conditioning and procedural ('implicit') learning are already operating after birth, while 'pre-explicit' working and long-term memory develop in the first months after birth, and improve within the first year of age; whereas working memory shows a protracted course of development (Nelson 1995). A special type of memory is prospective memory, which plays a major role in organising everyday life activities (Maylor and Logie 2010). Prospective memory refers to events and actions in the future. It entails forming a particular intention, keeping this intention in memory, and recalling it when needed, with initiation and execution of the intended action at the foreseen time or associated with future events or with persons. Thus prospective memory works at the intersection of memory and executive functions (Kliegel et al. 2008). Temporal lobe cortical structures, the hippocampus and thalamus appear crucial for episodic and semantic verbal (left hemisphere) and non-verbal (right hemisphere) memories; basal ganglia serve habit learning, and premotor/supplementary structures and basal ganglia process procedural memory (Squire and Wixted 2011), while prefrontal structures accord prospective memory (Burgess et al. 2011). Brain injury does not usually cause global memory impairment due to this functional and anatomical segregation of the memory systems.

The main developmental trajectories for the various forms of learning and memory are summarised below (after Reese 2002; Courage and Howe 2004; Barrouillet et al. 2009; Schwenck et al. 2009; Maylor and Logie 2010).

1st year. Classical and operant conditioning exist already at birth. In addition, basal capacities for the reception, processing and coding of olfactory, gustatory, somatosensory and acoustic stimuli are also developed. Within the first 12 months, vision develops rapidly such that learning through this modality can take place.

At the age of 6 months, visual observation learning is possible. At 9 months children can learn through imitation, one, or a series of two actions; by the age of 12 months this increases to 4, and by the age of 3 years, children can learn up to 25 action steps.

2nd–4th year: By the end of the second year of life, children can learn by insight. At the age of 2 years, children have access to episodic memory independent of the context. This flexible recall is a milestone in memory development because it demonstrates the detachment of the memory from the external world. The child is no longer dependent on external cues but can intentionally and voluntarily retrieve information from memory. However, at this age memories are still bound by their episodic context, i.e. memory for facts and procedures/actions are more or less coloured by the events in which they have been learned. The social context appears to play an important role, particularly the style of interactions with parents, brothers and sisters, and other relevant persons. Children need self-conception for the formation and development of an autobiographical memory; conversations with the mother or another relevant person support the building of the child's own experiences in proper order and context. Language capacities also play an important role in reporting episodes.

4th–6th year: At this age children possess reliable knowledge concerning similar and repeatedly occurring events, for example, regular journeys and restaurant visits (so-called script knowledge). In addition, children use learning strategies; these strategies are, however, still simple and cannot be improved so much by practice as at a later stage.

6th–16th year: Episodic memory shows a distinct increase in performance from the sixth year on, possibly from using more efficient strategies for encoding and recall. Working memory also improves markedly in terms of greater efficiency in parallel processing of information and flexible attentional control. At the age of 11 years children can report recent experiences (events) in great detail. At about the same age efficient and skilful learning strategies have been adopted and can be used, however, prospective memory is still developing until adulthood.

3.3 Executive Functions

Reasoning, planning and problem solving are among the most complex human mental abilities. The various cognitive processes and functions underlying these abilities are subsumed under the umbrella term 'executive functions' and represent a variety of components for guidance, regulation, control and monitoring of behaviour. These components render possible and ensure that actions can be adapted to particular stimulus and task conditions, involving changes in the various domains of perception, attention, memory, action and communication, modulated by motivation and emotion (Ardila 2008). Table 3.1 gives a summary of executive functions and their role in human behaviour. As can be seen, planning and problem solving consist of several components, which facilitate imagination of situations and tasks leading to action to solve problems, or a plan in mind before executing the action (thereby avoiding effortful, and largely frustrating, trial and error behaviour). Anticipation of real or

Table 3.1 Summary of executive functions

Functions	Behavioural significance
Regulation of cognition	
Initiation	Self-motivated and self-initiated actions
Shift	Shifting attention intentionally from one stimulus/information set/ action to another (cognitive flexibility)
Inhibition	Suppression of responses/actions
Planning and problem solving	Selection of goals, development of steps in an appropriate order, development of strategies, flexible execution, evaluation of action
Monitoring	Supervision of actions
Transient storing (working memory)	Maintenance and recovery of information relevant for action
Regulation of activity	Balance between activation and inhibition of intensity and selectivity of attention (in particular, alertness and concentration)
Regulation of emotion	(Condition- and task-dependent) control of affective state and affective responses
Regulation of social functions	Adequate social actions/behaviour (in particular in the context of communication)

possible difficulties and impediments, detection and correction of errors, development and actual use of alternatives, monitoring of provisional and final outcomes with respect to the intended goal, and learning from errors are also functions of the executive system. This rather complex structure and organisation of mental operations of the executive system is required to cope with its many roles. Relevant information is processed and coded by the perceptual systems, is maintained in working memory, attentional resources are allocated to the various executive action steps, irrelevant and false responses and actions are inhibited, while relevant and correct responses and actions are initiated and executed. It is still unclear, whether the executive system is in fact one big system, which comprises a high diversity of functions/capacities, or whether sub-systems act more or less independently. Each alternative appears possible (for a review, see Jurado and Rosselli 2007), although the dissociated nature of executive impairments tends to favour regional sub-systems, which despite a high degree of autonomy, interact closely with each other (Stuss and Alexander 2007). It is important to note that executive function influences the mapping of sensory information to motor activities via attentional bias toward rewarding stimuli and actions (Deco and Rolls 2005).

The development of executive functions continues until early adulthood, when the morphological development of the prefrontal cortex is complete (Jurado and Rosselli 2007). Working memory, response inhibition, and response and set shifting in elementary form, as well as their integration in behavioural schemes are available during the preschool period (Garon et al. 2008). However, tool use, which can be observed much earlier in childhood, reveals how the child behaves to achieve goals and thereby develops (simple) plans, practises problem solving, and brings about monitoring and error detection and correction (Keen 2011). Table 3.2 summarises the development of executive functions at different stages. While planning,

Table 3.2 Degree of developmental increase in four categories of executive functions

Age group	Planning	Cognitive flexibility	Inhibition	Working memory
5–8 years	+++	+++	+++	+++
8–11 years	++	+++	++	+++
11–14 years	+	++	+	++
14–17 years	++	++	–	–
>17 years	++	+	–	–

Modified after Romine and Reynolds (2005) during the age groups between 5 and >17 years
+++, large; ++, moderate; +, small; –, no change

cognitive flexibility, response inhibition and working memory show differing developmental trajectories, significant gender differences have not been identified.

Executive functions develop incrementally in the stages described below (after Colombo 2001; Anderson 2002; Romine and Reynolds 2005; Jurado and Rosselli 2007; Burrage et al. 2008; Garon et al. 2008; Sun et al. 2009; Best and Miller 2010).

1st year: Inhibitory responses within short intervals of about 5 s can be observed in children by the age of 4–6 months; at the age of 1 year, children can suppress learned responses, and show increased 'resistance' to distractor stimuli. In addition, children begin to develop their own emotional regulation, which is under the influence of the child's temperament and social (familiar) surroundings. Children at this age also show simple planning and problem solving activities, while working memory capacity increases considerably.

3rd–5th year: Control of inhibition increases, working memory capacity improves; explicit planning begins, for example, in the context of arranging many parts to a complex object or preparing for a birthday party. In addition, children gain insight into rule systems.

6th–10th year: In this period, executive functions show significant development, particularly because of more or less regular and systematic practice and use of executive function in school. Children learn how to develop and use learning and memory strategies, but also refine and optimise their planning and problem solving strategies. Furthermore, children also begin to use their strategies outside the original condition or task, i.e. they transfer their strategies to similar tasks, and try to apply them to comparable task conditions.

3.4 Language

Language capacity can be subdivided into the faculty of auditory verbal understanding, i.e. spoken language (speech comprehension), and the faculty of visual verbal understanding, i.e. written language (text comprehension: reading; see Sect. 2.3.9). Prosody ('melody of speech') plays an important role in understanding the emotional state of the speaker. The special type of communication used with babies and very young children is a special kind of prosody (higher

Table 3.3 'Milestones' of language development

Age	Language abilities
M 1	Production of brief guttural sounds
M 2	Production of longer vocal sounds ('oooh', 'aaah')
M 3	Spontaneous vocalisations
M 6	Vocalisation when addressed
M 7	Production of chains of syllables with consonants and vowels directly after (babbling)
M 8	Child gives verbal responses; learns new words and remembers them over weeks
M 9	Produces chains of syllables with 'a' ('wawa', 'baba')
M 10	Passive vocabulary of 11–145 words
M 11	Understanding of words during care activities
M 12	Intentional use of double syllables and short words ('mama'); imitation of verbal sounds, responses to simple verbal calls and interdictions
M 18	Analogous use of about 50 single words; daily learning of several new words
M 30	Child uses two-word sentences
Y 4	Child uses complete sentences, names himself as 'I'
Y 5	Language is acquired; child repeats and answers sentences, uses classification nouns and definitions; begins to decipher letters and short words and to write (copy) letters and short words
Y 6	Increasingly improving language analysis, further enlargement of vocabulary; correct repetition of longer sentences; continues to 'read' and 'write'
Y 7	Child can tell a 3-picture story; articulation and speech fluency improve; understanding of language increases further; reading and writing become skilful

Modified after Siegler et al. (2011)
M months of life, *Y* years of life

register of voice, larger range of tones, prolongation of elements), which supports semantic and social language acquisition (Siegler et al. 2011). Table 3.3 summarises important 'milestones' of language development in children. In the first 12 months, language development is characterised by an increasingly improving capacity of speech production (articulation, prosody); at the end of the first year children can produce short, simple words and can also understand simple calls. At the end of the second year children already use two-word sentences. By the age of 4–6 years children possess a good understanding of language, can use complete sentences, and employ this capacity to tell short stories.

3.5 Emotions

Emotions comprise feelings and moods that manifest themselves in overt behaviour including facial expressions, gestures, prosody, and so-called body language, but also in body responses, for example, changes in heart and respiration rates. Typical emotions include joy, sadness, fear, anger and disgust. Emotions also accord significance and guide behaviour, for example, approaching pleasant stimuli and avoiding unpleasant stimuli. Emotions can also arise from evaluations and depend, therefore, on perception and experience. Mood is understood as a long-term emotional state; positive mood is a crucial prerequisite for motivation and thus for all human activities. Mood not only influences perceptions, but operates also as a kind of filter, i.e. depending on the state of mood, positive or negative information is selected, processed and prioritised. In addition, information is better recalled when encoded in a similar mood state as the current one (Siegler et al. 2011).

For the development of emotions two dimensions seem important: the increasing differentiation of one's own emotions, and the increasingly differentiated understanding of the emotions of others. In early childhood, understanding of emotions is mainly based on the perception of facial expressions and of prosody. Also very young children can discriminate facial expressions, with finer facial discriminations beginning to develop at the age of 2 months (see also Sect. 2.3.8). The integration of visual facial and prosodic information begins at the age of 7 months (Grossmann and Johnson 2007). At the age of 3 years children can also label emotions. Happiness can be correctly labelled earlier than anger, fear and sadness, while pride, blame and shame can be labelled by the age of 8–10 years (Siegler et al. 2011).

3.6 Motivation

Motivation accords directed activation and modulation of mental processes and behaviour, and serves to satisfy an actual need. Without (intrinsic) motivation no intentional engagement is possible, nor is any visual engagement (Larson and Rusk 2011). Curiosity undoubtedly represents the most important motivation in perception, which serves to satisfy the need for information and thus for gaining experience and knowledge building. Curiosity is probably an innate type of motivation that can be enhanced and increased (or the contrary) by external factors, and guided by pleasure and reward seeking (Berridge and Kringelbach 2013). Curiosity enables the child, and the adult, to observe the surroundings with attention and interest, and to gain information about the physical and social environments, which can be used to both cope with and enjoy the demands that varying circumstances place upon the individual. The satisfaction of fulfilling curiosity is arguably the best reward, particularly in childhood. However, it is not only the external environment, with all its variety and diversity of stimuli, that evokes curiosity and offers reward, it is progressively the brain itself, which produces reward and forms a kind of reward 'memory'. Thus reward becomes more and more an 'internal affair' of the brain as a whole, which is also evidenced by the presence of a widespread particular reward system in the brain, served by structures including the prefrontal cortex, the basal ganglia, the amygdala, the hippocampus, the thalamus and the brainstem (Haber and Knutson 2010).

Visual curiosity also needs cognition. A reduced attention span can preclude or diminish observation of the surroundings and search for interesting and relevant stimuli. Distractibility impairs focusing on interesting and relevant visual items. Visual episodic memory is required for storing what is of interest and of relevance, and executive functions are needed for the allocation of resources, for co-operation, regulation and monitoring of the various processes involved. Thus, motivation is one partner in the orchestra of mental activities, which plays an important role in the context of successful interactions between the individual and the external world (Arnsten and Rubia 2012).

Conclusion

The development and function of the entire range of non-visual mental functions and capacities outlined are closely allied with vision. CVI in children therefore has the potential to impact adversely upon each aspect. Once the nature and degree of visual impairment has been ascertained, the impact that this has upon non-visual mental functioning and its development needs to be determined, recognised and ameliorated by sets of approaches and strategies matched to the individual needs and capacities of the child.

4 Visual Disorders

4.1 Preliminary Remarks

Disorders of brain function can be distinguished in relation to the time of occurrence of the pathological event in brain development, prenatal (before birth), perinatal (around birth) and postnatal (after birth). Such disorders may manifest as missing, incomplete or delayed development of the function(s) affected. Practically, all functional disorders that arise during the pre-, peri- and postnatal periods, irrespective of the underlying aetiology, can be subsumed under the term 'early developmental disorder'. For labelling of the pathological event, the global term 'brain injury' is used to subsume the wide range of conditions including cerebrovascular, hypoxic and traumatic events that lead to disorder and/or dysfunction of cortical and subcortical structures of the visual system, including the white matter that contains the inter- and intracortical fibre connections, being affected.

Early developmental disorders can affect only one functional system, for example, the visual system, but can also have consequences for other functional systems. For example, in the case of hypoxic or traumatic injury, much of the brain is affected; in contrast, in cases of more 'local' brain injury, the function subserved by this structure or region is impaired. However, secondary effects of brain injury have always to be considered, because the functional outcome of brain injury is not just limited to the functions or functional systems that belong to the injured brain structures, but also to linked functions or functional systems. In the extreme case of multi-system disorders, overall functional development is either limited or delayed.

As the child grows and develops, impaired visual functions due to the central visual system being affected result in a range of behavioural outcomes. Affected functions may be absent or deficient, leading to failure to respond to what cannot be seen, as well as a range of typical adaptive strategies, and under certain circumstances, typical reactive behaviours. Learning through vision tends to be impaired to a degree related to the limitations in accessing information and social cues, and in mobility dictated by each child's specific set of visual constraints, set in the context of the efficacy of the strategies put in place to avert these limitations.

J. Zihl, G.N. Dutton, *Cerebral Visual Impairment in Children: Visuoperceptive and Visuocognitive Disorders*, DOI 10.1007/978-3-7091-1815-3_4

Acquired disorders of brain function can occur in later childhood. The outcome of such loss of function, when it affects vision, differs from that due to early developmental disorder. Prior learning means that skills and memories acquired through the now lost functions can persist, and these may be identifiable and employed for rehabilitation.

Children with cerebral visual disorders and additional functional impairments present a special challenge for diagnostics and treatment, particularly in the various domains of cognition. Associated impairments can render objective reproducible assessment of the visual disorders and their diagnostic classification very difficult, particularly in the context of the more complex visual disorders (see Chap. 6). About 60 % of children with cerebral visual disorders also exhibit cognitive and (fine) motor impairments (Spreen et al. 1995; Dutton and Jacobson 2001). Difficulties with attention, learning, memory and motivation (curiosity) are among the most frequent associated disorders. The close interactions between vision, cognition and motivation mean that impairments in these domains can exaggerate the apparent degree of visual impairment or may secondarily affect any normally developed visual capacities. Lack of visual attention can manifest and be diagnosed as a visual disorder. For example, even detection and localisation and discrimination of simple visual stimuli require a critical minimum degree of attention (Brown 1990). A child with severely reduced attention will have great difficulties with gaining detailed visual experiences needed for detection, localisation, discrimination, identification, and storage of visual stimuli. Thus, a missing or delayed orienting response to a visual stimulus may indicate a severe degree of visual impairment, but may also result from pathologically reduced attention (Weiss et al. 2001), or both.

In this chapter, the concept of CVI is presented and developed, and the differences between cerebral visual disorders arising in (early) childhood and in adulthood are discussed. This section is followed by a more detailed presentation of the various visual disturbances manifesting in early development.

4.2 The Concept of CVI (Cerebral Visual Impairment)

Visual disorders as a sequel to injury to the central, i.e. post-chiasmatic visual system in adults are labelled cerebral visual disorders, but this is an umbrella term that does not indicate which visual functions or capacities are affected, and which are not (Zihl 2011, 2014). In most cases of cerebral visual disorders, the peripheral (pre-chiasmatic) part of the visual system is unaffected, but the optic nerves can be affected by presumed transsynaptic degeneration (Jacobson et al. 2003), or there may be associated pathology such as retinopathy of prematurity (Dutton 2013). The combination of peripheral (injury to the eye or optic nerve) and central visual disorder (posterior cerebral artery infarction) in traumatic injury is another example. For the diagnostic categorisation of visual disorders caused by post-chiasmatic injury in children the term 'cerebral visual impairment' (CVI) has been introduced. This term has, however, been criticised by several authors (e.g. Frebel 2006; Colenbrander 2009, 2010; Lueck 2010) for various reasons:

1. The purely anatomical reference is biased, because the term 'cerebral' does not refer exclusively to the central visual system; in addition children with CVI can also suffer from peripheral visual dysfunction, which can affect visual information processing;
2. The term CVI lacks diagnostic specificity and does not describe the visual functions/capacities that are affected and those that are spared;
3. CVI does not specify whether the visual disorder is of primary or of secondary origin;
4. CVI does not differentiate between 'lower' (for example, visual field, visual acuity, spatial contrast sensitivity) and 'higher' visual disorders, which also involve cognitive components (for example, visual spatial perception, visual recognition);
5. CVI does not include information concerning the possible functional consequences in terms of individual visual disability and handicap.

Of course, these arguments warrant serious consideration when using the term CVI. On the other hand, the similar term 'cerebral visual disorders', which is used for adults, is only used to discriminate central from peripheral visual disorders, and the same criticisms may hold true. Given the fact that before the introduction of the term CVI no diagnostic label existed to denote the full range of cerebral/cortical visual disorders in children, the term CVI may be useful to mark visual dysfunction due to brain injury of whatever aetiology. Of course, a better diagnostic definition of the critical issues mentioned above is not only useful but also crucial for a valid and reliable diagnostic classification, and the selection and application of habilitation/rehabilitation and treatment measures. The main difficulty may rest with the term 'impairment'. According to the WHO International Classification of Impairment, Disabilities and Handicaps (ICF), impairment is defined as 'any loss or abnormality in an anatomical structure or a physiological or psychological function'. Thus, visual impairment is defined as a limitation of functions and capacities of the peripheral and central components of the visual system, which subserve visually guided actions. According to the WHO, visual impairment considers visual acuity and visual field only, which is definitely too restrictive in the context of CVI. However, if experts in this field use the term CVI as a diagnostic category that denotes dysfunction of the post-chiasmatic visual system, then the term CVI can be used as in adults with cerebral visual disorders, because the same diagnostic criteria apply. Therefore, we would like to propose the use of the term CVI by specifying its significance in the following ways:

1. When referring to *cerebral* visual impairment, it should be accepted that the term 'cerebral' refers to the post-chiasmatic structures of the visual system. In this sense, the term 'cerebral' is more valid than the term 'cortical', because all aetiologies of posterior brain injury affect both the cortex and the underlying

white matter. Thus the term 'cortical' has been considered too restrictive (Frebel 2006; Colenbrander 2010; Lueck 2010). Furthermore, if a child also suffers from peripheral visual dysfunction, the appropriate diagnosis (e.g. cataract or optic nerve hypoplasia) and the potentially resulting visual impairment (e.g. reduced visual acuity or contrast sensitivity; visual field disorders; colour vision deficiencies) should be reported in addition (Lerner et al. 2006). The same diagnostic procedure is used in adults with combined pre- and post-chiasmatic visual dysfunction.

2. There should be agreement that a complete report on CVI includes both affected and spared visual functions as a standard. However, this supposes that all visual functions and capacities are assessed. Assessment of visual acuity and visual field is definitely insufficient, because visual acuity measures do not always reflect the degree of visual disability (Colenbrander 2009; Lim et al. 2005). Meanwhile, recommendations exist concerning standardised visual assessment in children with CVI (see Tables 4.1 and 6.4).
3. The specification as to whether a particular visual dysfunction is of primary or secondary origin is an important diagnostic demand. Hence it follows that for a valid and complete assessment of CVI, cognitive functioning has also to be assessed in regard to visual perception, and one should also consider interactions between vision and cognition (as well as motivation and emotion) (Dutton 2002, 2009).
4. Detailed diagnoses include refractive disorders and 'lower' as well as 'higher' visual disorders; however, because there is no accepted definition of 'lower' and 'higher' functions, it may be difficult to assign visual functions/capacities exclusively to one or other category. The best compromise seems therefore to screen then assess as appropriate, salient visual functions and capacities. In particular in the case of 'higher' visual disorders, it is important to differentiate between primary and secondary causation, i.e. visual recognition difficulties also arise from impairment in 'lower' visual functions.
5. Consideration of the possible functional consequences of individual visual disability and handicap is an important diagnostic issue, and it is essential to determine which visual capacity management measures are required. However, in the absence of research reports on functional consequences and their amelioration, this can sometimes be a difficult task, and only intuitive or 'common sense' provisions may be possible.

In conclusion, for a valid and reliable use of the term CVI as a diagnostic category a standard is needed, which not only defines which assessment tools should be used and how, but also takes into consideration (oculo-) motor and cognitive functions (see Table 4.1). CVI is still not defined and used consistently (Boot et al. 2010). It would, however, represent an important step forward to use the term CVI in a standardised form in all disciplines involved in the diagnostics, treatment and advice concerning CVI. We therefore adopt the recommendation raised by Boot et al. (2010) for a definition of CVI that 'is based on functional visual processing rather than anatomical landmarks' (p. 1149). In this book, we use the term CVI in this sense to denote cerebral visual disorders, which are then further specified.

Table 4.1 Visual disorders in children with CVI

Function/capacity	Disorders
Visual functions/capacities	
Visual field	Homonymous field disorders (hemianopia); bilateral lower quadrantanopia; unilateral upper or lower quadrantanopia
Visual acuity	Often reduced; may also be normal
Spatial contrast sensitivity	Often reduced; may also be normal
Colour vision	May be impaired, but often normal
Space perception	Position and distance perception may be impaired
Depth perception	May be impaired; visual navigation may be impaired
Movement vision	Detection of moving stimuli may be impaired
Visual identification	Objects, faces and facial expressions, places and routes may only partly or not at all, be correctly discriminated and/or identified (e.g. misidentification due to common features)
Overview	May be restricted (only local processing; see also Attention)
Figure-Ground-Discrimination	Often impaired
Visual search	Often impaired
Visual guidance of movement	Can affect upper limbs and/or lower limbs
Oculomotor functions	
Accommodation	Often impaired
Vergence	Strabismus
Nystagmus/tonic deviation	May be present
Fixation	Unstable; spontaneous nystagmus
Saccadic eye movements	Inaccurate (dysmetria: hypo-/hypermetria)
Pursuit eye movements	Inaccurate (jerky)
Visual search/exploration	Reduced (constricted) and unsystematic, exacerbated by fatigue
Other functions	
Attention	Field of attention is often restricted → reduced overview in one or both hemifields; global reduction of attention focused and divided attention are impaired (neglecting of stimuli)
Visual memory	Stimulus positions, places and paths are inaccurately stored in working and long-term memory Objects and faces (and proper features) are inaccurately stored in working and long-term memory
Visual curiosity	Reduced motivation for visual stimuli and visual cognition
Grasping, pointing	Often inaccurate when visually guided (see space perception)

Modified after Dutton (2002), Dutton et al. (2006), Roman et al. (2010)

Visual disturbances in CVI can vary markedly in degree. (1) The most profoundly affected children may show little evidence of useful functional vision apart from reflex 'blindsight' in some cases, which may only be intermittent in nature (Boyle et al. 2005). (2) In other cases there may be associated cerebral palsy and intellectual and attentional disorders related to extensive brain involvement. Indeed new classifications of cerebral palsy include CVI as a potentially integral element (Bax et al. 2007; Rosenbaum et al. 2007). (3) At the other end of the spectrum, perceptual visual dysfunction with normal or near normal visual acuities and abilities commensurate with mainstream education has also been described in relation to premature birth (Macintyre-Béon et al. 2013). Such 'minor' degrees of perceptual visual dysfunction may not be uncommon but may be going unrecognised (Williams et al. 2011).

While the manifestations of CVI can be seen as a spectrum, ranging from profound to mild, the pragmatic differentiation of affected children into the above three groups is arguably warranted because they tend to be managed and taught by different professionals in different environments, who may thus be unaware of the features and needs of children in the other two categories. Yet the lessons learned from children in one category can be conceptually transferred, to benefit children in the other two groups.

CVI in children can differ from patterns seen in adult patients with cerebral visual disorders. Knowledge of how the human higher visual system functions when damaged has been informed by the extensive literature describing the specific visual dysfunctions that occur following focal disorder of the adult visual brain, supported by experimental work studying the visual outcome in affected subjects. In children however, pathology affecting the developing visual brain leads to similar but significantly different features because:

- Early onset damage to the brain is frequently diffuse and affects a range of interacting and developing brain functions.
- Brain growth, neuroplasticity and development, following the injury, lead to variable degrees of recovery.
- Compensatory behavioural adaptations made by the developing child may mask the underlying deficit, unless that specific function is stressed, either by tiredness or by a scenario that isolates the disordered function.
- Reactive behaviours, for example, distress in crowded environments, are common.
- Habilitational strategies may facilitate and thus enhance both functional and behavioural adaptations.
- Young children have not knowingly experienced any other type of vision and so 'know' their vision to be 'normal'. They are therefore 'asymptomatic' and cannot describe their visual difficulties, as they are not initially aware of them, until they can make comparisons with their peer group. Their visual disorders need therefore to be inferred from their observed behaviours, and information needs to be sought from parents and carers by structured history taking.
- Performance in tasks requiring visual search, visual attention and visual guidance of movement can diminish in the context of tiredness, distraction and stress, perhaps due to diminished functional reserve. The resulting day-to-day variation in performance may be incorrectly attributed to lack of concentration, if an adult construct is inappropriately applied.

- Parents and professionals, such as teachers and psychologists may misinterpret a child's visual performance as a 'behavioural disorder'. This can lead to criticism, which can lower self-esteem and affect the behaviour of a child who cannot understand what is wrong, and cannot therefore 'improve'.

Adult models of interpretation of the features of perceptual and cognitive visual dysfunction in children therefore have significant limitations, and for children, a model of interpretation founded upon observation and interpretation of visual behaviour is needed, to provide the foundation for both diagnosis and management. This subject is in its infancy. Many psychological visual testing strategies are founded upon a presumption of normal visual acuities and visual fields (which is commonly not the case in children with damage to the visual brain). They are also designed to detect aberrance from the normal range, rather than applying a diagnostic model to identify and typify specific perceptual dysfunctions that result from brain injury. Thus there is a paucity of investigations designed to characterise the wide range of perceptual and cognitive visual problems that parents commonly describe. Detailed history taking is therefore essential to reveal the nature and degree of the visual dysfunctions, which can then be corroborated, by observation of the child's behaviour in salient contexts.

4.3 Visual Disturbances

In the first years, children are unable to report on visual difficulties or answer questions about them. Therefore, no visual 'anamnesis' can be recorded. However, expert/skilled history taking that characterises the visual difficulties provides typical patterns of visual behaviour, identifies disorders and skills, and determines the parents goals and ambitions for their child combined with systematic and detailed observation and analysis of visually guided behaviours, particularly at this age, allows important conclusions to be drawn concerning affected and spared visual functions and capacities (see Chap. 6). The analysis of these observations provides valuable information, which can be enhanced by systematic manipulation of stimulus and/or task conditions and determination of whether the features of a suspected visual disorder increase or decrease, respectively. This approach also provides useful insights to guide intervention, because any decrease in the impact of the visual disorder in question indicates that improvement may be possible (see Chap. 7).

In the following sections, the range of visual disorders in infancy is described. Where only few reports are available in the literature, descriptions of visual disorders are used from adults, because corresponding disorders in adulthood are of a similar nature. A significant difference exists, of course, between adults and children, in that children have not gained sufficient visual experience before the age of 2 years, and thus their mental representation of the visual world is still limited, and any injury to the central visual system during this period of life affects an incompletely developed visual system. Visual disorders depend on the site and extent of injury to

Table 4.2 Visual disorders in relation to the site of brain injury (see also Fig. 2.2)

Optic chiasm
Monocular or binocular visual field defects
Visual acuity and contrast vision may be reduced in one or both eyes
Optic tract
Homonymous visual field defects that tend to differ in extent and are therefore incongruous
Visual acuity and contrast vision may be reduced in both eyes when both sides are affected
Optic radiation, striate cortex (area 17, V1)
Homonymous visual field defects that tend to be similar in extent and are congruous
Visual acuity and contrast vision may be reduced and visual fields constricted when both sides affected
Visual association cortex (prestriate cortex)
Occipito-parietal visual areas (dorsal route; WHERE- pathway)
Impairments in spatial perception and perception of movement
Impairments in spatial orientation, and navigation
Impaired spatial guidance of motor activities (saccadic and pursuit eye movements; grasping and pointing, walking over steps, and through crowds or past obstacles)
Occipito-temporal visual areas (ventral route; WHAT- pathway)
Impairments in contrast sensitivity, form and colour vision, and stereopsis
Impairments in object and face perception, and route finding (identification and recognition)

the visual system. Persisting vision after brain injury is evaluated on the basis of its usefulness in everyday life activities; not all persisting capacities necessarily accord an advantage despite being demonstrated under examination conditions. Numbers and percentages, respectively, of children reported with CVI differ between studies because of different selection criteria, i.e. in groups with suspected visual dysfunction numbers are usually higher than in unselected groups.

Table 4.2 summarises typical visual disorders after unilateral or bilateral post-chiasmatic injury depending on the locus of injury. Most commonly, cortical and subcortical visual structures are affected; in this case, associations of visual dysfunction (e.g. absence of visual field, reduced visual acuity, oculomotor dysfunction) occur. For the classification and understanding of the various visual disorders it has to be recognised, that as a rule, a range of visual disorders tend to occur in association, and that they are only seldom isolated. Table 4.3 gives an overview of the frequency of visual disorders in 401 children. These data show that about 50 % of children exhibit a combination of reduced acuity, strabismus and/or nystagmus. In the individual case, this combination may make it very difficult if not impossible to disentangle estimated visual acuity values from fixation issues, especially in younger children.

The high variability in the frequencies of childhood cerebral visual disorders reported in the following sections may be explained by differences in inclusion/referral criteria, assessment methods, heterogeneity of aetiology, associated disorders, age at time of brain injury, age at time of testing, and group size. In Table 4.4,

Table 4.3 Summary of visual and oculomotor disorders in 401 children with mainly pre- and perinatal brain injury (age at assessment: 1–16 years)

Homonymous visual field defects	32.4 %
Reduced visual acuities	48.6 %
Strabismus	8.6 %
Nystagmus	3.9 %
Combinations	*50.1 %*

Modified after Groenendaal et al. (1989), Dutton et al. (1996), Jacobson et al. (1996) Mercuri et al. (1997) Stiers et al. (1998), Fazzi et al. (2007)

Table 4.4 Outcome of the Linz study (*A*) and the study of Fazzi et al. (2007) (*B*) (for details see text)

	A (*N*=82)	B (*n*=121)
Aetiology		
Hypoxia	9 (35.4 %)	81 (66.9 %)
Morphological brain disorders	23 (28.0 %)	15 (12.3 %)
Preterm	17 (20.9 %)	63 (52.1 %)
CV	08 (9.7 %)	
Encephalitis	06 (7.3 %)	
Traumatic brain injury	02 (2.4 %)	
Occipital tumour (operated)	01 (1.2 %)	02 (1.7 %)
Others	23 (19.1 %)	
Time of brain developmental disorder or brain injury		
Prenatal	23 (28.0 %)	28 (23.1 %)
Perinatal	50 (61.0 %)	81 (66.9 %)
Postnatal	09 (11.0 %)	12 (10.0 %)
Additional disorders		
Global developmental disorder	80 (97.6 %)	90 (74.4 %)
Reduced visual curiosity	61 (74.4 %)	
Motor disorders	74 (90.2 %)	88 (72.7 %)
Tetraparesis/-plegia	19 (25.6 %)	42 (34.7 %)
Hemiparesis/-plegia	06 (08.2 %)	46 (52.3 %)
Developmental delay	49 (66.2 %)	
Optic nerve atrophy (bilateral)	45 (54.9 %)	17/53 (32.1 %)
Epilepsy	26 (31.7 %)	55 (45.5 %)
Time of visual assessment		
≤3 years	22 (26.8 %)	
4 years	23 (28.0 %)	4.5 years (SD: 3.3 years)
5 years	19 (23.2 %)	
6–7 years	18 (22.0 %)	

Aetiology (multiple references possible), time of brain injury, additional disorders and age at time of assessment

CV cerebrovascular events (infarction, haemorrhage), *SD* standard deviation

results of visual assessment from 82 children with CVI and complete data sets are summarised. Data were collected between 1994 and 2002 in a study carried out in cooperation with Siegfried Priglinger, former head of the Unit for developmental visual disorders and early intervention, Hospital of the Hospitaller in Linz (Austria; in the following referred to as 'Linz study'). For comparison, data from 121 children (age: 3–180 months) with CVI from the study published by Fazzi et al. (2007) are shown. Among 186 children with visual dysfunction and complete assessment, the group with CVI represents 44 %. Nielsen et al. (2007a) found CVI in 48 out of 97 children; this corresponds to 49.5 %. The most frequent aetiologies for CVI in the Linz study was perinatal hypoxia or hypoxia in preterm children (56.3 %), followed by morphological disorders of brain development (28 %). In ~30 % the aetiology of abnormal brain development was of prenatal origin, in ~60 % of perinatal, and in ~10 % of postnatal origin. At the time of assessment, about 15 % of children were younger than 2 years; about 70 % of children were between 3 and 5 years old and about 15 % were older than 5 years. More than half of the children (55 %) showed optic nerve atrophy; about two-thirds suffered from epilepsy. The majority of children (~98 %) also suffered from global developmental disorder, mainly in the domains of cognition. In two children without associated cognitive developmental disorders, CVI was caused by bilateral occipital cysts and by an occipital tumour, respectively, the latter being removed at the age of 2 years. Visual curiosity (spontaneous exploration of the surrounding by eye movements) was reliably observed in only about 25 % of children; however, all children responded promptly and reproducibly to a peripheral light stimulus. About 90 % of children suffered from additional motor disorders, mostly cerebral paresis or delayed motor development. The combination of CVI, developmental cognitive and motor disorders is the typical constellation of features after chronic cerebral hypoxia (Dutton and Jacobson 2001). Our observations in the Linz study are in good agreement with the reported disorders in the study of Fazzi et al. (2007). Cerebral hypoxia and epilepsy were reported as being more frequent causes by Fazzi et al., while global developmental disorder, motor disorders, and atrophy of the optic nerves were less frequently reported. Table 4.5 shows the most frequent visual and oculomotor disorders in the Linz study. The proportion of children with homonymous visual field defects is in the region of 60 %. A high percentage of children (~75 %) had difficulties with discrimination of colours and with visual orientation; and the majority of children (~90 %) found it difficult to discriminate patterns, figures, and objects accurately and reliably. Strabismus (convergent and divergent) was found in about 60 % of children; a minority (<5 %) showed congenital nystagmus. However, about 60 % of children had difficulties with accurate fixation. In about half of the group (52 %) oculomotor abnormalities were associated with low visual acuity; this number is similar to other studies (Groenendaal et al. 1989; Dutton et al. 1996; Jacobson et al. 1996; Mercuri et al. 1997; Stiers et al. 1998; see also Table 4.3). Fazzi et al. (2007) found that in their group of 121 children with CVI of mostly perinatal origin only ~6 % manifested a homonymous visual field defect, but in ~87 % there was low visual acuity, and in 48 % inaccurate fixation. The relatively severe nature of the visual features described indicates that children with ostensibly

Table 4.5 Visual and oculomotor disorders in the Linz study (82 children with CVI; see also Table 4.4)

Homonymous visual field defects	48 (58.5 %)
Unilateral	09 (18.7 %)
Bilateral	39 (81.3 %)
Reduced visual acuity	82 (100 %)
Impaired colour vision	63 (76.8 %)
Impaired light adaptation (photophobia)	18 (2.0 %)
Impaired spatial orientation	61 (74.4 %)
Impaired form/object perception	76 (92.7 %)
Inaccurate fixation	48 (58.5 %)
Strabismus	50 (61.0 %)
Congenital nystagmus	03 (03.6 %)
Combination	*43 (52.4 %)*

Combination refers to low visual acuity (<0.30), inaccurate fixation, strabismus or nystagmus. Inclusion criterion: suspected CVI

perceptual visual dysfunction alone, that for example, may well be common but often undiagnosed sequel to premature birth (MacIntyre-Béon et al. 2013), and may be not infrequent in the general population (Williams et al. 2011), were probably not included in these studies.

4.3.1 Visual Field

Visual field defects are the most frequently identified visual disorders in adults with cerebral visual disorders (Zihl 2011). Vision is affected in homonymous regions of the left (after right-sided) and right hemifield (after left-sided brain injury), because of crossing of about half of the fibres in each optic nerve (arising from the nasal retina of each eye) at the optic chiasm. Typical unilateral visual field defects include loss of vision in one hemifield (hemianopia), upper or lower quadrant (quadranopia), and islands of blindness in the inner visual field (paracentral scotomata) (see Fig. 4.1, 1-4), which are identical or very similar in both eyes. Bilateral injury to the post-chiasmatic visual system can cause complete blindness in both visual fields ('cerebral blindness'). Less dramatic consequences are bilateral homonymous hemianopia but with sparing of central visual function or 'tunnel vision', bilateral upper or lower quadranopia leading to bilateral upper or lower visual field impairment, sometimes also referred to as upper or lower homonymous hemianopia, and central scotoma, i.e. loss of vision in the central visual field (Fig. 4.1, 5-8). While cerebral anopia and scotoma refer to total lack of vision, cerebral homonymous amblyopia refers to the homonymous depression of light vision, with lack of colour and form vision in the affected hemifield or in both hemifields (Fig. 4.1, 9-10). Figure 4.2 shows the effect of homonymous visual field loss on global perception of a scene.

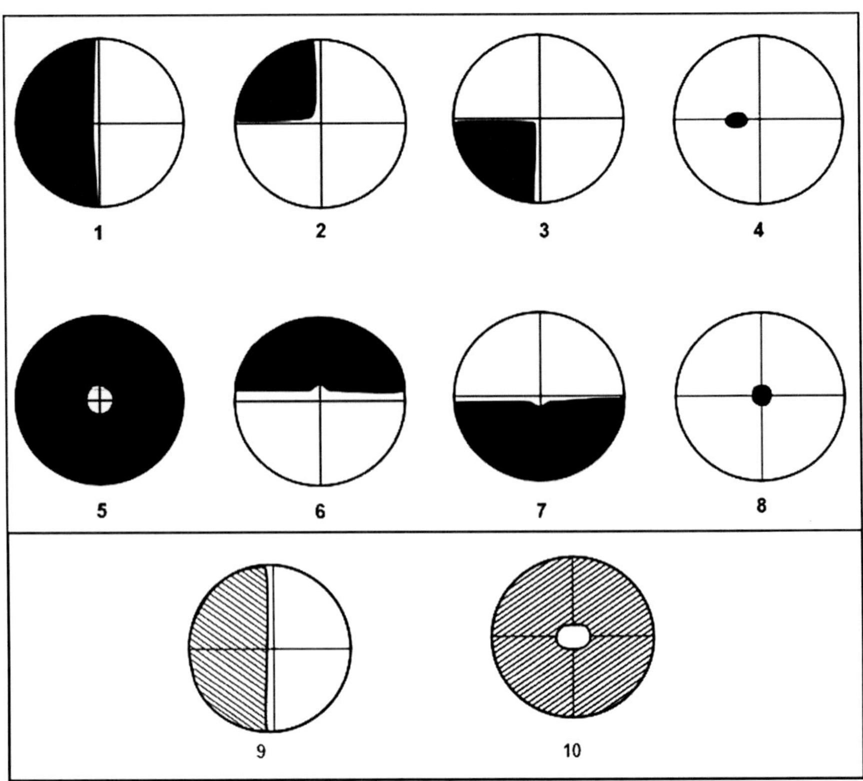

Fig. 4.1 Schematic illustration of homonymous visual field loss (binocular visual fields; spared parts are shown in *white*). *1–4* unilateral visual field loss, *5–8* bilateral visual field losses, *9–10* amblyopia. *1* left-sided hemianopia, *2* left upper quadranopia, *3* left lower quadranopia, *4* left-sided paracentral scotoma, *5* bilateral hemianopia ('tunnel vision'), *6* bilateral upper quadranopia (upper hemianopia), *7* bilateral lower quadranopia (lower hemianopia), *8* central scotoma, *9* left-sided hemiamblyopia, *10* bilateral cerebral hemiamblyopia

Homonymous visual field defects after post-chiasmatic brain injury of different aetiologies have also been reported in children (van Hof-van Duin and Mohn 1984; Flodmark et al. 1990; Ragge et al. 1991; Dutton et al. 1996; Jongmans et al. 1996; Mercuri et al. 1997; Jacobson et al. 2006; Fazzi et al. 2007). Bilateral homonymous visual field defects, in particular, bilateral hemianopia, are the most frequent type of homonymous visual field disorders in infancy, probably due to the high percentage of cases of the central visual system being affected, and being manifest at this stage of development (Table 4.6; see also Sect. 4.5). Bilateral lower visual field impairment is particularly common in children with periventricular white matter pathology (Jacobson and Dutton 2000).

Unilateral post-chiasmatic brain injury occurs less frequently in younger children (van Nieuwenhuizen and Willemse 1984), and, therefore, unilateral homonymous visual field defects are infrequent. In older children, unilateral

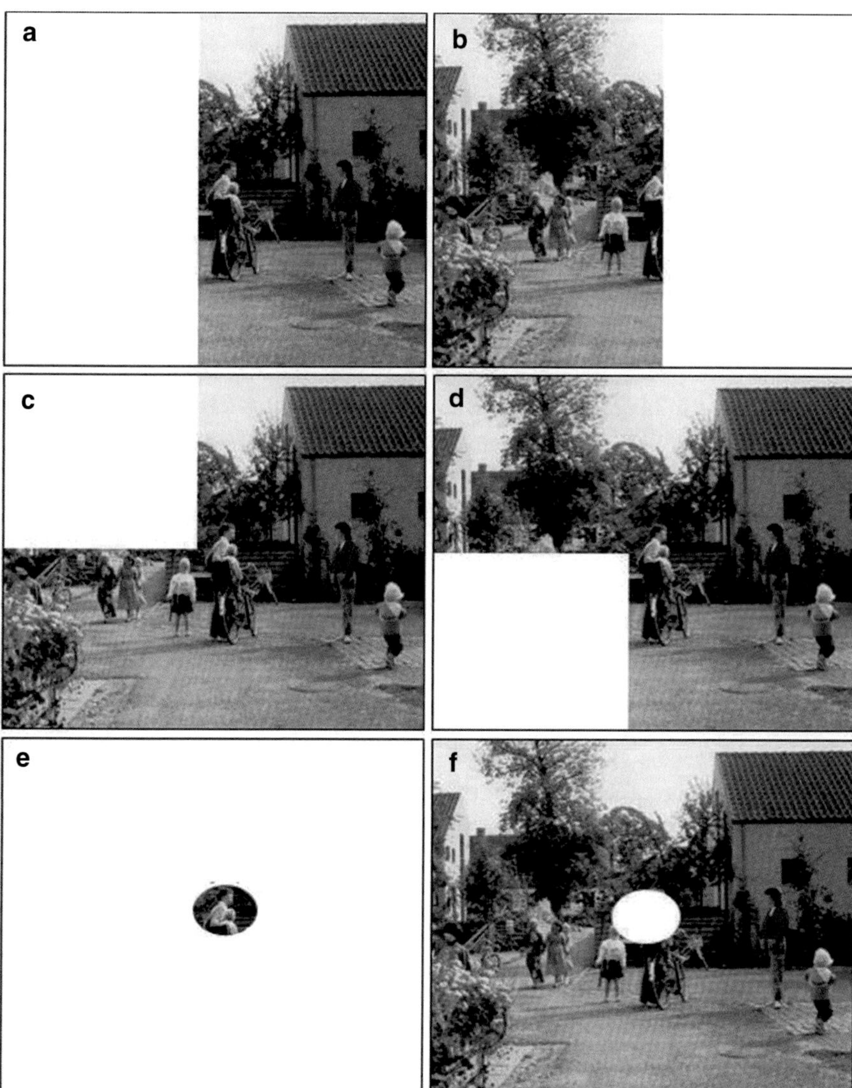

Fig. 4.2 Effects of homonymous visual field loss on global perception of a scene. Unseen portions of the scene are indicated in white. (**a**, **b**) left- and right-sided hemianopia; (**c**, **d**) left upper and left lower quadrantanopia; (**e**) bilateral hemianopia with central sparing, (**f**) central scotoma

homonymous visual field defects predominate and are as frequent as in adults (Kedar et al. 2006). Interestingly, children do not seem aware of their lack of visual field, when compensation tends to be efficient. Bajandas et al. (1975) investigated three children at the age of 10–14 years, who exhibited homonymous hemianopia because of congenital brain injury, but were never aware of their hemianopia. Possibly these children had developed compensatory strategies quite early in life

Table 4.6 Frequency of uni- and of bilateral visual field defects in childhood

Study	*N*	UNI	BIL
Van Hof-van Duin and Mohn (1984)	07	01	06
Jacobson et al. (1996)	13	00	13
Mercuri et al. (1997)	15	07	08
Total	*35*	*08*	*27 (77.1 %)*
Linz study	48	09	39 (81.3 %)

Numbers in brackets refer to bilateral visual field impairment
N number of subjects, *UNI, BIL* uni- and bilateral visual field loss

and had successfully adapted to their lack of visual field. Consequently, they had no (or only mild) difficulties in everyday life activities, at least no more 'difficulties' than children of the same age may also have. This report is supported by the observation of one author (JZ). In the context of neurological and neuroradiological examinations of an 11-year-old girl with suspected epilepsy, a small cystic lesion was detected in the left occipital lobe. She did not report any difficulties in school, in everyday life and in sports (for example, table tennis, cycling). Quantitative perimetry revealed right-sided homonymous hemianopia, with central sparing of 4°. Recording of oculomotor scanning during the inspection of scenes showed nearly normal scanning patterns (see Fig. 4.3). It may be assumed that this efficient spontaneous oculomotor compensation was possible, because visual curiosity, spatial guidance of attention and eye movements, and executive function, were not affected by the occipital cyst. About 80 % of adults with homonymous visual field defects do not usually show spontaneous compensation, probably because additional injury to brain structures involved in the visual-spatial guidance of attention and eye movements (thalamus, dorsal information processing route) and/or the underlying white matter, leading to disconnection from one another and from the prefrontal cortex. Typical consequences include time-consuming scanning patterns of the visual environment, or even smaller scenes, and – to a lesser extent – omission of stimuli on the affected side, in the absence of visual neglect. Scanning patterns are characterised by a considerably higher number of small saccades and fixations; in cases with bilateral visual field defects the range of visual search may in addition be restricted (Zihl 2011; see also Fig. 4.3).

Acquired homonymous hemianopia in later childhood is rare, but in one author's (GD) experience, is most commonly related to a vascular event (such as spontaneous rupture of an arterio-venous malformation). As in adults, this type of visual field loss tends to be problematic. One affected child (seen by GD), whose right-sided intra-occipital haemorrhage caused left hemianopia, discovered herself that reading was enabled by reading vertically upwards, so that the material that had been read moved into the hemianopic visual field. She disguised this behaviour by tilting her head to the right and the text to the left.

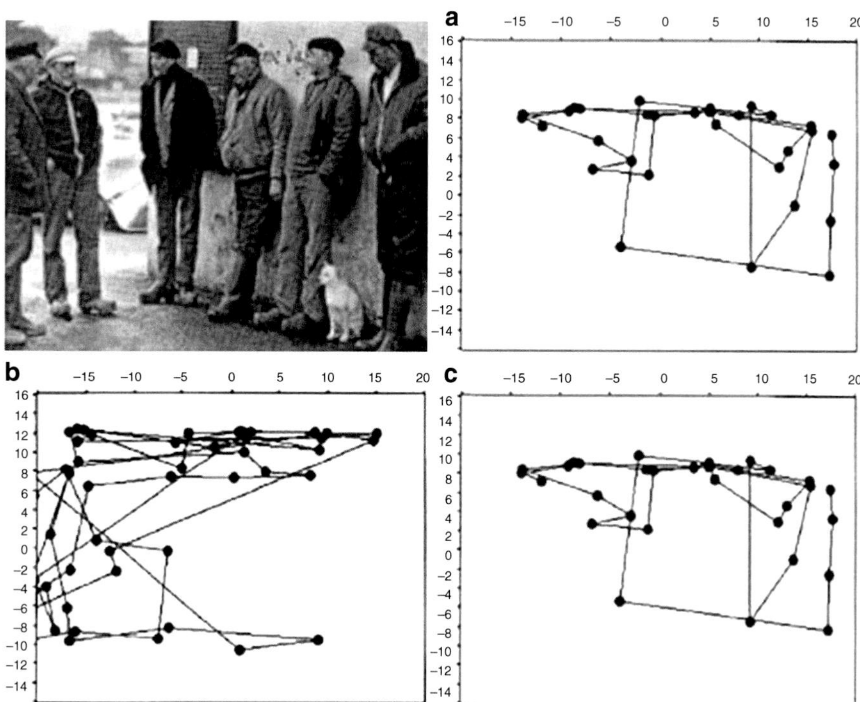

Fig. 4.3 Oculomotor scanning patterns during inspection of a scene in a normal 20-year-old subject (**a**), a 24-year-old patient with a right-sided hemianopia (sparing: 6°) after surgical removal of an occipital tumour (**b** 13 weeks 'post-op'), and an 11-year-old girl with a right-sided congenital hemianopia (**c** sparing: 4°). *Black dots*: fixation positions, *lines*: saccadic movements. Scanning times were 17.7 s in **a**, 43.3 s in **b**, and 19.3 s in **c**. All patients reported all relevant items of the scene. Note the efficient oculomotor compensation in the case of congenital hemianopia in **c**

It is possible that in some cases, the development of divergent strabismus develops and becomes compensatory for the hemianopia, and care has to be taken when considering cosmetic strabismus surgery (Jacobson et al. 2012).

Dutton et al. (2004) found in children with occipito-parietal brain injury and bilateral lower quadranopia a limitation of downward gaze, indicating that children with injury to the superior radiation can exhibit a combination of homonymous lower visual field impairment and reduced spontaneous oculomotor compensation in the same way as adults.

Homonymous quadrantic and hemianopic visual field deficits potentially draw attention to associated perceptual disorders. A unilateral or bilateral lower quadrantic visual field deficit points to possible contralateral unilateral or bilateral posterior parietal dysfunction respectively, while a unilateral or bilateral upper quadrantic

Table 4.7 Frequency of reduced visual acuity in children with CVI reported in different studies

Study	*N*	Frequency (%)
Jan et al. (1986)	236	82
Schenk-Rootlieb et al. (1994)	49	73
Dutton et al. (1996)	90	30
Fazzi et al. (2007)	121	87
Linz study	82	100

N number of children tested. Inclusion criterion was suspected CVI

deficit points to possible contralateral unilateral or bilateral temporal lobe pathology (if the visual field deficit relates to damage to the optic radiations as they pass through these structures).

4.3.2 Visual Acuity, Contrast Sensitivity, Optics and Accommodation

4.3.2.1 Low Acuity and Contrast Sensitivity

After unilateral post-chiasmatic injury *visual acuity* in adults is not at all or only moderately impaired. After bilateral post-chiasmatic injury, visual acuity can be completely preserved, or impaired to varying degree; in the extreme case only finger counting may be possible (Zihl 2011).

Bilateral reduced visual acuity is the most frequently reported visual dysfunction in children with CVI (see Table 4.7); reported frequencies vary between 30 and 100 %. Acuity values range between normal acuity and 2.0 logMAR, i.e. visual form discrimination impairment varies between moderate and very severe, with only coarse discrimination between black and white, or light and dark, respectively (Jan et al. 1986; Dutton et al. 1996). Many children with CVI and reduced visual acuity in addition exhibit myopia, hyperopia, or astigmatism, which may also contribute to low acuity and should, of course, be corrected by optical means. Refraction anomalies have been reported by Khetpal and Donahue (2007) in 20 % of 98 children with CVI; Fazzi et al. (2007) reported such anomalies in 80 % of 121 children with CVI. In the Linz study all 82 children with CVI had reduced visual acuities; 31 children (37.8 %) also had hyperopia, 32 children (39 %) myopia, and 54 children (65.8 %) astigmatism. Of course, visual acuity values depend on test conditions; results are therefore, not always comparable. In addition, acuity values also depend on a child's fixation accuracy and attentional capacities and compliance; an accurate and reliable measurement outcome can only be expected, if both are sufficient (see also Sects. 4.4.2 and 6.4.2).

Adults with impaired spatial *contrast sensitivity* ('contrast vision') after brain injury report 'unclear' or 'foggy' vision, stimuli appear 'blurred', in particular details of patterns, figures and objects, letters and faces; it often produces considerable visual discomfort. The explanation for this visual phenomenon may be reduced acuity or difficulties with accommodation and convergence (fusion capacity is reduced), or may not be explained by these factors. Contrast sensitivity may be reduced mainly for the higher spatial frequencies (Bulens et al. 1989), but can also

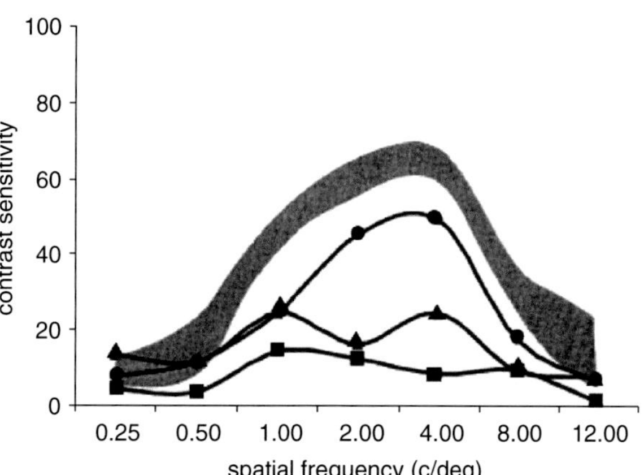

Fig. 4.4 Impaired spatial contrast sensitivity in a 5-year-old boy with central amblyopia and reduced visual acuity (0.9 near vision; *circles*), a 4-year-old boy with CVI and near visual acuity of 0.1 (*triangles*) and in a 5-year-old boy with CVI and near visual acuity of 0.1 (*squares*). *Grey profile* indicates range of contrast sensitivity in five normal children aged 5–6 years

be depressed in the entire range of spatial frequencies (Bodis-Wollner and Diamond 1976; Hess et al. 1990; Zihl 2011).

In children with CVI, contrast vision is probably as often impaired as visual acuity (Fig. 4.4). Jacobson et al. (1996) reported impaired contrast vision in 11 out of 13 children with CVI; Mercuri et al. (1997) found this visual dysfunction in 12 out of 31 children with CVI, while Stiers et al. (1998) found it in 21 of 22 children with CVI. Fazzi et al. (2007) reported impaired contrast vision in 58 (47.9 %) of 121 children. Good et al. (2012) reported reduced contrast sensitivity in 30 children and impaired grating acuity in 32 out of 34 children with CVI. It is important to note that contrast sensitivity is perceived more easily for single stimuli, and much more difficult to perceive for regular patterns of, for example, vertical stripes. Children with reduced single-stimulus contrast sensitivity may also show reduced visual acuities, while children with reduced pattern stimulus contrast sensitivities may show better acuity values for optotypes. Furthermore, it should be mentioned that peripheral dysfunction causing amblyopia may also be associated with reduced contrast sensitivity because of visual deprivation effects (Lerner et al. 2006). Central image crowding also disturbs visual processing of fine details and of reading (Martelli et al. 2009; Huurneman et al. 2012).

4.3.2.2 Refractive Error

Refractive errors comprise short (or near) sightedness, long (or far) sightedness and astigmatism. The greater the refractive error, the greater is the degree of correctable visual impairment.

Newborn children have a wide range of refractive errors. These progressively diminish during the first few months of life, as growth and development of the eyes brings about emmetropisation. However, persistent refractive errors are common in children with cerebral palsy (many of whom also have CVI), probably due to impaired emmetropisation (Saunders et al. 2010). Initial refraction is carried out in at risk children (Das et al. 2010), having first paralysed accommodation using a cycloplegic agent such as cyclopentolate to ensure accurate refraction. In most cases of identified refractive error, the full spectacle correction is prescribed. For large refractive errors spectacles may not improve vision initially, because of superadded ammetropic amblyopia, for which full time spectacle wear leads to subsequent gradual improvement of vision over a period of weeks.

4.3.2.3 Lack of Accommodation

Lack of accommodation also compounds CVI in more than 50 % of those with cerebral palsy (Leat 1996; McClelland et al. 2006). Lack of the pupil constriction that normally takes place when looking at a near target gives a reliable indicator that accommodation may be lacking (Saunders et al. 2008). This leads to impairment of near acuity. In those who are hypermetropic, accommodation overcomes the refractive error, but when accommodation is poor or absent, both near and distance visual acuities are impaired. The presence and degree of accommodative function are determined clinically by a procedure known as dynamic retinoscopy, in which refraction is measured while the child looks at targets at different distances and the degree of resulting myopia is elicited. When accommodation is impaired, this myopia is less than expected or absent, and the requisite near spectacle correction is provided. Either varifocal or bifocal lenses are given for children who are able to elect to use down gaze to view near targets through the lower part of the spectacles, or as separate (well labelled) spectacle corrections for those who cannot.

Refractive error and accommodative dysfunction are common in children with CVI of early onset. Refraction is warranted for all cases, and optimal spectacle correction needs to be worn by those with refractive error, prior to assessment of functional and perceptual vision (Das et al. 2010).

4.3.2.4 Hypermetropia Causing Convergent Strabismus (Accommodative Esotropia)

Another indication for spectacle wear is convergent strabismus due to hypermetropia. The accommodative effort needed to bring the near scene into focus brings about the synkinesis of convergence, which is less likely to be inhibited in those whose damage to the brain has caused CVI, rendering accommodative esotropia more likely. Spectacle wear that corrects the hypermetropia eliminates the need for the increased accommodative effort. This in turn eliminates the stimulus for the eyes to converge, and immediate diminution in the angle of strabismus takes place. In many cases gradual, progressive further improvement of eye alignment is observed during the ensuing months. If surgical intervention is needed for this type of strabismus, it is deferred until the eye alignment has normalised as much as possible.

4.3.2.5 Spectacle Wear

Spectacle wear corrects the blurred distance vision of myopia, but a side effect of the required concave lenses is to reduce image size, especially when the myopia is marked. Children with additional low visual acuities due to CVI, or associated pathology of the eyes or optic nerves may choose to remove their spectacles when looking at books or when viewing near objects, because they can instead focus upon material held close to the eyes. This gives the magnification due to proximity, diminishes visual crowding, and helps compensate for the low vision.

Visual crowding due to CVI can impair reading. For children who are long sighted and in those who have impaired accommodation, positive lenses both magnify text, and allow it to be read closer to the eyes, bringing about additional magnification due to proximity. This can in turn reduce crowding of text on the printed page, which can enhance access to the printed word and story-book images. Correction of only one or two dioptres of hypermetropia can benefit some children with CVI.

Children who have CVI associated with visual crowding often choose to remove their spectacles when they are tired, presumably because the resulting blur serves to diminish the degree of image crowding. However, unlike in myopia, this does not lead to any improvement of vision.

4.3.3 Visual Adaptation

Visual light and dark adaptation can be impaired in (even moderate) retinopathy, as a sequel to dysfunction of retinal light receptors (Hansen and Fulton 2000), as a result from chiasmal compression (Kawasaki and Purvin 2002) and following injury to the post-chiasmatic visual system (Zihl 2011). Patients with impaired light adaptation, which can manifest with increased light sensitivity when changing from a defined scotopic level to a defined mesopic or photopic level, complain of blinding effects even under normal daylight conditions. This can particularly impair reading and discrimination of fine visual pattern. In addition, patients can report visual discomfort, with a sense of eye burning and headache. Patients with impaired dark adaptation, as demonstrated by reduced or absent enhancement of light sensitivity after a change from a defined photopic level to a defined mesopic or scotopic level, tend to report that lighting is insufficient even under normal daylight conditions; again, reading and fine visual discrimination may be secondarily affected. Particularly unpleasant is the combination of impaired light and dark adaptation, because patients need more light for clear vision, but at the same time suffer from photophobia when the lighting is enhanced. In such cases, patients have difficulties with fine visual discrimination under mesopic, photopic and scotopic light levels.

For methodological reasons, the course of light and dark adaptation cannot be measured in young children. However, impaired central light adaptation in young children is also associated with visual discomfort, and they may therefore exhibit shunning of light and avoid light sources by head shifting and eye closure (so-called central photophobia). Jan et al. (1993) found this type of avoidance behaviour in 35 (42 %) of 83 children. The majority (77 %) had shown this behaviour from birth, so that it was probably the consequence of pre- or perinatal brain injury. In the Linz study, 22 (26.8 %) out of 82 children experienced central photophobia. Some children with profound CVI show evidence of improved visually evoked potential grating acuity thresholds under low luminance conditions indicating a greater sensitivity at lower levels of ambient lighting (Good and Hou 2006), a feature consistent with the parental observation of better vision under low lighting, and one that can be sought, and integrated into habilitation plans if identified.

4.3.4 Colour Vision

Impairments in colour vision after acquired brain injury (e.g. following severe hypoxia) can either affect colour perception in the contralateral hemifield (homonymous hemiachromatopsia; see also Sect. 4.3.1), or in both hemifields, also including central vision (cerebral achromatopsia), or hue discrimination in the central field of vision can be affected (cerebral dyschromatopsia). The other visual functions, for example, light and form vision, are usually not affected (Zihl 2011) but if they are, difficulties recognising what is seen can be profound. In contrast to congenital colour vision deficiencies of peripheral origin, e.g. red-green colour blindness, cerebral colour vision difficulties are not characterised by specific patterns of deficiency. Patients with complete cerebral achromatopsia report even saturated colour stimuli as appearing pale, or sometimes as dark brownish; colour naming is incorrect or impossible. Those affected may have difficulties with visual object recognition, if colour is a characteristic property for the particular object.

Impaired colour vision in children with CVI has not often been reported. This may be explained by the difficulty of standardised assessment in young children; alternatively, one may assume that colour vision is not as often impaired after brain injury as are other visual capacities (Jacobson et al. 1996; Korkman et al. 1996). Connolly et al. (2008) have found impaired colour hue discrimination in adults who have suffered from moderate cerebral hypoxia. Because cerebral hypoxia is the most frequent aetiology for CVI in infancy, it appears likely that cerebral dyschromatopsia may be more frequent than reported (Adams et al. 2005). In the Linz study, colour discrimination was assessed using a standardised preferential looking technique (see Sect. 6.2); the systematic screening of children may explain the high rate of impaired colour vision (63/82 children, 76.8 %).

There is preliminary evidence that identification of colours may be chronically impaired despite normal colour hue discrimination; because this impairment exists from birth, it has been labelled congenital colour agnosia (Nijboer et al. 2007; Van Zaandvort et al. 2007). Adult subjects with this 'higher order' visual dysfunction have difficulties with the association of colours and objects or colour names.

Difficulty or inability to name colours is not uncommon in children with CVI in our experience, and is therefore a differential diagnosis that warrants consideration.

4.3.5 Stereopsis

Stereopsis is the mental facility to see in three dimensions brought about by the disparity of image data provided by the two eyes. Its development starts to become evident at the age of 4 months (see Sect. 2.3.5). The commonest cause of lack of stereopsis is absence of vision or low visual acuity and/or contrast sensitivity in one eye, often related to strabismus and amblyopia. This affects over 3 % of the general population (Ying et al. 2014).

Systematic studies on stereopsis in very young children with CVI do not exist. The additional visual and oculomotor dysfunctions mentioned may also impair development of monocular depth perception, because depth cues cannot reliably be processed and used. Fazzi et al. (2007) reported impaired stereopsis in 74 of 82 (90.2 %) children with CVI. Dutton et al. (1996) found in 4 of 90 children with congenital brain injury striking difficulties to reach correctly in depth to grasp objects, although no motor problem was present. These children systematically over- or underestimated distances and grasping movements fell short or long of target. It is possible that optic ataxia was a contributory element.

After unilateral posterior brain injury, stereopsis may be only moderately impaired; in contrast, bilateral posterior brain injury in adults may cause severe impairment (Miller et al. 1999). Patients with moderately impaired stereopsis may not report difficulties although stereoacuity is reduced when tested. However, patients with severely impaired stereopsis associated with brain injury can experience the three-dimensional world as two-dimensional (so-called astereopsis); staircases appear flat, and stairs can be difficult to go up and down; faces may look very 'strange', because the 'plasticity of expression' is less evident. In contrast to patients with moderately impaired stereopsis, patients with severe impairment typically may also lose monocular depth perception cues, and can, therefore, not compensate for their astereopsis. Distance perception may also be secondarily affected; distances are under- or overestimated. This change in distance perception may also influence object perception. In case of underestimation of distance, objects may appear larger (macropsia), in case of overestimation they may appear smaller (micropsia) (Zihl 2011).

4.3.6 Perception of Movement

The centres serving perception of movement comprise the middle temporal lobes located at the occipito-parietal temporal junction. Bilateral damage can cause impaired or absent visual perception of movement (akinetopsia) (Zihl et al. 1983). Only the static visual world can be seen and appreciated in this situation.

Children with periventricular white matter damage commonly show reduced perception of movement, which has been demonstrated with visual evoked potentials to global motion and motion onset (Weinstein et al. 2012; Kuba et al. 2008). Impaired motion perception is common in children born before 34 weeks, and is more marked in those who manifest periventricular white matter lesions (Guzzetta et al. 2009). Specific aspects of motion perception can be deficient, for example the perception of linear motion, while other aspects, such as seeing radial and circular motion may be intact in children with evidence of periventricular white matter pathology (Morrone et al. 2008). Children born extremely prematurely may also have difficulties with motion-defined form processing, but may in addition exhibit problems with visual search, stereopsis, and with visuo-spatial tasks

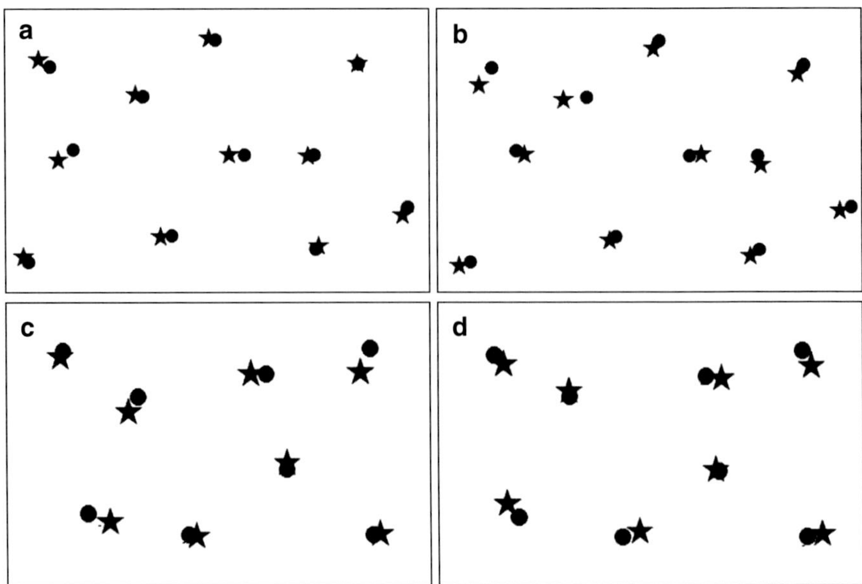

Fig. 4.5 Difficulties with visual localisation in a 56-year-old patient with right-sided occipito-parietal injury (**a** 11 weeks post-injury), a 52-year-old patient with bilateral occipito-parietal injury (**b** 13 weeks post-injury), in a 9-year-old boy with CVI (**c**), and in a 10-year-old boy with CVI (**d**). Patients in **a** and **b** were asked to cancel out the dot stimuli as accurately as possible, while the two boys in **c** and **d** were asked to match positions of pairs of dot stimuli. *Stars and dots* indicate cancellations and matches, respectively. Note the consistent deviations of localisation responses from target positions

(construction, mental rotation) (Jacobson et al. 2006). In the authors' experience older children can volunteer that a ball that has been kicked disappears, reappearing when it slows down.

Impaired recognition of biological movement has also been described in relation to periventricular white matter damage (Pavlova et al. 2003). The behavioural features indicative of possible impaired perception of movement are described in Chap. 5.

4.3.7 Visual Localisation and Visual Direction Perception

In adults, disorders of visual localisation and perception of visual direction (main spatial axes) have been reported mainly after right-sided occipito-parietal brain injury, i.e. after injury to the right dorsal route. Unilateral right-sided brain injury is associated with moderate inaccuracy in visual localisation (Fig. 4.5); horizontal and vertical spatial axes of perception may be shifted to the contralateral (i.e. left) side, while what appears as the straight ahead direction can be shifted contralaterally, i.e. to the left after right-sided injury and to the right after left-sided injury (Fig. 4.6). In addition, visual orientation may be moderately impaired; this becomes particularly

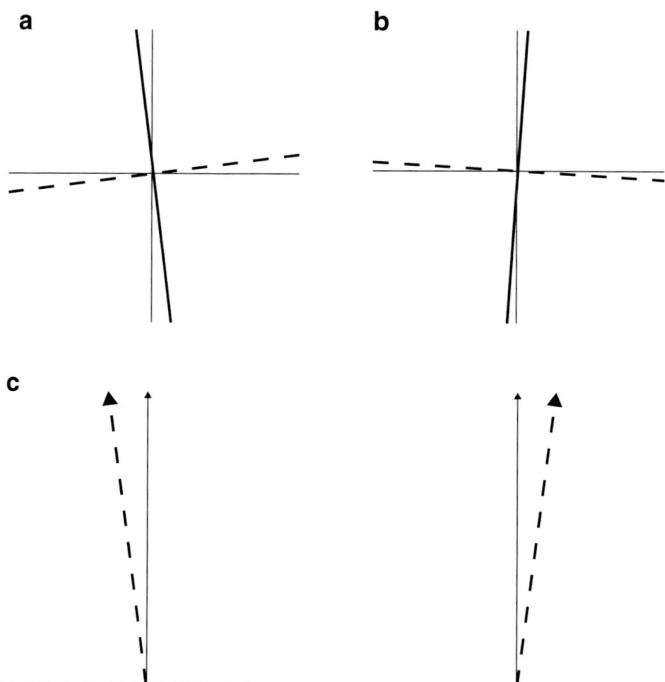

Fig. 4.6 Shift of vertical and horizontal spatial axes (*broken lines*) to the left-sided in a 58-year-old patient with right-sided occipito-parietal injury (**a** 14 weeks post-injury) and in a 44-year-old patient with left-sided occipito-parietal injury (**b** 12 weeks post-injury). Note contralateral shifts of subjective axes; shift is typically larger after right-sided brain injury. (**c**) Shows contralateral shifts of subjective visual midline (*broken lines*) in a 51-year-old patient with right-sided occipital injury (7 weeks post-injury; *left figure*), and in a 54-year-old patient with left-sided occipital injury (8 weeks post-injury; *right figure*)

manifest with scanning of a scene or with reading, because patients 'lose' lines and paragraphs. After bilateral superior posterior brain injury, the visual-spatial dysfunctions mentioned are more severe; in the extreme case, patients can lose the ability to localise a stimulus (so-called space blindness), cannot navigate in rooms or buildings, and are unable to read (Zihl 2011; Fig. 4.7).

In children with CVI, 'pure' disorders of visual space perception have only rarely been reported, which may be explained by the fact that visual spatial capacities can be assessed reliably only after the age of 3–4 years. Stimulus localisation can be similarly impaired as in adults (Fig. 4.5). Riva and Cazzaniga (1986) found impaired discrimination of line length and orientation of objects in 6- to 12-year-old children who had sustained brain injury in early childhood. Similar observations were reported by Meerwaldt and van Dongen (1988) in two 7-year-old children with early brain injury; in some children the degree of impairment decreased with increasing age. The outcome of both studies indicates that early brain injury can cause persistent visual-spatial deficits, but advancing visual experience may ameliorate severity. In the Linz study (see Table 4.5) we found

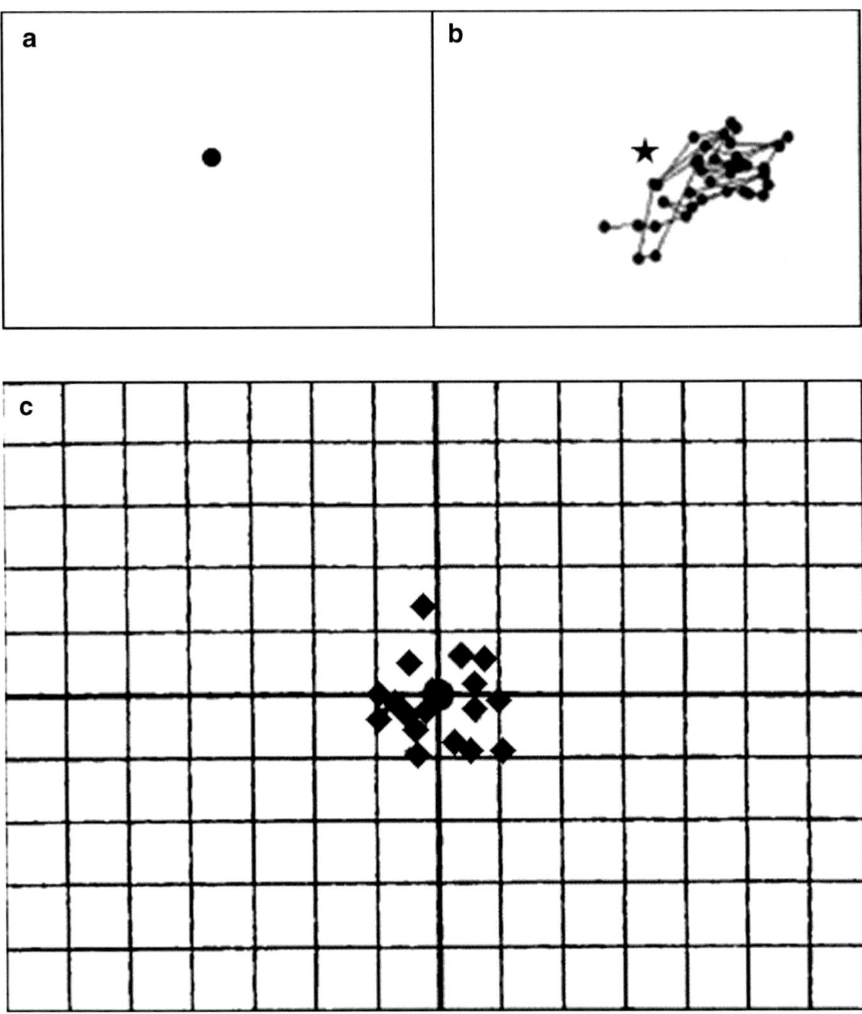

Fig. 4.7 Fixation in a normal 51-year-old subject (**a** *dot* indicates fixation position) and fixation attempts in a 52-year-old patient with bilateral occipito-parietal injury (**b** star indicates position of fixation stimulus). (**c**) Pointing responses (recordings with a touch screen) of the same patients as in **b**. Note inaccuracy of visual localisation in both oculomotor and limb movement systems

visual-spatial impairments in about 75 % of 82 children, which became mainly manifest as inaccurate grasping and pointing and in difficulties with spatial orientation in rooms. Visual spatial difficulties may also affect copying and drawing of figures (Fig. 4.8), whereby it often remains unclear, whether visuo-constructive difficulties are primarily caused by visuo-spatial impairments, or by visuo-motor deficits (optic ataxia), or both. Dutton et al. (1996) found in 6 of 90 children with CVI significant difficulties with accurate and reliable spatial and topographical orientation. In addition, children also found it difficult to learn routes. This observation

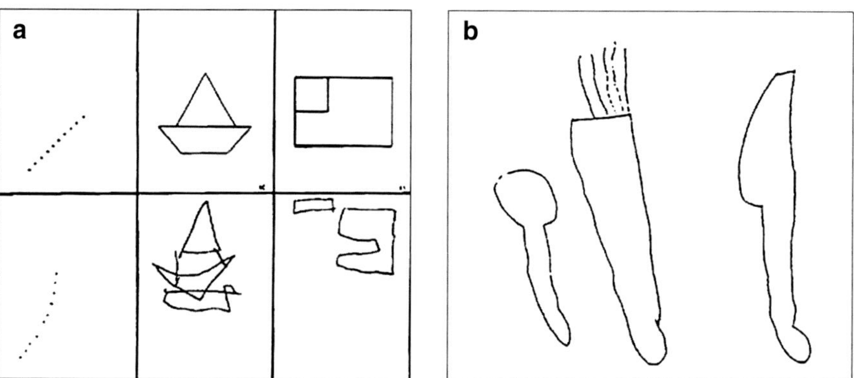

Fig. 4.8 Copying by a 9-year-old boy with Williams syndrome (**a**; Eriksson et al. 2003. © Elsevier reprinted with permission) and drawing from memory of an 8-year-old boy with developmental visual agnosia (**b**; Ariel and Sadeh 1996. © Elsevier reprinted with permission). Note difficulties with the spatial arrangement of figure elements in **a**, and oversimplification of figures in **b**

is supported by the study of Pavlova et al. (2007). These authors tested 14 young people at the age of 13–16 years with periventricular leucomalacia (PVL; see Sect. 4.5.3) using a maze and found considerable deficits in visual-spatial orientation. There is evidence that the learning of so-called landmarks, which allow accurate and reliable spatial and topographical orientation, can be specifically affected in children with CVI (Brunsdon et al. 2007). In addition, impaired ordering of landmarks properly with respect to spatial axes can also affect the acquisition of a reliable spatial reference system (McCloskey 2004).

4.3.8 Form Vision, Object and Face Perception

Form vision is an important prerequisite for visual identification, because figures, objects, faces and also letters consist of forms or parts of forms. The discrimination of forms and figures is important for *figure-ground separation*, which supports spatial structuring of complex objects and scenes. Patients with impaired form vision and figure perception, and impaired figure-ground separation, respectively, have difficulties differentiating and separating objects from each other. Similar forms, figures and objects are confounded and overlapping parts intermingled; sometimes only parts of figures or objects are used for identification and recognition. Impaired *visual identification* is known as visual agnosia, which is defined as the inability to identify and visually recognise objects, faces, places and letters despite sufficient visual capacities (visual field, visual acuity, contrast sensitivity, colour and form vision), oculomotor functions (fixation, accommodation, vergence, saccadic eye movements, visual scanning) and cognitive functions (attention, executive function). Identification/recognition in another modality, i.e. by hearing sounds or voices, or by tactile exploration, is preserved; thus visual agnosia is a modality specific 'higher-order' visual disorder (Zihl 2011). Visual recognition concerns familiar stimuli, i.e. objects, faces, places, letters, etc. that have been known by the patient for a long time, which ensures that they are reliably and accurately represented in visual memory. A stimulus is first identified on the basis of its features; the outcome of this analysis can be used in a second step for recognition, when properties are available, which allow more or less perfect matching with its mental representation. In the context of developmental visual agnosia, it is important to consider whether the child has had sufficient visual experience, i.e. systematic and repeated visual perceptual learning with complex visual stimuli before brain injury. If this is not the case, then visual recognition cannot take place, because no match can be performed between the seen stimulus and its mental representation in visual memory.

It has been found useful to classify visual agnosia according to the affected visual category. Visual object agnosia refers to the loss of visual recognition of objects; prosopagnosia to the loss of visual recognition of faces; topographagnosia is the inability to recognise and navigate places, and paths; letter agnosia (also known as pure alexia) means the loss of recognition of letters. Each category of visual agnosia can occur in isolation, but a combination is the rule (Farah 2000). In contrast to prosopagnosia and agnosia for letters, which have been reported frequently in adults as isolated forms of visual agnosia, object agnosia has not. Lissauer, who published the first detailed single case report on visual agnosia in 1890, pointed out that the typical error is misidentification of objects, i.e. his patient used features that are also shared by other objects. It seems as if this patient still possessed the capacity to identify visual stimuli, but neither monitored the identification process (what are the significant features of the object in question?) nor controlled the outcome of his visual analysis. Thus, visual agnosia may consist of two components: a failure in identification, because specific object properties are no longer known and are therefore not discovered, and a failure in monitoring and controlling the process of recognition and its outcome; the latter capacities belong to executive functions. However, this is not a global inability to recognise, monitor and control identification and recognition of stimuli, but a modality-specific one, because these capacities are still normally operating in other modalities. Of course, for diagnosing a failure in visual recognition, it is essential to assess all prerequisites mentioned above; only if they are sufficiently available can the diagnosis of visual agnosia be made. Thus, one should carefully differentiate between visual agnosia as a primary visual disorder, and impaired visual recognition secondary to visual, oculomotor or cognitive disorders, as outlined above (see also Serino et al. 2014). Furthermore, difficulties with naming visual stimuli are not necessarily due to visual agnosia, they can also result from disconnecting visual naming from visual perception (visual anomia). In the author GD's practice the most frequently occurring visual anomia relates to the inability to name colour in children of an age where this would be universally expected, colour anomia.

Impairments in visual form perception and in visual recognition in children with CVI may be expected in association with reduced visual acuity and inaccurate fixation, both occurring frequently in combination (see Table 4.3, p. 69). According to the definition of visual agnosia given above, these impairments are classified as secondary disorders. There exist, however, also genuine ('primary') disorders of visual recognition. In a study on 90 children with early brain injury, 20 % exhibited low visual acuity, and 10 % severe impairment of all visual functions/capacities (Dutton et al. 1996). Six children in this group showed evidence of a primary impairment in visual recognition. Stiers et al. (1998) assessed 22 children with early brain injury at the age of 4–14 years, and found difficulties with visual recognition in 17 children, independently of visual acuity values. The main problems were integration of features to a whole (Lissauer's 'synthesis'), object constancy, i.e. recognition of the same object under different conditions (perspective, context; see Sect. 2.3.7) and checking the outcome of recognition for plausibility (controlling the outcome of recognition) by referring to the context. Brain injury had typically occurred in occipito-temporal structures (ventral route) in both hemispheres, but it cannot be excluded that unilateral injury to these brain regions may also cause such deficits, as is known to occur in adults (Landis et al. 1988; Barton 2008). In the Linz study (cf. Table 4.5, p. 71) visual recognition difficulties were found in 76 out of 82 children (92.7 %). However, because all children also exhibited low visual acuity, it seems plausible to assume that in many cases visual recognition was (also) secondarily impaired. All children with impaired visual recognition, either of primary or of secondary origin, had difficulties visually identifying objects, faces and scenes. Difficulties with face recognition, including familiar faces (parents, brothers and sisters) comprised the most frequent type of recognition disorder (see also Eriksson et al. 2003). Selective developmental agnosia for objects but normal processing and recognition of faces has been reported by Germine et al. (2011) in a 19-year-old female indicating that visual recognition memory for faces is independent of object recognition and storage.

Face perception and recognition in children can be impaired in different ways. Global processing of faces may be impaired but local processing of facial features is preserved and more or less exclusively used (Avidan et al. 2011; Palermo et al. 2011). Visual imagery for faces may be difficult while visual imagery for objects may be normally developed (Tree and Wilkie 2010). An illustrative example of developmental visual agnosia has been reported by Ariel and Sadeh (1996). An 8-year-old pupil, LG, who had normal cognitive, language and motor development, was assessed. He complained of having had 'peculiar problems' with his eyes since his sixth year, especially in school. His mother reported that LG had had difficulties from early childhood, in recognising his grandparents' faces and putting together even simple puzzles. Detailed ophthalmological and neuropsychological assessment did not reveal any visual, oculomotor or cognitive impairment. However, LG had difficulties in visual identification of letters and partly also of words; in contrast, writing and (mental) calculation were normal. Form vision was not impaired; discrimination of grey and colour hues was normal, but LG required more time to do this than his peers of the same age. No signs of visual spatial impairments were found, but visual object, and face identification and recognition were considerably impaired (see Table 4.8). LG found integration (synthesis) of parts of objects and recognition of real familiar objects difficult, but he could recognise them easily after

Table 4.8 Visual performance in a case (LG) with congenital visual agnosia and prosopagnosia

Stimuli	Number	Correct responses (%)
Real objects	45	77.8 (100)
Object drawings	30	90.0 (100)
Animals made of plastic	22	63.6 (100)
Single letters	23	60.9 (96.7)
Object photographs	30	56.6 (100)
Complex scenes (photographs)	28	53.6 (96.4)
Object constancy	23	30.4 (100)
Integration of parts of object	30	13.3 (73.3)
Overlapping objects	20	10.0 (100)
Familiar faces (family)	26	38.5 (*)
Discrimination of faces	15	87.7 (66.7)
Face constancy	78	30.8 (92.0)
Discrimination of age and gender	25	28.0 (92.0)
Identification of face parts	10	00 (100)
Identification of facial expression	21	02.1 (*)

Modified after Ariel and Sadeh (1996)
Number refers to the number of stimuli shown in the respective task; percentages (in brackets) indicate performance of four age-matched peers (*: not assessed)

tactile exploration. Particularly difficult for LG was recognition of object drawings and objects presented in different perspectives (object constancy). LG also exhibited great difficulties with discriminating and identifying unfamiliar and familiar faces in photographs, including his own face, but also identification of age, gender and expression (anger, sadness, joy) of the face holder. Interestingly, LG outperformed his peers in face discrimination, which may indicate that discrimination was better developed possibly because LG had to use fine facial differences to discriminate between faces, i.e. he had (spontaneously) gained more efficient special visual experience with faces. Asked why he had visual difficulties, LG commented that he did not exactly know what the pictures or objects signified. Thus LG appeared to have never experienced sufficiently the (particular) significance of complex visual stimuli, like objects and faces. Furthermore, similar to Lissauer's patient, LG misidentified objects with similar features. Copying of objects and figures was characterised by a slavish mode of procedure: each line was exactly copied. Drawing of objects from memory was possible, but representations of objects (comb, spoon, fork, etc.) looked highly simplified (Fig. 4.8), resembling drawings from a much younger child, who uses basic prototypes to draw familiar objects. LG used highly efficient auditory (voice) and tactile recognition strategies for people and objects in his everyday life. His excellent adaptation to the visual demands of everyday life may be explained by the fact that LG had all the mental capacities fully available for developing and optimising efficient compensatory strategies to cope with his visual difficulties. LG provides an excellent example of the development of functional brain plasticity in terms of adaptation to functional anomalies in early visual development. Although no evidence was found in LG for morphological brain

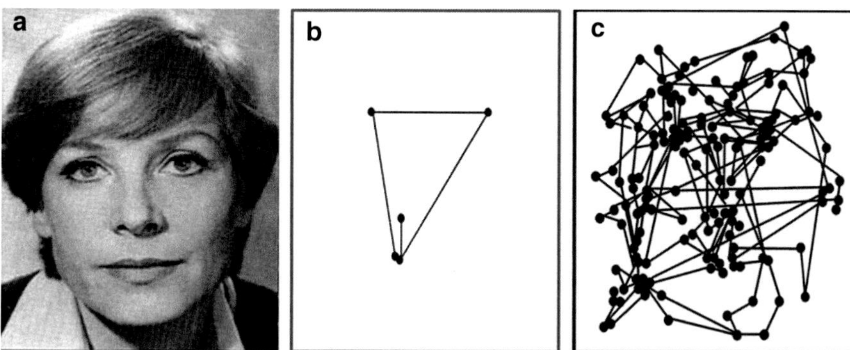

Fig. 4.9 Oculomotor scanning patterns during inspection of a face (*centre*) in a normal subject (**a**) and a 62-year-old patient with acquired prosopagnosia after bilateral occipito-temporal injury (**b** 17 weeks post-injury). *Dots*: fixation positions, *lines*; saccadic movements. Note detailed local processing in **b**

alterations, and his developmental agnosia and prosopagnosia may be attributed to genetic abnormalities (Wilson et al. 2010), one is inclined to classify his visual disorder as a form of CVI.

Developmental visual agnosia and prosopagnosia have also been reported in other single case studies (Duchaine and Nakayama 2006; Dalrymple et al. 2012; Susilo and Duchaine 2013). A common symptom of all children with this 'higher-order' visual disorder is difficulty integrating parts of objects or faces into a whole (Behrmann et al. 2005). When confronted with the picture of a face, it is very laborious for children to put all the pieces of the face together; this is akin to the effortful scanning of faces in adult patients with acquired prosopagnosia (Zihl 2011; Fig. 4.9). Processing of faces is assumed to be a process of integration of both global and local information (which is less important for many objects). This idea is supported by the notion that children with developmental prosopagnosia may show normal visual object recognition (Duchaine and Nakayama 2005) indicating that processing and coding of both stimulus classes are functionally segregated. But even within developmental prosopagnosia, diversity exists. Some children find it difficult to identify some but not all parts of faces on photographs (Brunsdon et al. 2006); others can correctly identify parts of faces, but cannot recognise faces they have seen very often (Joy and Brunsdon 2002). Children with prosopagnosia may also exhibit difficulties with discriminating and using abstract forms, figures and symbols; additionally, contrast vision (Barton et al. 2003; Lee et al. 2009) and processing of relative distances between facial and non-facial visual features may be reduced (Ramon and Rossion 2010). Finally, it appears that identification of facial expression is more often spared in developmental compared with acquired prosopagnosia (Humphreys et al. 2007).

Impaired processing of faces, including identification of face identity and facial expression, may result from either left or right posterior brain injury in the pre-, peri- or early postnatal period without accompanying visual dysfunction (de Schoenen et al. 2005). Developmental prosopagnosia can also result from familial transmission, but symptoms are similar to developmental prosopagnosia caused by brain injury (e.g. Lee et al. 2009; Wilson et al. 2010; Susilo and Duchaine 2013).

4.3.9 Text Processing and Reading

Developmental visual dyslexia is defined as impairment in the acquisition of visual identification and recognition of written characters (letters and digits), not only concerning differences in their form, but also their significance. It is assumed in this context that visual, oculomotor and cognitive (e.g. visual-verbal working memory) capacities that are required for text processing and reading are sufficient and available. In this sense, developmental visual dyslexia is a specific form of developmental agnosia, similar to acquired agnosia for letters (pure alexia) in adults (Valdois et al. 2004).

In recent years, research on developmental dyslexia has mainly focussed on the specificity of this visual disorder recognising that in earlier studies, the various functional components at the level of text processing and semantic coding have not been addressed in detail. In particular, pre-semantic visual processing has been assessed in children with developmental dyslexia, e.g. parallel processing, low-level processing (form discrimination and analysis, also for non-verbal stimuli), interference phenomena (misidentification of similar letters and symbols), processing of letter position, text-dependent guidance of eye movements (regular sequences of fixation and saccadic jumps), and working memory for words (so-called word-length effects). It was found that children with developmental dyslexia very often exhibited difficulties in one or more of these components (Martelli et al. 2009; Handler and Fierson 2011; Peterson and Pennington 2012). For example, Jones et al. (2008) assessed visual search performance and processing accuracy for symbols in children with developmental dyslexia, and found lower accuracy for both stimulus categories compared with normal age-matched children. Furthermore, children with developmental dyslexia may perform normally in serial search tasks, but show lower performance in parallel search tasks, although the latter condition is much easier for controls (Lassus-Sangousse et al. 2008), indicating that parallel processing capacity is impaired. Sireteanu and colleagues (2006, 2008) found evidence that both modes of visual search may be impaired. Impaired oculomotor function and spatial shifts of attention, which can hinder learning of efficient text processing and reading, have also been reported (Boden and Giaschi 2007; Bosse et al. 2007; Shaywitz and Shaywitz 2008). Insufficient fusional convergence may also impair text processing, because binocular fixation cannot be shifted accurately along words and lines (Ponsonby et al. 2009). Reading acquisition and reading performance may also be impaired secondarily because of refractive and or/vergence difficulties (Quaid and Simpson 2013), immaturity of saccade and vergence interaction (Bucci et al. 2012), deficient binocular saccade coordination in strabismus (Lions et al. 2013), and unstable binocular fixation (Jainta and Kapoula 2011). However, abnormal eye movement patterns may also be the consequence, rather than the cause of impaired reading (Medland et al. 2010). Moreover, Ferretti et al.

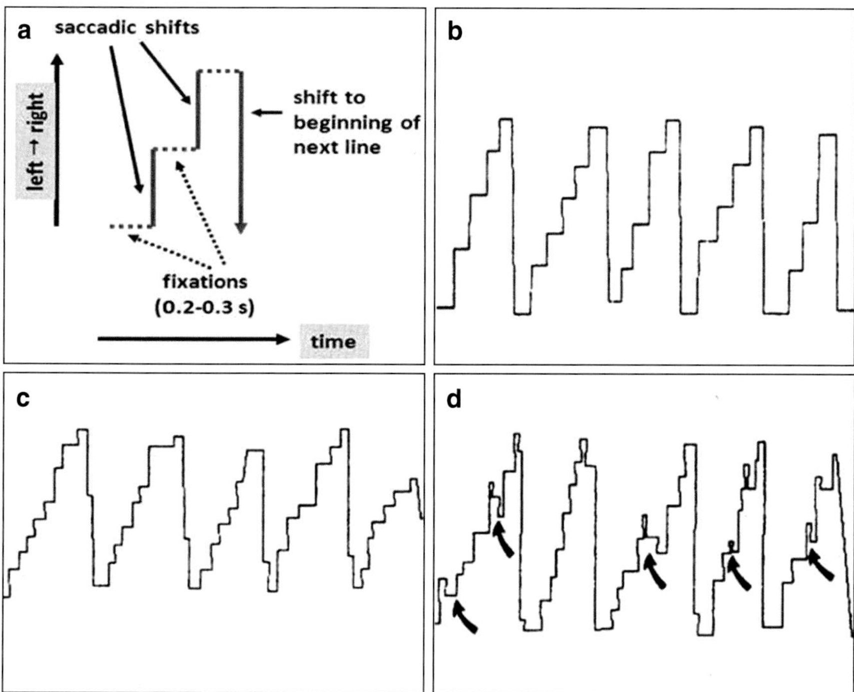

Fig. 4.10 (**a**) Schematic illustration of the sequence of saccadic shifts and fixation reading eye movements; (**b**) reading eye movement pattern in a 46-year-old normal subject (five lines with six words each), (**c**) reading eye movement pattern in a 44-year-old patient with left-sided homonymous hemianopia (9 weeks post; central field sparing: 2°), (**d**) reading eye movement pattern in a 47-year-old patient with right-sided homonymous hemianopia (7 weeks post-stroke; central field sparing: 3°). Note the difficulty shifting fixation from the (*right*) end of line to the beginning of next line in **c**, and with shifting fixation in a regular fashion for text processing direction in **d**. Return eye shifts to the left are indicated by *arrows*

(2008) found difficulties with shifting of fixation in reading direction, i.e. fixation shifts were considerably slowed, which may either indicate visual-oculomotor dysfunction, or may also be explained by less accurate and thus slowed processing of text stimuli, integration of letters to words, or coding of words to semantic units. Sequence of saccadic jumps and fixations may be disorganised in terms of spatio-temporal relationships (Mackeben et al. 2004; see Fig. 4.10). Furthermore, eye movement abnormalities may not be specific for processing of text stimuli, as they may also affect non-reading tasks indicating a more fundamental difficulty with coordination of eye movements in all aspects of visual processing (Eden et al. 1994). In addition, reduced attentional or reading span, i.e. the number of letters processed in parallel (Prado et al. 2007) may cause difficulties with text processing. Information processing speed (Heiervang and Hugdahl 2003) and working memory may also be impaired in children with developmental dyslexia, either with respect to capacity or concerning coding and matching processes (Smith-Spark and

Table 4.9 Factors that can impair acquisition of text processing and reading in childhood

Parallel processing capacity ↓ (limited by crowding of text)
'Low level' processing (forms, figures) ↓
Processing of letter position in word ↓
Interference by similar symbols and letters ↑
Working memory for symbols and letters ↓
Text-dependent guidance of fixation shifts ↓
Fusion ↓
Vergence ↓
Refractive errors and impaired accommodation
Visual acuity ↓
Contrast sensitivity ↓
Attention ↓

Fisk 2007), all factors that can impede learning of to read efficiently. Table 4.9 summarises the various factors that can impair acquisition of text processing and reading skills. Children with developmental visual dyslexia at the age of 14–16 years, i.e. after several years of school, show persisting reduced activation in the left occipito-temporal cortex during reading (Kronbichler et al. 2006), a region which is crucial for text processing and reading (see Sect. 2.3.9). This observation has been verified in many other studies; interestingly prefrontal and cerebellar activities were not affected (Maisog et al. 2008). Familial developmental dyslexia is a genetic disorder, which however is characterised by abnormal neuropsychological profiles, including associated cognitive deficits, and morphological alterations in occipito-temporal brain structures similar to developmental dyslexia caused by external events (e.g. hypoxia, cerebrovascular events, or traumatic injury) (Brambati et al. 2006; van der Mark et al. 2009, 2011).

4.3.10 Field of Attention

Visual perception and attention do not operate in isolation, but are intimately interconnected (see Chap. 1). This does not only hold true for visual information processing in general, but relates also to the visual field. The even distribution of attention in the field of vision enables the individual to detect stimuli in the corresponding sector of the surroundings. The complex interplay between visual field, spatial attention and oculomotor scanning depends on posterior and anterior brain systems, in particular the dorsal and ventral routes and their reciprocal prefrontal partners; injury to these systems and their fibre connections impairs this interplay in a specific way (Zihl and Hebel 1997; see also Sect. 4.4.3). After acquired posterior brain injury, the field of attention can be altered in an even more dramatic way. Part of the field of attention may be missing, i.e. stimuli in the hemispace contralateral to the side of brain injury (in the adult it is typically the left hemispace) are no longer processed despite a normal visual field on this side (so-called visual neglect). As a consequence, the external visual world is neglected left of the line of sight, which

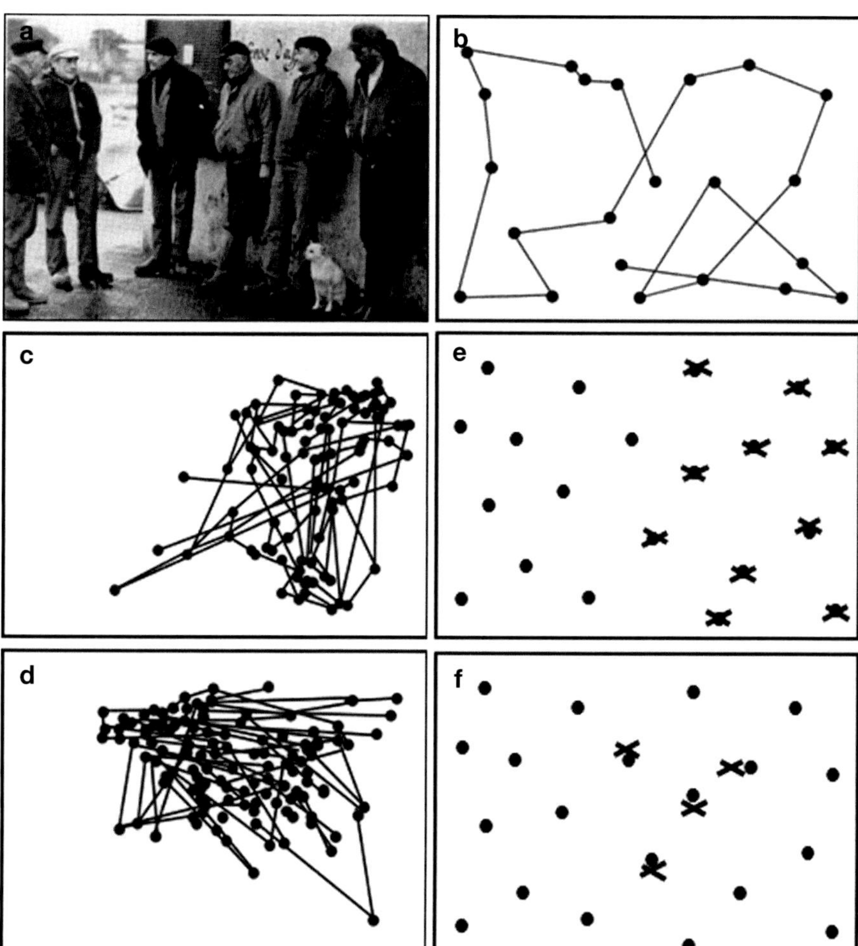

Fig. 4.11 Oculomotor scanning patterns in a 54-year-old normal subject (**b**), 56-year-old patient with left-sided visual neglect (**c**) and in a 64-year-old patient with Balint syndrome (**d**) during inspection of a scene (shown in **a**) and performance in a cancellation test (**e** visual neglect, **f** Balint syndrome). Note absence of visual scanning and cancellation in the left hemispace in the patient with visual neglect and bilateral limitation of scanning and cancellation in the patient with Balint syndrome

is shifted to the right. Patients also no longer search intentionally for stimuli on the affected side, and the same holds true for reaching and grasping movements (e.g. Milner and MacIntosh 2005). Bilateral posterior brain injury can cause bilateral restriction of the field of attention, sparing – depending on the degree of severity – only a small area for visual information processing (the so-called Balint syndrome, in the severe condition; Zihl 2011). In both conditions, patients do not respond to external stimuli, but are also unable to shift attention intentionally to the affected parts of visual space (Fig. 4.11). It seems that they have also lost much of the 'compartmentalised' internal representation of entities in surrounding space. The external world appears to be represented internally by far fewer elements in either the contralateral part (visual neglect) or to both, the ipsilateral and the contralateral parts (Balint syndrome), so that only a minimal number of entities can be appreciated at once in the affected attentional field, and shift of attention leads to loss of perception of the previously attended entity, rendering visual search, for example, profoundly difficult if not impossible.

In children with congenital brain injury similar forms of impaired field of attention have been reported. It appears, however, that such children more often show bilateral limitation of the field of attention than adults, associated with reduced responses to visual stimuli and decreased spontaneous shifts of attention and of gaze. Consequently, stimulus driven and intentional oculomotor scanning is limited to a smaller part of the external world (oculomotor apraxia) (Craft et al. 1994; Mercuri et al. 1997). Only when visual stimuli are exactly positioned in the children's line of sight, are they fixated and can be processed. Apart from this bilateral restriction, single case studies have revealed that *visual neglect* may also exist in children (Ferro et al. 1984; Billingsley et al. 2002; Laurent-Vannier et al. 2003; Kleinman et al. 2010; Fig. 4.12). Most affected children have suffered brain injury after the third year of life (infarction, haemorrhage, tumour excision). Visual neglect recovered in all cases within several weeks. Trauner (2003) found symptoms of visual neglect in 37 out of 59 children (62.7 %). The age of children at the time of assessment was 6–48 months (younger group) and 28–75 months (older group), respectively; some children also exhibited homonymous hemianopia. Interestingly, in the younger group the percentage affected by left-sided visual neglect was 59 %, and for right-sided visual neglect it was 82 %. In the older group, the corresponding numbers were 54 and 62 % affected, indicating a decrease in likelihood of right-sided neglect with age. Thus, the 'dominance' of the right hemisphere for spatial perception and space representation seems not be established before the age of 6 years (see also Johnston and Shapiro 1986). Reports of both spontaneous recovery and the higher proportion with right-sided visual neglect in children are in contrast to adult patients suffering from visual neglect. Adult patients exhibit a much higher frequency of left-sided neglect (Suchan et al. 2012). However, after recovery children still showed some attention difficulties on the affected side, because latency for shifts of attention and of gaze remained increased. Fig. 4.13 shows examples of impaired parallel visual processing in two children with CVI due to PVL, which is mirrored by the oculomotor scanning pattern.

In the children we have seen, the inability to search and find relates to the midline of the body, and unlike hemianopia which moves with the head and eyes, hemianopic visual inattention, particularly to the left is not compensated for by search with the head and eyes, but is compensated for by a body turn to that side (fitting well with the concept that visual guidance of body movement must be body but not head centric). Some mobile-affected children tend to adapt by, for example adopting a body turn at table so that the attended hemifield encompasses both knife and fork; while rotating the chair helps others empty their plate, when previously food was left on one side. In our paediatric clinical experience, left-sided neglect tends to be more severe, and body rotation to the left is needed as part of management to allow these children to encompass the central scene on both sides. In contrast, the features of right-sided neglect tend to be more subtle, such as telling the time wrongly more often when the hands of the clock are on the right side of the clock face, or having difficulties with the right

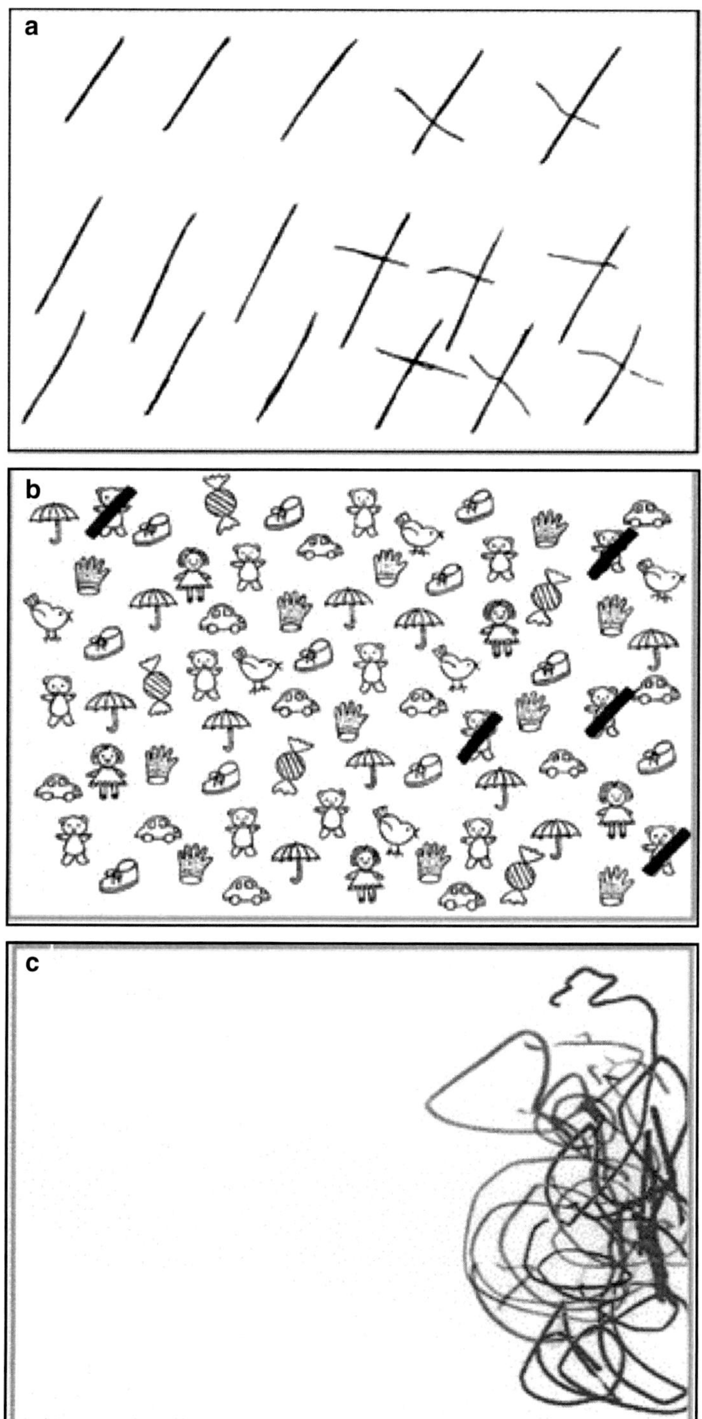

Fig. 4.12 Neglect in children: cancellation of line stimuli by a 9-year-old boy (**a**; Ferro et al. 1984. © Wiley reprinted with permission), and of teddy bears by a 2-year-old boy (**b**). (**c**) "Drawing" from memory (*line figures*) by the same boy (Laurent-Vannier et al. 2003. © American Academy of Neurology reprinted with permission)

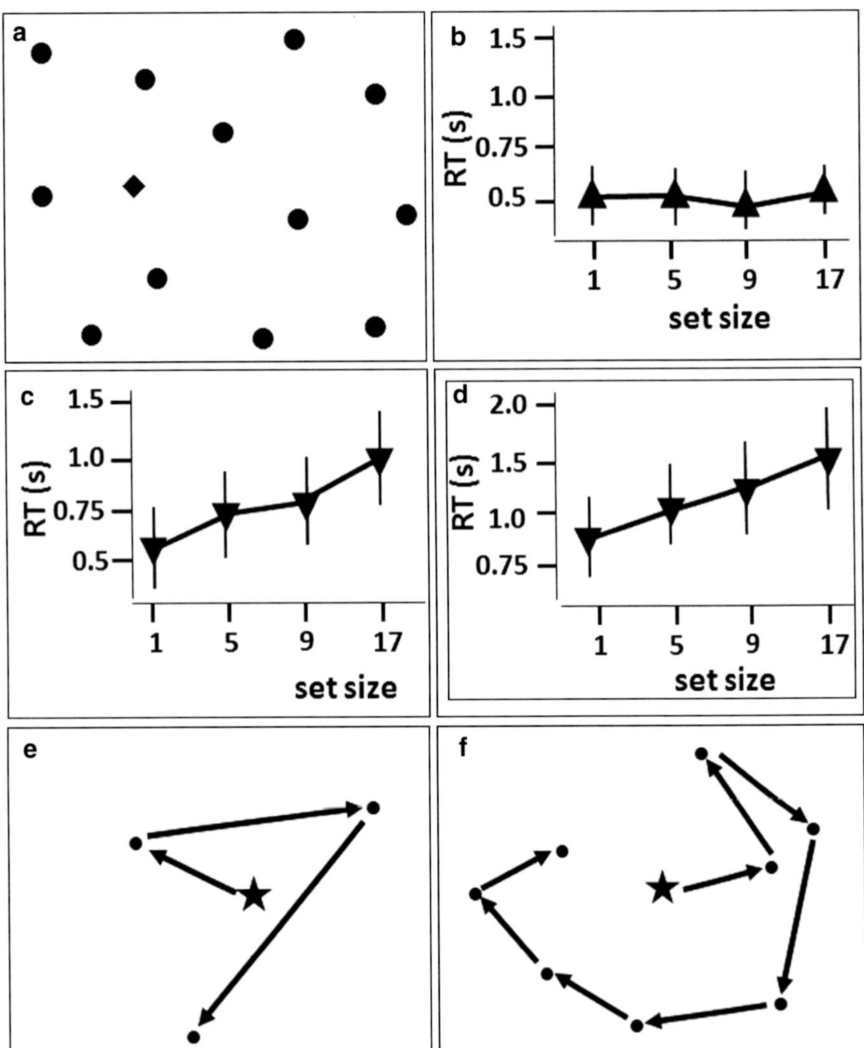

Fig. 4.13 Visual search performance in normal children, and in children with CVI. (**a**) Example of parallel search condition (task: search for the diamond) with set size (number of total stimuli in the array) of 13 (1 target, 12 non-targets). (**b**) Mean search times (20 measurements, target was present in 12 trials) and ranges of response times (*RT*; vertical lines) in five children (age: 8–10 years) for set sizes 5,9,13 and 17. (**c**, **d**) Search performances in an 8-year-old boy and an 11 year-old boy, both with CVI, respectively, in the same search condition as in **b**. While normal children show the typical parallel search mode (no increase in RT with increasing set size), both children with CVI show a serial mode of search, which is characterised by an increase in RT with increasing stimulus density. (**e**) Oculomotor scanning pattern in a normal child (**b**) for search condition shown in **a** (scanning time: 5.2 s); (**f**) oculomotor scanning pattern in the same search condition of the child shown in **c** (scanning time: 18.3 s). *Dots* indicate fixation positions (with start at the position of the star), *arrows* show the direction of saccadic movements. Note the increased number of fixations in **f** indicating prominent local processing of the stimulus array, with serial processing

side of drawings (that can be rectified by turning the paper upside down to complete the right side of the drawing). These are however clinical observations under busy clinical working conditions, rather than being founded on systematic study.

Balint syndrome has been reported in children in case reports. Gillen and Dutton (2003) presented a 10-year-old boy who had suffered cerebral haemorrhage at the age of 3 years. He recovered well, but presented with difficulties with parallel visual processing ('simultanagnosia'), optic ataxia and symptoms of acquired oculomotor apraxia. He found it difficult to read longer words, writing words in the correct order, copying from blackboard, avoiding people when walking, etc., symptoms that can be explained in terms of restricted field of attention. Drummond and Dutton (2007) reported a 7-year-old boy who was born preterm and had suffered perinatal hypoxia, and demonstrated a similar typical Balint syndrome symptomatology. Saidkasimova et al. (2007) reported seven cases with CVI after posterior periventricular white matter injury. Case 3, a 5½-year-old girl with perinatal injury exhibited difficulties with (visually guided) walking and reaching for objects, finding her mother in a group of people, and topographical orientation. Despite recovery, all children showed great difficulties with global vision, parallel processing, and visual guidance of eye, hand and body movements, indicating rather persistent symptoms of the Balint syndrome. Dutton et al. (2004) report very similar clinical findings in a further 40 children out of 364 attending a vision clinic over a period of 9 years. In many of the cases described there was accompanying peripheral lower visual field impairment, leading to inability to see the feet or the ground immediately ahead without looking down, a common symptomatic feature in children with periventricular white matter pathology (Jacobson and Dutton 2000). Conversely in our experience, structured history taking of parents and caregivers of children who do not see their foot unless it is raised high (indicative of peripheral lower visual field impairment), commonly reveals the cluster of typical visual behaviours (see Chap. 6).

For the sake of completeness, it is mentioned that uni- and bilateral neglect of visual stimuli has also been reported in children with attention-deficit disorder (ADD) (Voeller and Heilman 1988; Ben-Artsy et al. 1996). The authors speculate a parietal dysfunction as the basis for this visual-attentional dysfunction. It is, however, unclear, whether it is in fact a specific alteration of the field of attention, or is better explained in the framework of a more general attentional disorder, possibly of attention intensity (see Sect. 3.1), which affects all components of attention similarly.

4.3.11 The Dorsal/Ventral Stream Dissociation of Visual Processing

Some authors have found it useful to assign visual disorders according to the two main visual processing routes in the brain (see Sect. 2.2). While the dorsal/ventral stream model of visual processing as promulgated by Milner and Goodale (Milner and Goodale 2006, 2008; Goodale and Milner 2010) may have limitations in conceptually embracing the plethora of normal visual brain functions (e.g. Schenk 2006; Schenk and Mcintosh 2010; De Haan and Cowey 2011), it affords a practical approach that can be applied in the context of cerebral visual dysfunction related to damage to the brain, the context from which it was developed. However, it should be considered that 'dorsal' and 'ventral' are anatomical and not functional terms. In addition, selective visual disorders that can unequivocally be attributed to either stream are the exception rather than the rule (Zihl 2011, 2014), which is explained by the facts that (1) brain injury is usually not restricted only to the visual cortical area in question, and (2) coherent visual perception, which includes both visual spatial information and visual object attributes, also depends on the reciprocal interconnections between both streams of visual processing (Goodale and Westwood 2004). Considering the typical aetiology of injury to the central visual system particularly in pre- and perinatal periods, which is diffuse/multifocal rather than localised (see Sect. 4.5), selective visual disorders are expected to a much lesser extent in children.

The dorsal stream integrates occipital lobe and posterior parietal lobe function. It affords subconscious analysis of the visual scene integrated with analysis of data from other sensory inputs such as hearing. This brain area is thought to continuously map the components of the visual scene, providing a real-time, constantly refreshing, virtual, multimodal mental representation of the surroundings. This facilitates visual attention and visual guidance of movement by emulating the 3D spatial coordinates of what is being looked at and what is heard, probably combined with what is contextually remembered, to plan and bring about movement of the body, and, via the frontal eye fields, to generate rapid, accurate gaze (eye and head) movements to chosen targets in the visual scene. When a locus of the scene is chosen, for example a knife on a dining table, the fronto-parietal pathway facilitates the choice to move the head and eyes to look at it, by mapping it to its internal representation. The knife's coordinates can then be passed to the motor cortex, to initiate and bring about hand movement and accurate reach with 'in-flight' pre-adjustment of finger position, to accurately grasp the knife (Milner and Goodale 2006). This process is automatic, 'on line', accurate, rapid, is not afforded conscious awareness, and is not founded in memory, and thereby facilitates movement through and interaction with the surrounding world with immediacy and accuracy.

By integrating the internal map of the surroundings with the visual recognition centres in the temporal lobes, the posterior parietal cortex contributes significantly to attentional visual function via the fronto-parietal pathways. Severe bilateral posterior parietal pathology gives rise to lack or loss of simultaneous/parallel processing ('simultanagnosia') in which there is profound difficulty registering the presence of any object that is not being given direct attention. Affected individuals are unable to interpret the totality of the scene despite a preserved ability to see individual portions of the whole picture (Cuomo et al. 2012; Thomas et al. 2012). It is not possible to move the eyes from one element of a scene to another, probably because the multiple elements are not seen. This inability to move the eyes volitionally from one element of the scene to another, despite having a normal substrate for bringing about eye movement, is called apraxia of gaze, and is commonly accompanied by impaired visual guidance of movement of the upper and/or lower limbs (optic ataxia). At an extreme level, only one item at a time can be seen, and visual guidance of movement is profoundly impaired. This phenomenon is well reported in soldiers sustaining bilateral posterior parietal disruption due to shrapnel wounds (Holmes 1918; Luria 1959), but has also been described in patients after bilateral vascular, demyelinating, or infectious diseases with varying degree of severity (Hécaen and de Ajuriaguerra 1954; Moreaud 2003). The descriptions of their visual features closely resemble those seen and described in affected children (Gillen and Dutton 2003; Drummond and Dutton 2007). The acquired severe condition in adults is known as Balint syndrome (Rizzo and Vecera 2002). In multiply disabled visually impaired (MDVI) children who have quadriplegic cerebral palsy associated with cerebral damage, the posterior parietal cortex is affected as well as the other parts of the brain. These children may only raise their heads and look around, when covered by a bed sheet, or surrounded by a monochromatic tent, or when inside a sensory room with only one item on display. This behaviour is consistent with the hypothesis that they also have a profound form of Balint syndrome as part of their clinical condition, and in our experience the elimination of surrounding pattern and clutter in this way can be the first step towards significant habilitation (Little and Dutton 2014). A similar pattern of visual behaviour but of lesser severity has been accorded the term 'dorsal stream dysfunction' (Dutton et al. 2006; Jacobson et al. 2006; Saidkasimova et al. 2007; Van Genderen et al. 2012; Macintyre-Béon et al. 2013). When an affected adult or older child is asked to look briefly at a large group of people, then asked how many people they saw, the answer is usually less than ten. As a simile, the vision is akin to looking through a colander. As gaze shifts, a different small group of people are seen, but the original group cannot easily be re-located. Not surprisingly, search is difficult, and attention cannot be given to what has neither been seen nor located, as the posterior parietal brain substrate that serves attentional function is limited in the number of entities that can be simultaneously perceived. The visual behavioural characteristics that are typical of dorsal stream dysfunction are described in Chap. 6.

The ventral stream integrates occipital lobe functions with those of the temporal lobe structures that serve as the brain's 'visual library', serving conscious recognition and visual memory. Recognition of faces is served by the fusiform gyrus (commonly the right). If there is a match, the face is recognised. Recognition of shape and form and the ability to recognise and follow routes are likewise temporal lobe functions.

Dorsal stream dysfunction can occur in isolation but ventral stream dysfunction, when it occurs, usually accompanies dorsal stream dysfunction (Dutton 2009). However, when there is extensive bilateral occipito-temporal pathway damage from an early age, the affected person may not recognise nor know what he or she is looking at, despite remarkably good visuomotor abilities (Lê et al. 2002), giving a clinical picture akin to that described in the adult with acquired damage in the same area (Milner and Goodale 2006).

Table 4.10 Consequences of injury of particular brain structures involved in the control of saccadic and smooth pursuit eye movements

Brain structure	Saccadic eye movements	Smooth pursuit eye movements
Cerebellum	Dysmetria	Slow phases jerky
Midbrain	Restriction in the vertical direction	Restriction in the vertical direction
Cortex	Hypometria with catch-up saccades	Slowing (decreased velocity)
	Slowing	Slow phases jerky
	Latencies increased	Latencies increased

Modified after Leigh and Zee (2006)

4.4 Eye Movements

The oculomotor system produces eye movements that serve to fixate stationary or moving (pursuit movements) stimuli; fast eye jumps (saccades) are available to transport the fovea to the position of the stimulus, while pursuit eye movements serve to maintain fixation upon the moving stimulus. Accuracy of saccades depends on accuracy of visual localisation, visual spatial control, and eye muscle function. Saccades are generated in the frontal eye field territory, and are contralateral (the right-side generating saccades to the left and vice versa). They are either triggered by external stimuli, or brought about intentionally, for example, when the individual elects to shift fixation within a scene. Pursuit eye movements are generated in the occipital territory and originate ipsilaterally (Leigh and Zee 2006). They always need an external moving stimulus to 'guide' them (see Sect. 2.7). These movements are integrated within the brainstem at the level of the ponto-medullary junction. Convergence eye movements maintain binocular vision while viewing near static or moving targets, while divergence movements facilitate return to distant viewing. These functions are served in the upper midbrain.

After brain injury, alterations in oculomotor parameters (latency, amplitude, speed, accuracy) occur quite frequently, which is not surprising, given the fact that many different brain structures are involved in oculomotor control (Leigh and Zee 2006). Table 4.10 summarises the main consequences of injury to various brain structures serving saccades and smooth pursuit eye movements. Unilateral frontal brain injury usually impairs saccadic eye movements directed to the contralateral side, while the intact contralateral frontal territory tends to involuntarily drive the head and eyes to the opposite side, with spontaneous (but not always complete) improvement taking place over the ensuing months after acute brain injury. Extensive occipital pathology can impair ipsilateral pursuit, in association with contralateral hemianopia. After bilateral frontal brain injury, control and execution of saccadic eye movements to both sides may be impaired. Similar oculomotor disturbances have also been reported in children with congenital or early brain injury; typically, saccades, fixation and smooth pursuit eye movements are impaired in combination.

4.4.1 Fixation

An elementary form of impaired fixation is congenital or fixation nystagmus, which is most marked when a distant stimulus is fixated; it beats mostly in the horizontal direction and decreases when the subject converges for near (Leigh and Zee 2006). Children with congenital nystagmus often also show low visual acuity, but they tend to perceive the world as more or less stable (Bedell 2000) and do not see their nystagmus in a mirror (as the eyes and their reflections move in equal register, and therefore do not appear to move). Time to fixation is significantly increased and fixation accuracy is significantly reduced in children with congenital nystagmus (Pel et al. 2011).

Fixation inaccuracy may also be caused by insufficient visual acuity or contrast sensitivity, and by impaired concentration; under these conditions fixation is unstable and children may not be able to maintain fixation long enough for complete and accurate processing.

Jacobson et al. (1996) found horizontal gaze direction nystagmus in 12 of 13 children with bilateral PVL (see Sect. 4.5.3) when assessed by nystagmography. Stiers et al. (1998) reported fixation nystagmus in 10 of 22 children with perinatal hypoxia, who were tested at the age of 3–14 years. Thus, fixation nystagmus tends to persist. In the study of Fazzi et al. (2007), 40 % of 121 children exhibited impaired fixation. Khetpal and Donahue (2007) found spontaneous nystagmus in 21 % of 98 children. Children with nystagmus often adopt a compensatory head posture to suppress it, particularly when demands on visual acuity are high (Jacobson et al. 1996). However, this form of 'compensation' when marked may warrant treatment by surgical measures, not only because of the unfavourable effects on neck and shoulder muscles (stiffness, torticollis), but also because visual space and body perception may in rare cases become altered by biased unilateral vestibular and sensorimotor activities, and body control may be affected.

Congenital or fixation nystagmus has recently been identified in children whose mothers took opiates, benzodiazepines and other agents during pregnancy (Mulvihill et al. 2007). This is associated with reduced visual acuities (Gupta et al. 2012), abnormal visual evoked potentials (Hamilton et al. 2010) and neurodevelopmental abnormalities (McGlone et al. 2013).

4.4.2 Saccadic and Smooth Pursuit Eye Movements; OKN

Jacobson et al. (1996) found in 5 of 13 children with bilateral PVL, impaired saccadic and pursuit eye movements in both horizontal directions. In the study by Mercuri et al. (1997), 19 of 31 children (61 %) with perinatal uni- and bilateral hypoxic-ischaemic brain injury showed dysmetric saccades and 11 children (34 %) manifested impaired pursuit eye movements. Fazzi et al. (2007) reported 41 children of 121 (34 %) with dysmetric saccadic movements and 94 children (78 %) with impaired pursuit eye movements. Difficulties with attention may also contribute to

Table 4.11 Oculomotor alterations in 82 children with CVI (Linz study; see Tables 4.4 and 4.5)

Oculomotor function	Normal	Partially normal	Abnormal
Fixation	34 (41.5 %)	35 (42.7 %)	13 (15.8 %)
Saccades	38 (46.4 %)	27 (32.9 %)	17 (20.7 %)
Pursuit movements	26 (31.7 %)	25 (30.5 %)	31 (37.8 %)
OKN	37 (45.2 %)	28 (34.1 %)	17 (20.7 %)

OKN optokinetic nystagmus

impairments in saccadic and pursuit eye movements, leading to superadded apraxia of gaze; in addition, for accurate smooth pursuit eye movement, sufficient visual acuity and contrast vision are essential (Jan et al. 1986). Furthermore, accurate smooth pursuit eye movements also require sufficient movement vision for pursuing the stimulus at different speeds. Very preterm and preterm infants with CVI may show delayed development of smooth pursuit and, therefore, find it difficult to keep fixation on a moving stimulus particularly at higher speeds, because vision for moving targets is only possible for lower speeds (Jakobson et al. 2006; Gronqvist et al. 2011; Strand-Brodd et al. 2011). Delayed development of smooth pursuit may be exaggerated by perinatal risk factors, for example, retinopathy of prematurity, periventricular leucomalacia, and administration of prenatal corticosteroids (Strand-Brodd et al. 2012).

OKN comprises pursuit movements in the direction of a moving pattern and a reflex saccadic jump back again to take up fixation of the moving stimulus once more. OKN can be impaired because of increased saccadic latencies or dysmetric saccades, or because of impaired smooth pursuit, or of impairment in movement vision, which may be limited to lower stimulus speeds (see above). Typically OKN is more impaired for movement in the direction contralateral to the brain injury (van Hof-van Duin and Mohn 1984; Mercuri et al. 1997). Fazzi et al. (2007) found impaired OKN in 73 % of 121 children; this percentage was higher than for impaired fixation (50 %) or saccadic dysmetria (34 %), but lower than for pursuit eye movements (78 %). In Table 4.11 frequencies of oculomotor disorders in the Linz study are shown. Fixation was impaired in 58 %, saccadic dysmetria was present in 54 %, and pursuit eye movements in 68 % of children. More than half of children (55 %) exhibited abnormal OKN.

As already mentioned above (Sect. 4.4.2), visual acuity requires accurate fixation; this applies also to OKN. In Table 4.12, data from the Linz study on the relationship between eye movements and visual acuity in children with CVI are shown. As expected, children with inaccurate fixation also show very low visual acuities (2.0 – 1.0 LogMAR). On the other hand, accurate fixation is not always associated with higher visual acuity; more than half of children (54.3 %) showed sufficiently accurate fixation, but visual acuity was <1.0 logMAR. This indicates that specific impairment of visual acuity also exists in CVI. A similar picture emerges for saccadic accuracy. Pursuit eye movements and OKN may be observed even at low (<1.0 logMAR) visual acuity (~21 %); of course, size and contrast of visual stimuli used, as well as the child's attention and co-operation also play an important role. However,

Table 4.12 Oculomotor functions and visual acuity in a group of 72 children

	n	A	B	C
Fixation +	35	04 (11.4 %)	15 (42.9 %)	16 (45.7 %)
Fixation (+)	32	19 (59.4 %)	12 (37.5 %)	01 (3.1 %
Fixation –	15	15 (100 %)	00	00
Saccades +	39	08 (20.5 %)	16 (41.0 %)	15 (38.5 %)
Saccades (+)	24	12 (50.0 %)	10 (41.7 %)	02 (08.3 %)
Saccades –	19	18 (94.7 %)	01 (05.3 %)	00
Pursuit movements +	29	03 (10.3 %)	14 (48.3 %)	12 (41.4 %)
Pursuit movements (+)	25	10 (40.0 %)	10 (40.0 %)	0 (20.0 %)
Pursuit movements –	28	25 (89.3 %)	03 (10.7 %)	00
OKN +	40	10 (25.0 %)	15 (37.5 %)	15 (37.5 %)
OKN (+)	27	15 (55.5 %)	10 (37.0 %)	02 (07.5 %)
OKN –	15	13 (86.7 %)	02 (13.3 %)	00

A children with visual acuity ≤0.05 (n=38; 46.3 %), *B* children with visual acuity 0.06–0.1 (n=27; 34.9 %), *C* children with visual acuity >0.1 (17; 20.7 %). +, normal; (+), partially normal; – abnormal

a higher (>1.0 logMAR) visual acuity does not always imply that pursuit eye movements and OKN are preserved, indicating that associations and dissociations exist between visual acuity, fixation, saccades, pursuit eye movements and OKN.

4.4.3 Oculomotor Scanning Patterns; Visual Exploration and Visual Search

Eye movements, in particular saccades, are also used for scanning complex visual stimuli, for example, visual objects, faces and scenes. Efficient scanning patterns are adapted to the spatial structure of the complex visual stimulus or stimulus array being viewed, so that spatial–temporal integration of continuous processing of information in the context of the global structure of the stimulus and thus entire perception is ensured. This efficiency is guaranteed by accurate coding of the spatial properties of a scene, planning the sequence of fixation and fixation duration, and monitoring the scanning process. Brain structures subserving oculomotor scanning efficiency are located in the posterior parietal and the prefrontal cortices; the posterior parietal cortex is particularly engaged in coding of spatial properties, the prefrontal cortex in planning and executing scanning eye movements on the basis of spatial coding outcome. In adults, uni- and bilateral injury to posterior parietal structures can impair processing and coding of the spatial properties of a scene, while injury to prefrontal structures impairs adaptation of the scanning pattern to the global and local spatial structure of the scene (Zihl and Hebel 1997; Fig. 4.14).

To date, few studies on the effect of congenital or early brain injury on oculomotor scanning exist. However, it can be assumed that children with posterior parietal and/or prefrontal dysfunction may find it difficult to efficiently scan a scene, to

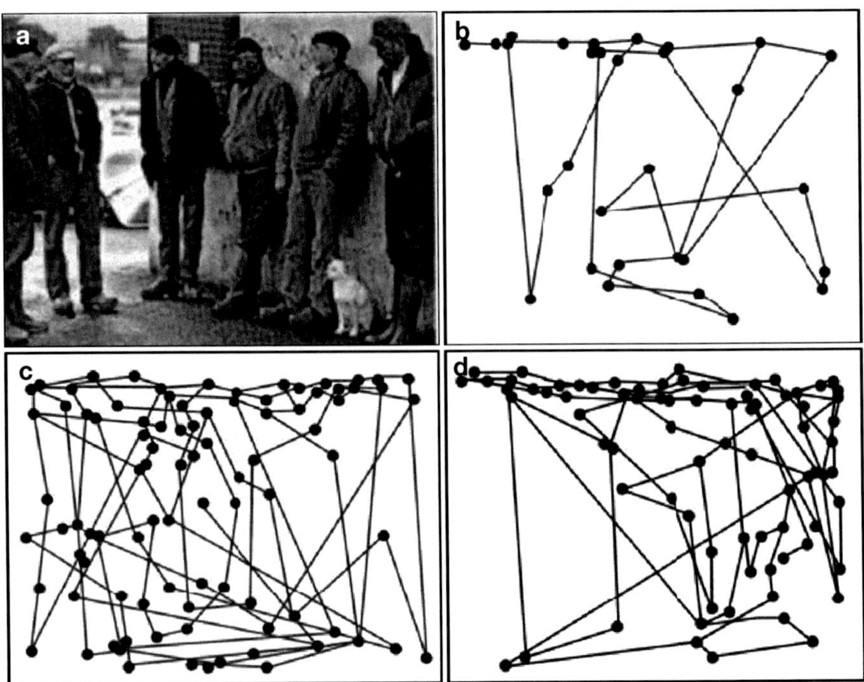

Fig. 4.14 Oculomotor scanning patterns during inspection of a scene (**a**) in a normal subject (**b** search time: 19.2 s), a patient with right-sided posterior parietal injury without visual neglect (**c** 44.8 s), and in a patient with a right-sided prefrontal injury (**d** 33.2 s). *Dots* indicate fixations positions, *lines* denote saccadic movements. All patients reported all the significant items (seven men and a dog), but note the increased number of fixations and small saccades in **c** and **d**

learn, how to adapt the scanning pattern to the global and local spatial properties of the scene, and to integrate successively processed information to a whole. Salati et al. (2002) found impairments in visual exploration in 48 of 56 (85.7 %) older children, characterised by requiring more time, omitting information, difficulties with integration of information into a whole and, therefore, difficulties with comprehending the overall significance of scenes. Netelenbos and Van Rooij (2004) reported prolonged search times in 6- to 10-year-old children with early right-sided brain injury of various aetiologies mainly affecting anterior cerebral structures. Visual search may also be secondarily impaired because of immaturity of saccade and vergence interaction (Bucci et al. 2012). Objectively measured visually attracted and guided eye movement is prolonged in children with CVI (Pel et al. 2011), and children with spastic diplegia make fewer anticipatory scanning saccades than normal children (Fedrizzi et al. 1998). Whether this results from defective dorsal stream visual processing (as a mild form of the apraxia of gaze seen in Balint's syndrome), or whether it reflects defective anticipatory control (Fedrizzi et al. 1998), is unknown. (Conceptually, the fewer items that are mapped due to deficient posterior parietal function, the fewer there are to attract attention and bring about eye movements.)

A range of supra-nuclear disorders of gaze can be seen (Salati et al. 2002). Paroxysmal ocular deviations are common in more severely affected children. Horizontal conjugate gaze deviation, often with exotropia, occurs with cortical damage, while tonic down-gaze and esotropia are more frequently associated with subcortical damage in prematurely born infants with additional spastic quadraplegia or diplegia (Brodsky et al. 2002), and can slowly improve (Yokochi 1991).

The eye movement disorders seen in cerebral palsy are likely to impair access to visual information, but the relative contributions of visual impairment and dysfunction of ocular motility can be difficult to dissociate. It is likely that paroxysmal and tonic ocular deviations, and disorders of pursuit and saccades all limit the speed of access to information, leading to visual information being missed, and contributing to attentional visual dysfunction.

A particular form of impaired oculomotor scanning is the so-called congenital ocular (or oculomotor) ataxia (also known as Cogan syndrome), which is characterised by the absence or severe reduction of intentionally generated horizontal saccades, but stimulus-elicited saccades and pursuit eye movements are preserved (Fielder et al. 1986; Borchert et al. 1987; Harris et al. 1996). Children with this syndrome mainly use head movements in visual exploration and scanning, which are understood as compensatory features (Goncalves Carrasquinho et al. 2008). Externally triggered saccades are typically hypometric (too small) and may also be transiently absent ('intermittent saccadic failure'). Clinically, spontaneous gradual resolution tends to take place by late teenage years. Congenital ocular motor apraxia may also exist for vertical eye movements (Hughes et al. 1985).

4.4.4 Head Movements

Children with CVI with significantly impaired visual acuities often show an altered head position (see Table 4.13). In the study of Jan et al. (1986), only 17 % of 70 children with CVI were able to properly control their head in an upright position (providing an index of the severity of cerebral dysfunction in the population described). Control of an upright head posture and visual acuity were related; the higher the visual acuity, the better the head control and vice versa (Jan et al. 1986). Inaccurate control of an upright head position may be associated with inaccurate fixation or even loss of fixation; consequently, central vision is not available for information processing, particularly concerning spatial resolution and form vision. In addition, accurate visually guided saccadic and smooth pursuit eye movements and normal oculomotor scanning also require sufficient head control. Head turning towards the contralateral side of brain injury and an associated shift of fixation may also be observed in children with homonymous hemianopia developed early in life, and may represent adaptive behaviour to enlarge the useful field of vision (Donahue and Haun 2007), but could also represent the tonic head and eye deviation seen with asymmetric frontal pathology.

Table 4.13 Head posture in children with CVI due to congenital or early brain injury

Head position	A (n=70)	B (n=226)
Head upwards	12 (17.1 %)	201 (88.9 %)
Head downwards	45 (64.3 %)	00
Variable head position	13 (18.6 %)	25 (11.1 %)

Modified after Jan et al. (1986); N=296
Children without any head control are not included. *A* children with no or no useful vision; *B* children with useful vision

4.5 CVI and Aetiology of Brain Injury

In this section, common aetiologies of brain damage or dysfunction associated with CVI in children are described, as are visual functions and capacities, and oculomotor functions and dysfunctions, which are impaired in the context of particular syndromes, and causes of brain injury.

4.5.1 Disorders of Brain Development

Genetically caused, or early onset disorders of brain development, can occur in combination with eye and optic nerve disorders and can affect the development of visual and non-visual brain functions. Such disorders include:

ADD (attention deficit disorder): Restricted field of attention and/or inaccurate fixation are probably secondary to a more general attention disorder, but may manifest as a concentrically restricted binocular visual field and/or as reduced binocular visual acuity (Martin et al. 2008). Reading may also be impaired (Germano et al. 2010; Sexton et al. 2012). In addition, analysis of visual social stimuli and/or their evaluation as social signals may be impaired (Williams et al. 2008).

Autism spectrum disorder: Facial configuration and eye gaze processing (Barton et al. 2007; Hoehl et al. 2009), facial identity recognition, and general visual recognition (Wilson et al. 2010, 2012), biological motion perception (Nackaerts et al. 2012), visual exploration (Ozonoff et al. 2008) have all been described as being deficient. Features of 'dorsal stream dysfunction' have also been described (MacIntyre-Béon et al. 2010).

4.5.1.1 Embryological Errors

Holoprosencephaly results from failure of differentiation of the forebrain. It can be due to teratogenesis for example maternal diabetes, and genetic disorders such as Patau's syndrome (trisomy 13) and Edwards syndrome (trisomy 18). Disordered formation of the corpus callosum and optic nerve hypoplasia, affecting vision, are common accompaniments (Brodsky 2010; Hoyt and Taylor 2013).

Occipital encephalocele describes the extracranial extension of occipital lobe tissue. A wide range of visual impairments including perceptual visual impairment can result.

4.5.1.2 Malformations of Cortical Development (Brodsky 2010)

Aicardi syndrome (Aicardi 2009) is likely to be an X-linked dominant condition (Aicardi 2009). It is fatal in males. It causes a range of different types of anomalous development of both retina and brain. Vision is often profoundly impaired due to both ocular and cerebral involvement.

Lissencephaly (or smooth brain) results from impaired early migration of developing brain neurones.

Pachygyria is a sequel to impaired migration of brain neurons later in development. Unilateral occipital involvement can cause hemianopia.

Polymicrogyria is the commonest disorder of brain development and focal unilateral occipital involvement is a cause of hemianopia.

Porencephaly is a smooth-walled fluid-filled cavity in the brain resulting from resorption of damaged tissue due to brain injury during the first two trimesters of pregnancy. It can be associated with visual dysfunction when the posterior brain is involved.

Schizencephaly describes full thickness brain clefts, often associated with polymicrogyria. Occipital cortical involvement can result in hemianopia.

These conditions need to be managed with kindness, competence, professionalism and sensitivity, with the aim of ensuring that throughout the child's management, families are informed of the child's visual capacities, so that they can try to ensure that their child is able to use vision to best advantage, notwithstanding progressively failing visual functions.

Down syndrome is commonly associated with impaired visual acuity and contrast vision (John et al. 2004), hypermetropia, impaired accommodation as well as strabismus (Cregg et al. 2001; Stewart et al. 2007; Creavin and Brown 2009). Stereoacuity may also be reduced (Little et al. 2009). Visual attention may be more focused for social than for object stimuli (Ruskin et al. 1994).

Fragile X syndrome: Decreased accuracy in perception of gaze direction is commonly seen in those affected (Garrett et al. 2004).

Turner syndrome: Visual space perception (Kesler et al. 2004; Hong et al. 2009) and visual-spatial working memory (Hart et al. 2006) have been found to be impaired.

West syndrome (infantile spasms): Lack of visual attention manifesting as lack of visual eye movements may precede the onset of epilepsy (Guzzetta et al. 2002), and it is essential to suspect this diagnosis in all infants who appear not to see from birth.

Williams syndrome (Williams-Beuren syndrome; WS): Impaired visual acuity, stereopsis and space perception may be accompanied by strabismus in children with Williams syndrome (Atkinson et al. 2001; Van der Geest et al. 2005; Palomares et al. 2008). Impaired global visual information processing (Porter and Colheart 2006), disordered visual search and scanning (Scerif et al. 2004; Nagai et al. 2011), deficient topographical orientation (Nardini et al. 2008) and developmental dyslexia (Grinter et al. 2010) have all been described. The often reported visuo-constructive impairments are not explained in all cases by visual-spatial difficulties (Farran and Jarrold 2003). In addition, children and young adults with WS may have difficulties evaluating peoples' faces as to whether they are approachable. They evaluate happy faces as highly approachable, while people with other facial expression are rated as less approachable. This difference may demonstrate heightened salience of social stimuli and is associated with disinhibition of social interaction, along with a strong compulsion to engage (Frigerio et al. 2006). Interestingly, children with WS may benefit from looking at whole face stimuli in motion when inferring the mental states of others (Riby and Back 2010).

Neurodegenerative disorders: There is a large number of rare neurodegenerative disorders which lead to progressive cerebral visual impairment (Brodsky 2010). These include disorders of different intracellular elements such as mitochondria, lysosomes and peroxisomes. Seizures, motor impairment, hearing loss and abnormal cognitive development are other consequences.

4.5.2 Preterm Birth

Preterm, i.e. birth before the 32nd gestation week, is considered a risk factor for the development of CVI, because maturation of the central visual system is delayed or because the post-chiasmatic components are injured, particularly at the subcortical level (Ball et al. 2012), or both (so-called encephalopathy of prematurity), (Volpe 2009a); or periventricular leucomalacia, (PVL), (Dutton and Jacobson 2001; Bassi et al. 2008; see also Sect. 4.5.3). The consequences include homonymous visual field (Jacobson et al. 2006), lack of stereovision (Geldof et al. 2014) and impaired movement vision (MacKay et al. 2005), but mostly delayed development of visual functions and capacities and/or a variety of visual dysfunctions in the visual and oculomotor systems. Compared with normally developed children, children with 'delayed visual maturation' show delayed development of visually guided behaviour. In most cases visual pattern-evoked potentials are normal and presage a good prognosis, but in some they may develop late. Delayed development of attentional capacities or attentional dysfunctions may cause delayed maturation of vision (Mellor and Fielder 1980; Fielder et al. 1985; Lambert et al. 1989; Rose et al. 2001). Gronqvist et al. (2011) have reported impaired smooth pursuit ability in preterm children, associated with a higher frequency of substituted saccades. Table 4.14 summarises visual and oculomotor dysfunction reported in the literature. At the time of assessment, most children were at least 6 years old; thus, dysfunctions are assumed to be persistent. In addition, preterm children may exhibit difficulties with attention, learning, memory and executive functions, as well as motor dysfunction (cerebral paresis; see Sect. 4.5.7). In some cases, learning disability may be present (Dutton and Jacobson 2001; Rose et al. 2001; Tommiska et al. 2003; Atkinson and Braddick 2007; Hellgren et al. 2007). Low visual acuity and impaired contrast vision may relate to CVI (Dutton 2013) or retinopathy of prematurity (ROP) (Dogru

Table 4.14 Visual and oculomotor dysfunction in preterm children

Vision
Homonymous visual field defects, mostly bilateral (frequently inferior)
Reduction of visual acuity (bilateral)
Reduction of contrast vision (bilateral)
Impaired stereopsis
Impaired space perception and visual search
Impaired visual guidance of movement
Impaired ability to see movement
Impaired visual identification/recognition
Oculomotor functions
Impaired/inaccurate fixation (nystagmus); impaired fixation shifts and oculomotor scanning
Strabismus

Modified after Dowdeswell et al. (1995), Dutton and Jacobson (2001), Jacobson et al. (2002), Rudanko et al. (2003), Cooke et al. (2004), MacKay et al. (2005), Atkinson and Braddick (2007), Hellgren et al. (2007), Fazzi et al. (2009)

et al. 2001; Ramenghi et al. 2010), which is also a risk factor for impairment of subsequent visual development (O'Connor et al. 2004). Jacobson et al. (2009) found a higher incidence of visual impairment in 114 preterm children due to CVI and/or ROP in boys (32.6 %) than in girls (9.2 %). More subtle visual impairment, identified through cluster analysis of structured history taking for evidence of typical behaviours, corroborated by impaired performance on tests of visual perception and attention has been identified in 33 % of 46 children (aged between 5 and 12 years) born between 24 and 34 weeks gestation. The pattern of perceptual deficit was consistent with dorsal stream dysfunction (MacIntyre-Béon et al. 2013). Preterm children who have sustained intraventricular haemorrhage may show poorer visual (grating and recognition) acuities and a smaller average visual field extent (Harvey et al. 1997).

4.5.3 Periventricular Leucomalacia (PVL)/Periventricular Brain Injury[1]*/White Matter Damage of Immaturity

The term PVL comprises consequences of cerebral disturbances of blood supply, which preferentially affect the white matter around the ventricles but also subcortical structures, e.g. thalamus and basal ganglia and cortical regions (Deng et al. 2008; Volpe 2009a, b). The post-chiasmatic visual pathways, occipito-parietal

[1] 'Periventricular leucomalacia' is primarily a neuropathological term. There has therefore been a move towards less specific descriptors like 'periventricular brain injury' in more recent publications that describe features seen on MRI scanning.

(dorsal) and occipito-temporal (ventral) structures may each be affected. Depending on the location of injury, children with PVL tend to exhibit homonymous, mostly bilateral visual field defects, reduced visual acuity, impaired visual motion processing (Weinstein et al. 2012), pursuit eye movements (Porton-Deterne et al. 2000) and impaired development of visual-spatial capacities and of visual identification (Lanzi et al. 1998; Cioni et al. 2000; Porton-Deterne et al. 2000; Jacobson et al. 2002; Fazzi et al. 2009; Ortibus et al. 2009). In the extreme form, PVL can cause blindness. Lanzi et al. (1998) reported blindness in 9 of 23 children (26 %) with PVL, without peripheral causes attributing to the absence of vision, while in the least severe form, a characteristic pattern of impaired visual search, attention and visually guided movement (particularly of the lower limbs) associated with lower visual field impairment can be identified (Jacobson et al. 1996; Dutton et al. 2004). Oculomotor dysfunction in children with PVL includes strabismus, nystagmus and inaccurate saccadic eye movements (Jacobson et al. 2002). A common association is optic disc hypoplasia, or cupping, resembling that of glaucoma, which has been ascribed to transsynaptic degeneration (Jacobson et al. 2003).

4.5.4 Hypoxia

Hypoxia usually affects not only the visual system, but also other parts of the brain, resulting in a combination of visual, cognitive and motor dysfunction (Stiers et al. 2002). Table 4.15 summarises visual, oculomotor and other dysfunctions in children who have primarily suffered perinatal hypoxia; at the time of assessment, children were 2–16 years old.

4.5.5 Epilepsy

4.5.5.1 Epileptiform Visual Aura

Focal epilepsy affecting visual areas of the brain can give rise to symptoms of seeing coloured forms and shapes when the occipital lobes are involved, with more complex imagery being seen when the temporal lobes are affected. Sometimes this condition can progress to the development of generalised seizures. Referral to paediatric neurology, with a view to further investigation by electro-encephalography and treatment if required, is indicated in symptomatic children, who commonly already have known prior cerebral pathology. The condition has to be differentiated from the visual aura of migraine (Brodsky 2010).

4.5.5.2 Ictal and Post Ictal Blindness

Epileptic activity in the occipital lobes can also give rise to acute cortical blindness, and is a cause of intermittent blindness in children. Children with this history also warrant referral to paediatric neurologists.

Children tend to develop transient visual loss as a sequel to generalised seizures more frequently than adults. Sometimes the loss of vision can be hemianopic in

Table 4.15 Visual, oculomotor and other dysfunctions in children who have sustained cerebral hypoxia

Vision
Homonymous visual field defects, mostly bilateral
Reduction of visual acuity (bilateral)
Reduction of contrast vision (bilateral)
Impaired stereopsis
Impaired space perception and visual search
Impaired visual guidance of movement
Impaired perception of movement
Impaired visual identification/recognition
Oculomotor functions
Impaired/inaccurate fixation (nystagmus); impaired fixation shifts
Inaccurate and delayed saccades
Impaired pursuit eye movements
Visual exploration/visual search impaired
Strabismus
Other capacities affected
Attention
Learning/memory
Executive function
Motor functions (CP)

Modified after Salati et al. (2002), Stiers et al. (2002), Atkinson and Braddick (2007), Fazzi et al. (2007)

nature. The loss of vision can last from minutes to days, with a period of gradually improving vision during the recovery phase. Rarely, loss or reduction in vision due to seizures can be longstanding or even permanent (Brodsky 2010).

4.5.5.3 Photosensitive Epilepsy

Generalised epilepsy can occur in those who have poor cerebral control of contrast gain for high intensity, low temporal frequency flickering light. This is thought to be the explanation why television and video games can cause this condition in those who are susceptible (Brodsky 2010).

4.5.6 Other Aetiologies

Cerebrovascular disease affecting the posterior and middle cerebral artery territories can give rise to homonymous visual field defects (Kedar et al. 2006; van der Aa et al. 2013). Occlusion of a middle cerebral artery causes contralateral hemiplegia, while damage to the optic radiations leads to hemianopia. Occlusion of a posterior cerebral artery infarcts the occipital lobe, leading to hemianopia, often with sparing of central visual function. In children, however, rupture of an arteriovenous malformation leading to intracerebral haemorrhage is a more common event, the extent and severity of the visual outcome being dependent upon the extent and distribution of the resulting haemorrhage.

Cerebral blindness can occur following successful resuscitation from prolonged cardiac arrest, which may have been spontaneous or as a complication of cardiac surgery. Gradual spontaneous recovery of vision tends to take place culminating in reduced visual acuities often accompanied by perceptual and cognitive visual dysfunction.

Closed head trauma can lead to impaired visual acuities and homonymous visual field defects. Impairment of convergence can occur but commonly resolves spontaneously (Poggi et al. 2000; Barlow et al. 2005; Kedar et al. 2006). In the so-called Shaken Baby Syndrome, and non-accidental injury in older children retinal injury (haemorrhages) and traumatic brain injury may cause visual impairment (Brown and Minns 1993; Kivlin et al. 2000). The spectrum of severity ranges from total loss of vision, to any degree of impairment of visual acuity and visual field loss, through to visual perceptual dysfunction, notably in our experience, the typical pattern of 'dorsal stream dysfunction' due to bilateral posterior parietal dysfunction, culminating in impaired visual search, which may be associated with impaired visual guidance of movement. Features of cerebral palsy may also be manifest. Changes in volitional saccadic eye movements may be present after mild closed head injury in children, which may persistently impair visual processing (Phillipou et al. 2014).

Congenital and childhood myotonic dystrophy type 1: visual acuity, astigmatism, hyperopia may be present (Ekstrom et al. 2010).

Fetal alcohol spectrum disorders have been described as giving rise to supranuclear disorders of gaze including increased saccadic latencies, as well as inaccurate visually guided saccades (Green et al. 2009).

Hydrocephalus has a wide range of causes. It can lead to impaired visual acuities. In severe cases downward deviation of the eyes (the setting sun sign) can persist after successful treatment. Expansion of the lateral ventricles into the temporal lobes can be associated with visual field constriction (Rudolph et al. 2010), impaired recognition and identification, sometimes associated with topographic agnosia, while 'dorsal stream dysfunction' manifesting as impaired visual guidance of movement accompanied by impaired parallel processing ('simultaneous vision') is described by parents in over 50 % of cases of shunted hydrocephalus. Strabismus is also common (Houliston et al. 1999; Andersson et al. 2006).

Shunt blockage in children with hydrocephalus can cause acute cerebrospinal fluid retention in the brain leading to brain distortion and high intracranial pressure. Despite successful shunt replacement, profound visual impairment due to either optic nerve or brain ischaemia can develop as a consequence in some cases.

Neonatal hypoglycaemia can give rise to focal damage affecting the occipital lobes and posterior parietal territories. Uni- or bilateral homonymous visual field defects often associated with reduced visual acuities can result (Tam et al. 2008). The typical picture of 'dorsal stream dysfunction' is not uncommon as an additional feature in affected children in our experience.

Neurofibromatosis (type 1) is associated with glioma affecting the optic nerves, chiasm and hypothalamus. In cases where the tumour is post-chiasmatic impaired visual acuity, colour vision and contrast sensitivity, may be accompanied by homonymous visual field deficits (Balcer et al. 2001; Dalla Via et al. 2007; Ribeiro et al. 2012).

Posterior reversible encephalopathy syndrome is rare. It is associated with a range of causes including severe anaemia and hypertension, reflecting the susceptibility of this highly active part of the brain to impaired metabolic function. Manifestations range from reversible bilateral homonymous loss of visual function to cortical blindness (Endo et al. 2012). Recovery tends to be gradual, with perceptual visual dysfunction being evident in some cases during the recovery phase.

Tumours affecting the anterior visual pathway: Such tumours can impair visual acuity in one or both eyes. Strabismus is common and can also be a presenting feature (Caldarelli et al. 2005; Defoort-Dhellemmes et al. 2006). Measurement of visual acuity is the most reliable parameter to monitor children with low grade gliomas of the anterior visual pathways (Avery et al. 2012). Posterior visual pathway tumours are rare, but visual field deficits may often go unrecognised (Harbert et al. 2012).

Thyroid hormone insufficiency: may be associated with reduced contrast vision (VEP responses) and impaired visual attention (Mirabella et al. 2005; Rovet and Simic 2008).

Viral encephalitis and presumed viral encephalitis: Rapid onset blindness in children can be a harbinger of sub-acute sclerosing panencephalitis resulting from measles (Senbil et al. 2004; Ekici et al. 2011). The author GD has seen two teenage children who developed presumed viral encephalitis which, following recovery culminated in severe impairment of visual recognition, owing to presumed temporal lobe involvement.

4.5.7 Visual Disorders in Children with Cerebral Palsy (CP)

In children with CP the motor dysfunction is evident, but many children also have difficulties with vision that are less evident, and can go unidentified (Dutton et al. 2014). Visual field, visual acuity, stereopsis, space perception and visual identification can be impaired (Fedrizzi et al. 2000; Stiers et al. 2002; Kozeis et al. 2007). In addition, children with CP may also exhibit refractive errors, impaired accommodation, strabismus, and abnormal saccadic eye movements, whereby tetraplegia is associated with a more severe profile of visual impairment (Fazzi et al. 2012). Because vision is a crucial prerequisite for the development of body control (Porro et al. 2005) and guidance of motor activities, including independent walking (Fedrizzi et al. 2000), CVI may represent an unfavourable condition in the context of physiotherapy, given that about 60 % of children with CP also show impaired vision (Kozeis et al. 2007; Fazzi et al. 2012). Children with less severe forms of CP show visual impairment less frequently (Ghasia et al. 2008), or they may manifest perceptual visual impairments, associated with more subtle attentional or visual field deficits (Jacobson et al. 1996; Dutton et al. 2004). In older children with CP, homonymous visual field impairment may persist particularly when the underlying brain injury occurred later in the developing brain. Jacobson et al. (2010) found homonymous visual field loss in 18 out of 29 children with unilateral CP, with severe field restriction in 6 cases; interestingly 5 children with unilateral injury to the post-chiasmatic visual system during gestation (white matter damage of immaturity, malformations) exhibited normal visual fields.

4.5.8 Acquired in Later Childhood

There exist significant differences between congenital or early onset CVI, and later acquired CVI in children. Children who have been born with CVI, or who developed CVI very early in life, have never been aware of what it might be like to have vision like their peer group. When they are young they tend to use their vision to best advantage, but are, of course, not aware of what they do not see. On the other hand, damage to the visual brain later in childhood, although rare is important to understand and manage well. The visual deficits that result tend to be different from those due to very early onset brain injury because:

- A range of skills have been learned when vision was intact;
- Learned skills have a prior memory and concept framework;
- Language and concepts have been learned in a visual context;
- Knowledge and memories related to vision have been gained, and this can afford an understanding of what is not being seen.

The nature of the impact of visual brain injury, with respect to age of onset in childhood, has yet to be investigated in depth. However, from our experience, three patterns are evident:

1. Pre- and perinatal visual brain injury leads to a wide variety of patterns of visual dysfunction from early life. The child's development can therefore be wholly influenced by the degraded visual functions, compounded by the effects of injury to other parts of the brain.
2. Early year's visual brain injury impacts upon the aspects of development that remain incomplete (see Chap. 5).
3. Patterns and outcomes of visual brain injury over the age of 10 years more closely resemble those seen in adults, because the developmental impact is minimal.

It has been argued that potentially, the earlier the brain injury the more amenable the child is to habilitational approaches capitalising upon potential neuroplasticity (Cioni et al. 2011). On the other hand, later onset pathology means that prior skills acquired through vision can be ascertained and optimally employed by rehabilitative strategies aimed at facilitating recovery.

These aspects of prior knowledge, the potential for recovery of vision, and the fact that residual vision can be employed to great advantage by learning adaptations (such as visual search to compensate for loss of visual field) make it possible to apply previously acquired skills and knowledge in the rehabilitation of these children.

4.5.9 Non-organic ('Functional') Visual Dysfunction

Non-organic visual dysfunction in children is rarely reported in the literature, but occurs in the context of non-organic overlay or rarely in association with abuse. Therefore, apart from detailed visual and oculomotor assessment, psychiatric and clinical psychological evaluation is essential (Moore et al. 2012). Adults with non-organic ('psychogenic' or 'functional') visual loss show tunnel vision and/or reduced visual acuity and contrast sensitivity and accommodation (Barnard 1989; Liu et al. 2001; Vuilleumier 2005; Pula 2012). It has been found to be associated with (reversibly) decreased activation in visual cortex, but increased activation in limbic regions (Vuilleumier 2005; Schoenfeld et al. 2011) indicating a kind of 'exclusion of sensory representation from awareness through attentional processes' that is 'mediated by dynamic modulatory interactions between limbic and sensory networks' (Vuilleumier 2005, p. 309). Children may show the similar patterns of visual dysfunction, but functional visual loss may also be limited to one eye (Leaverton et al. 1977). The presentation of functional visual impairment may, however, be different to that of adults. In addition, poor cooperation or understanding of instructions may bias diagnosis, and one should consider that children are also more suggestible (Liu et al. 2011), which facilitates management through positive consultation strategies. It is essential to exclude organic pathology of early onset, such as Stargardt's disease, that does not initially manifest objective clinical signs. Identification of normal visual acuities by means of visual evoked potentials is sensitive and specific for the diagnosis (Hamilton et al. 2013). Toldo et al. (2010) analysed retrospectively 58 patients younger than 16 years old with non-organic visual loss who underwent at least a 3-month follow-up assessment of their visual acuity and visual field. The majority of patients (76 %) exhibited reduced visual acuity, and about half (48 %) visual field defects. Brain imaging and VEP recordings were normal. Complete spontaneous resolution of all visual symptoms was found in 85 % of patients after 1 year. The authors did not find significant correlation between the duration of visual symptoms and age at onset, gender, time to diagnosis, or type of visual symptoms, but psychosocial stressors may play a significant role.

On the Coexistence of CVI and Mental and Motor Dysfunctions

5

5.1 Some Introductory Remarks

As outlined in Chap. 2, a large proportion of the information concerning our physical and social worlds is processed in the visual system (Goldstein 2010; Yantis 2013). The close integration with cognition, language, emotion, motivation and the motor systems, as well as the importance of visual information for these functional systems, also means that visual impairment can affect them. Thus, the normal development of vision depends on the corresponding development of cognitive, linguistic, emotional, motivational and motor capacities, and vice versa (see also Chap. 3); hence, visual perception, cognition and mental capacities are closely associated.

Visual disorders can have different consequences for mental and motor functions; often, children with CVI show combined impairments in vision, cognition, social-emotional and motor difficulties; the exact proportion of children with cerebral palsy who have CVI is unknown, but may be in the region of 60–80 % (Mervis et al. 2002; Venkateswaran and Shevell 2008; Barca et al. 2010). In everyday life, visual impairment may cause difficulties with finding a particular toy on a patterned floor or in a toy box, with learning to read, with recognising people or finding the way (Dutton 2009). Thereby, aetiology, severity and extent of brain injury or brain dysfunction play a crucial role: the more brain structures affected, typically, the more severe the resulting disability, vision impairment included (van den Hout et al. 1998). In children with PVL, CVI is typically associated with cognitive impairment (Jacobson et al. 1996). Additional functional impairments may not only exaggerate the degree of visual disability but perhaps also impede spontaneous improvement (Bonnier et al. 2007; Tadic et al. 2009) or improvement following treatment and require greater effort to manage, particularly if cognition and motivation and mood are affected. Cioni et al. (2000) have found that in children with PVL the degree of visual impairment correlates significantly with the child's general development; nearly all Griffiths developmental subscales (hearing and talking, motor functions, eye-hand coordination) showed moderate to high correlations with the degree of visual impairment. In addition, CVI has been shown to be a significant predictive

J. Zihl, G.N. Dutton, *Cerebral Visual Impairment in Children: Visuoperceptive and Visuocognitive Disorders*, DOI 10.1007/978-3-7091-1815-3_5

Table 5.1 Functional impairments in 30 children (age of assessment, 3–16 years) with perinatal brain injury

Fine motor functions	100 %
Vision	80 %
Cognition (attention, learning and memory)	60 %
Gross motor functions	50 %
Language	23 %

Modified after Fedrizzi et al. (1996)

factor for a child's further development. The same interdependency has been found in children with hypoxic-ischaemic brain injury (Mercuri et al. 1999). The higher the degree of visual impairment at the age of 5 months, the more pronounced the delay in development in the motor domain, and for general development, by the age of 3 years. Table 5.1 shows the rates of visual and nonvisual impairments in a group of 30 children with perinatal brain injury, who were assessed at the age of 6–15 years. Although this group is small, the data can be taken as evidence, that the combination of visual impairment and at least one additional dysfunction in the cognitive, motor or language domain, is the rule, i.e. most children with CVI suffer from dysfunction in another functional domain.

Developmental trajectories of children with CVI differ, in particular qualitatively, from those of children with normal development (van Braeckel et al. 2010); moreover, developmental differences may increase with increasing age. In addition, children with early brain injury more frequently exhibit (~60 %) psychopathological symptoms compared to children with normal development in the sense of an increased psychological vulnerability (Spreen et al. 1995). However, as Stiers and Vandenbussche (2004) have reported, children with CVI may also show normal cognitive development.

In conclusion, CVI can influence nonvisual functional systems in an unfavourable way and can cause secondary functional impairments. However, in cases of combined dysfunction, it is important to also differentiate between primary and secondary impairments in the nonvisual domains. In the following sections, interactions between vision and nonvisual domains and secondary effects of CVI on these domains are described in more detail.

5.2 Cognition

Visual disorders can impair development of direction and maintenance of *attention*, both externally triggered and by intention (Cavezian et al. 2013). Intentional guidance of attention depends on prior visual experience of objects, faces, scenes, etc. If visual-spatial appreciation is insufficient, visual attention cannot be accurately shifted to locations in space that contain relevant information. Attention can, however, also support vision and gaining of visual experience. Children with impaired but still useful vision often engage attention and perceptual learning highly efficiently and develop special strategies to enhance capture of visual information by attention. The price for this higher engagement of attention is fluctuating concentration and earlier and more rapid onset of fatigue, along with greater expenditure of time. These impairments in attention are typically associated with reduced visual performance thereby accentuating the features of CVI (Das et al. 2007).

If visual information cannot be processed accurately and completely, stored information in visual *memory* is incomplete and inaccurate and may even be false, as is the experience gained; use of vision for action will cogently be less successful. Examples of effects of visual impairment on visual memory include difficulties with identifying and recognising landmarks for visual-spatial/topographical orientation, or incomplete or incorrect drawing of objects from memory (Dutton 2002). For the acquisition of reading skills, learning of an efficient strategy of text processing is essential, including optimal eye movement patterns for reading. If, however, letters and words cannot be processed accurately (see Sect. 4.3.9), the development of an efficient reading strategy will be impaired (Fellenius et al. 2001).

Executive functions also need visual information for the execution of superordinate functions for the guidance of behaviour, for monitoring and controlling, and for flexible adaptation to changes in the stimulus and task conditions (see Sect. 3.3). In the presence of visual impairment, executive functions cannot develop and operate properly (Tadic et al. 2009) unless supplementary or compensatory skills are developed and employed.

5.3 Language and Reading

In language development, assigning names (labels) to visual stimuli, e.g. forms, figures, colours and objects, but also animals, flowers, faces and places may be difficult and inaccurate, if visual stimuli are not processed and identified correctly. The same problem applies to spatial directions and references (e.g. left-right, up-down, forwards-backwards). Furthermore, learning to read may also be impaired in children with CVI (see Sect. 4.3.9). This is exemplified in children with PVL (see Sect. 4.5.3), who may have low visual acuities but also may have difficulties with discrimination of symbols and letters presented in a line (Pike et al. 1994) and (as mentioned above) difficulties due to visual crowding. Possibly, impaired organisation and guidance of eye movements in text processing (e.g. oculomotor apraxia; see Sect. 4.4) may additionally render learning to read difficult (Lanzi et al. 1998). The probability that children with this combination of visual and oculomotor disorders will be able to learn to read depends crucially on their verbal intelligence, their verbal memory capacity and their attentional and executive capacities (Fellenius et al. 2001; Sireteanu et al. 2006; Menghini et al. 2010; Vidyasagar and Pammer 2010). Thus, successful acquisition of reading requires visual, oculomotor, perceptual, cognitive and linguistic capacities, which have to interact in an optimal way; any dysfunction in one of these domains, or their interplay, can impair reading acquisition. In children who cannot interpret written symbols, despite being able to pronounce, identify and put letters together to synthesise words by sound, reading of print may be unattainable (Jacobson and Dutton 2000).

5.4 Emotions and Affective and Social Behaviour

Correct identification of affective (social) signals is essential to 'read' emotions of other people (social perception; see Sect. 2.3.10). Impaired vision can affect social perception and can influence social behaviour, which depends on social perception. As a result, social responses may be inadequate or even absent, which may be interpreted as missing or defective social understanding (empathy) or lack of social interest, i.e. as an affective disorder. If social experience is limited in the way described, the risk of developing inadequate social behaviour in the long term may be increased, and persistent psychopathological symptoms may develop (Max et al. 1998). It is our experience that children, whose lack of vision is recognised, understood, handled optimally and not criticised, are least likely to manifest such difficulties.

However, emotions may also be affected independently of impaired vision. Children with developmental disorders due to brain dysfunction or early brain injury often show increased motor restlessness, enhanced irritability and emotional lability (Max et al. 1998; Janssens et al. 2009).

5.5 Motivation

It is easy to understand that low visual capacities will also impair visual curiosity, which can be understood as a *motivating factor* for visual information. Lack of visual curiosity may also occur in the context of a more global reduction of motivation; in this case, the child is not interested in any modality of stimulus, visual or otherwise (Max et al. 1998; Janssens et al. 2009).

5.6 Motor Activities

Because the visual system plays an essential role in the guidance and control of actions and motor activities, visual dysfunction can impair these operations and their development, and thus motor development can be secondarily affected. For example, difficulties with space perception (position of objects, distance and depth) and texture perception (floor) may impair mobility and postural control (Porro et al. 2005). Visually guided grasping, pointing and touching, and fine motor activities, and visually guided gaze shifts may also be impaired (oculomotor apraxia) as well as fixation (Koeda et al. 1997; Fedrizzi et al. 2000; Kozeis et al. 2007). Children with motor clumsiness often also have visual impairments, which interfere with motor control and guidance (optic ataxia) (Sigmundsson et al. 2003). Children with CP (see Sect. 4.5.7) may also show visual and oculomotor dysfunction (Guzzetta et al. 2001, 7–9 %; Ghasia et al. 2008, 16 %; Fazzi et al. 2012, 60–70 %, when studied prospectively). Interestingly, reduced visual acuity was most often found in children with quadriplegia and diplegia, while children with hemiplegia typically had normal visual acuity, but had the highest proportion of altered visual fields (Fazzi et al. 2012). Moreover, children with CP often have difficulties integrating visual and proprioceptive information (Guzzetta et al. 2001). Furthermore, motor problems in preterm children are associated with visual impairments, particularly low visual acuity (Evenson et al. 2009).

Finally, vision has been found to be a good predictor for developmental trajectories in general (see also Sect. 5.1). Guzzetta et al. (2008) assessed both visual development and cognitive, motor and social development in a longitudinal study in 21 children suffering from West syndrome (a particular form of epilepsy, which can also occur after brain injury). Children with this syndrome and normal cognitive, social and motor development also showed normal vision and audition. In contrast, in the children who developed CP, visual and cognitive development was similarly impaired, irrespective of the degree of motor dysfunction.

6 Diagnostic Assessment

6.1 Some Preliminary Notes

Diagnostic assessment of CVI in children is an interdisciplinary task, which needs close cooperation between the disciplines of (neuro-)ophthalmology, neuropaediatrics, developmental neuropsychology, orthoptics as well as early intervention and special education specialists. Observations reported by parents, brothers and sisters and other reference persons about the child's visually guided behaviour such as grasping for toys, visual exploration, fixation, responses to display of toys and other objects and play behaviour can provide significant indications concerning spared and affected visual capacities. In principle, it has to be acknowledged that when assessing children, who do not possess sufficient language competence and, therefore, cannot report or comment on what they can see and why vision is problematic, behaviour-based methods are used. Even for older children with CVI, it might be difficult to report in detail what they can see and can make out, in terms of useful vision. Language development may be delayed, and naming may be impaired because of semantic problems or because visual accuracy is (was) not sufficient to learn reliable associations between visual stimuli and their labels. Delayed language development may also make understanding of instruction and giving the proper verbal response difficult for the child. In these cases, behaviour-based assessment methods should be given preference. The reliable assessment of visual capacities, and their impairments, respectively, supposes at least sufficient cognitive, in particular attention, motor capacities and motivation, including visual curiosity. It is important to note that responses to visual stimuli, or performance in a visual task, which cannot be replicated, should not be taken for granted as contributing to a diagnosis.

Apart from the conventional criteria for tests, validity, reliability and objectivity, the so-called ecological validity plays an essential role in both the diagnostic assessment and treatment of functional impairments. Ecological validity comprises three dimensions, the nature of the setting, stimuli and response, and signifies (1) the degree to which the observed and recorded behaviour/performance reflects the

J. Zihl, G.N. Dutton, *Cerebral Visual Impairment in Children: Visuoperceptive and Visuocognitive Disorders*, DOI 10.1007/978-3-7091-1815-3_6

behaviour/performance that a subject shows/possesses in the 'real world and (2) the degree to which findings based on standardised test instruments can be generalised (or extended) to natural, everyday life settings (Schmuckler 2001). Of course, ecological validity varies between functional domains and thus assessment instruments. The diagnosis of homonymous hemianopia, for example, possesses a rather low ecological validity, because it does not include any information concerning the degree of compensation and thus the associated visual impairment. In contrast, impaired visual search performance will allow a good prognosis concerning a child's behaviour in everyday life conditions, because reduced accuracy tells us that the child will omit targets and reduced speed indicates that the child needs much more time for the visual search process, with limited search time also resulting in neglecting parts of the actual scene.

For the acquisition of valid, significant and reliable diagnostic data as well as for comparisons in follow-up (longitudinal) assessments of the same child and between children, it is essential to keep testing conditions comparable, i.e. to assess vision in standard conditions. Standardisation includes lighting conditions, equipment of the testing room (friendly atmosphere, but not too many pictures and furniture, because the child may be distracted), type and duration of stimulus presentation and verbal and nonverbal interaction with the child. Any effective means of stimulation of the child's motivation by the investigator is welcome, but this may also be too much for the child to cope with, due to information overload with visual, auditory and tactile stimuli; therefore, 'less is sometimes more'. In addition, it is important to consider breaks as often and as long as required. New visual stimuli may increase attention and enhance motivation; it seems sensible, therefore, not to show the same stimulus too often successively, because the child may show habituation to this stimulus and thus fail to respond (Fantz 1964). Results, which are obtained under conditions that do not guarantee examination, can be used for preliminary screening, but not for diagnostic reports.

The examination of the various functional capacities of the central visual system should always seek not only impaired visual capacities but also those that are spared. The so-called positive and negative picture of performance is not only important to understand the quality and degree of visual disability but also for the planning of therapeutic interventions and the benefit of these interventions. The use of standardised assessment tools is, therefore, recommended; in addition, data from children with normal development of the same age, gender and socio-economic status should be available for comparison.

There is still a lack of standardised diagnostic tools. Many assessment measures that are used in developmental research cannot easily be translated into diagnostic practice; on the other hand, proven tests, for example, to assess visual acuity or contrast vision, are not very helpful for the evaluation of (the degree of) visual disability in individual everyday life conditions of the child, i.e. ecological validity is rather low (Colenbrander 2009, 2010; Boot et al. 2010; see Sect. 7.3) when other visual disabilities are evident. The verification of spared manifest visual capacities often meets with difficulties, because assessment standards designed for typical children may have limited salience for the child whose visual system has developed differently. Here, a quasi-experimental procedure may be helpful: one factor is manipulated in a systematic and reproducible way, for example, the use of coloured instead of 'black' symbols and forms may be used to estimate visual acuity, because coloured stimuli can have higher salience for the specific child (exceptions: congenital colour deficiencies or cerebral dyschromatopsia). Visual acuity can also be estimated by means of moving stimuli that differ in size, because accuracy of smooth pursuit eye movements depends crucially on visually acuity (Atkinson and Braddick 1979; see Sect. 6.5.4). This quasi-experimental approach may be especially helpful if 'normal' assessment procedures do not produce useful results. Such deviations from the standardised assessment should, however, always be documented. In addition, it should be clearly understood that such procedures do not possess the same diagnostic quality in terms of validity, although reliability and objectivity can, however, be achieved by using this type of approach in a standardised form. Diagnostic assessment tools presented in this chapter, which have been standardised, accord with the outcome from developmental studies in children with normal development (e.g. Granrud 1993; Slater 1998a, b). Finally, it should be added that measurements of visual functions and capacities should be repeated by the examiner, and in doubtful cases by another examiner; this can increase the reliability of measurements considerably and thus also the validity of the test used (Mash and Dobson 2005).

6.2 The Method of Preferential Looking (PL)

The method of PL was developed by Fantz and Oddy (1959) to assess visual capacities at the behavioural level in babies and young children. The method is based on the observation that newborn infants show 'natural' preferences for particular visual stimuli, i.e. they favour such stimuli above others and, therefore, fixate upon them longer (see Sect. 2.3.6). This preference behaviour underlies many assessment methods in visual development, for example, for visual acuity, contrast sensitivity, discrimination of colour hues and of forms, figures and complex visual stimuli and size and number of stimuli (Miranda 1970; Fantz and Fagan 1975; Clavadetscher et al. 1988). Estimation of the corresponding visual capacity is based on fixation times, whereby the particular stimulus of a stimulus pair (e.g. that has been preferred by at least 75 % of normal children) is taken as the cut-off score for discrimination (Fantz 1964). It is, however, important to avoid habituation effects by presenting the same stimulus pair too often.

The method of PL has been proven reliable for the assessment of visual acuity in children with CVI (Chandna et al. 1989; Birch and Bane 1991; Schmidt 1994). It is, however, important to mention that the behavioural response in question must be attainable by the child. Table 6.1 summarises typical visual activities of children aged 1–12 months, which may also serve as a guideline for diagnostic assessment in children with CVI. For determination of the so-called difference threshold, pairs of stimuli are shown, whereby one stimulus remains unchanged (so-called standard stimulus), while the other stimulus is approximated (variable stimulus), so that the

Table 6.1 Typical visual activities during the first 12 months in children with normal development

Months 0–1
Looks at light stimuli, turns eyes and head
Blink responses as avoidance behaviour to bright light
Eye contact with others
Slow and jerky horizontal pursuit eye movements
Months 2–3
Intensive eye contact
Interest in mobiles
Vertical pursuit eye movements
Months 4–6
Grasps at moving objects
Observes falling and rolling away of objects
Shifts fixation across midline
Extends visual field of search (attention)
Begins to decouple eye from head movements
Pursuit eye movements are smooth
Months 7–10
Becomes aware of and detects small objects
Touches and later grasps at stationary objects
Is interested in pictures and scenes
Keeps eye contact with others over a distance of several metres
Months 11–12
Good visual orientation in familiar surroundings
Looks through window and recognises familiar persons
Can visually recognise pictures; plays hide and seek
Observes and examines objects in detail
Communicates visually in an efficient way (understands and uses facial expressions and gestures)

Modified after Hyvarinen (2000); see also Table 2.14

difference between the two stimuli decreases progressively. If no preference for either stimulus can be observed, i.e. the frequency of orienting responses, and duration of fixations are more or less equal, the limit of stimulus discrimination has been reached, and this value can be taken as the difference threshold. To avoid too high a demand on visual memory, the time between pair presentation should not be longer than 3–5 s. Apart from direct observation of oculomotor and grasping responses, video recordings of responses may be very helpful, because they allow repeated analysis and are, in addition, very suitable for individual longitudinal assessments, as well as for comparisons between children (e.g. children with different manifestations of CVI, or children with CVI and those with normal visual development). Eye movements to visual stimuli can also be recorded using video- and infrared-registration techniques. Further sources for getting information about visual capacities include the systematic observation of visually guided everyday life activities and the use of electrophysiological methods, which allow recording of physiological correlations of visual capacities (Lundh 1989; Hartmann et al. 1990; Bane and Birch 1992; Bravarone et al. 1993; Katsumi et al. 1995, 1997, 1998; Lewis et al. 1995; Rydberg and Ericson 1998).

6.3 Visual Evoked Potentials (VEPs)

Registration of VEPs facilitates determination of the quality and speed of processing of visual stimuli, e.g. patterned black-and-white stimuli, which are transmitted from the retina to the primary visual cortical area (striate cortex, Brodmann area 17, V1), where the electrical responses are generated (Barnikol et al. 2006). Latency and amplitude of the first positive wave (P1) are the most commonly used parameters to evaluate the electrophysiological responses. However, it must be recognised that the amplitude and form of the VEP depend crucially on fixation accuracy and concentration upon the stimulus pattern during the recording, because the major contribution to the amplitude of P1 stems from the central visual field (Cannon 1983). Furthermore, even if the form, amplitude and latency of P1 are optimal for analysis, a fundamental problem remains. These parameters characterise the electrophysiological response to a defined visual stimulus, which means that it is a kind of correlate of vision, but is neither a measure of true vision nor an assessment of visual capacity, e.g. visual acuity or contrast sensitivity (Arroyo et al. 1997). Fortunately, there exist highly positive correlations in children (and adults) between the amplitude of P1 responses to a pattern reversal checkerboard or grating stimulus and visual acuity and spatial contrast sensitivity, respectively, if an adequate range of spatial frequencies is used (0.1–30 cycles/degree; Ridder 2004; Lenassi et al. 2008; Mackay et al. 2008; Iyer et al. 2013). Pattern-evoked visual potentials have also been proved to possess high sensitivity and specificity in children with suspected functional visual acuity loss (Hamilton et al. 2013), in preterm children with subtle visual dysfunction (O'Reilly et al. 2010) and in children with spastic cerebral palsy (Costa and Ventura 2012). In addition, pattern-evoked visual potentials may also be useful in longitudinal assessment of visual function in children with CVI (Watson et al. 2007), but besides parallel courses of PL, visual acuity and VEP development, disparities in PL and VEP can also be found (Lim et al. 2005). Unfortunately, however, a sufficient quality of P1 can occur in the context of cerebral blindness. Nearly normal P1 responses after pattern stimulation have been recorded in adults with bilateral destruction of V1 and resulting severe visual disability, characterised by a visual acuity 1.3logMAR (<0.05). Apparently, a smaller number of spared neurons in V1 is required for generating P1 than are needed to 'see' the same stimulus pattern and discriminate pattern components (Celesia et al. 1982; Wygnanksi-Jaffe et al. 2009). Thus, the preserved P1 does not always allow a valid conclusion to be drawn about visual acuity or contrast vision; the only correct conclusion that can be drawn is that there is good transmission of visually triggered retinal signals to V1 and that there is still some neuronal activity in this visual cortical area, which taken positively could provide evidence for persisting cortical visual function. Despite the methodological and interpretational difficulties, VEP recordings may be useful in children with severe forms of CVI (van Genderen et al. 2006). In some cases, it is the only way to get diagnostic information about the morphological and physiological 'state' of the visual system (Taylor and McCulloch 1992), which in addition, allows a prognosis concerning the development of visual acuity in preterm children and in children with CVI (Atkinson et al. 2002a; Watson et al. 2010). Measurements can also be used as a guide to the dimensions of habilitational and educational materials to evaluate for responses and use. However, VEP vernier acuity appears more affected in subjects with CVI and is more associated with behavioural measures of grating acuity than is VEP grating acuity (Skoczenski and Good 2004; Watson et al. 2009). It should be added here that flash-evoked visual potentials are not useful to assess cortical visual function, because they are mainly generated by subcortical structures of the visual system and thus do not reflect acuity-equivalent visual processing (Schroeder et al. 1989).

6.4 Diagnostic Procedures in Children with CVI

In this section, assessment methods are presented for visual and oculomotor functions and capacities, which play a prominent role in visual perception and its development and which can be assessed with high validity and reliability: visual field, spatial contrast sensitivity and visual acuity, colour and form discrimination, localisation of visual stimuli, stereopsis, object and face perception and oculomotor functions including visual exploration and visual search. Thus, a comprehensive set of visual and oculomotor tools should not solely comprise visual field, visual acuity, contrast sensitivity and eye movements, although such a tool set can serve as a valid basic standard with high availability and simple use by practitioners (Powers 2009). Emphasis is on children in the first 3–4 years; for older children, assessment standards exist or neuropsychological assessment methods can be applied, which are also used with young adults (see Fischer and Cole 2000; Hyvarinen 2000; Topor and Erin 2000; Zihl 2011; Lezak et al. 2012). In older children who show severe multiple disabilities, particularly in cognition, the tests described can also be used. It should be mentioned that not all tests are sufficiently standardised and for some tests data from normal children for comparison are missing.

In cases of suspected CVI, it appears reasonable and useful to follow a standard scheme. After making the first contact with the child, including systematic observation of the child's behaviour (which often gives the first indication of visual difficulties), the medical history, head and body posture, eyelids, poisition of the eyes and possible spontaneous eye movements (e.g. spontaneous nystagmus and gaze dependant nystagmus) are elicited. After checking the ability of the child to participate sufficiently in the assessment, anterior parts of the eye, pupil function, accommodation, vergence, ocular motility (saccades and pursuit eye movements) and eye, head and grasping movements to a simple visual stimulus are examined. Systematic assessment of visual and oculomotor functions and capacities is then performed.

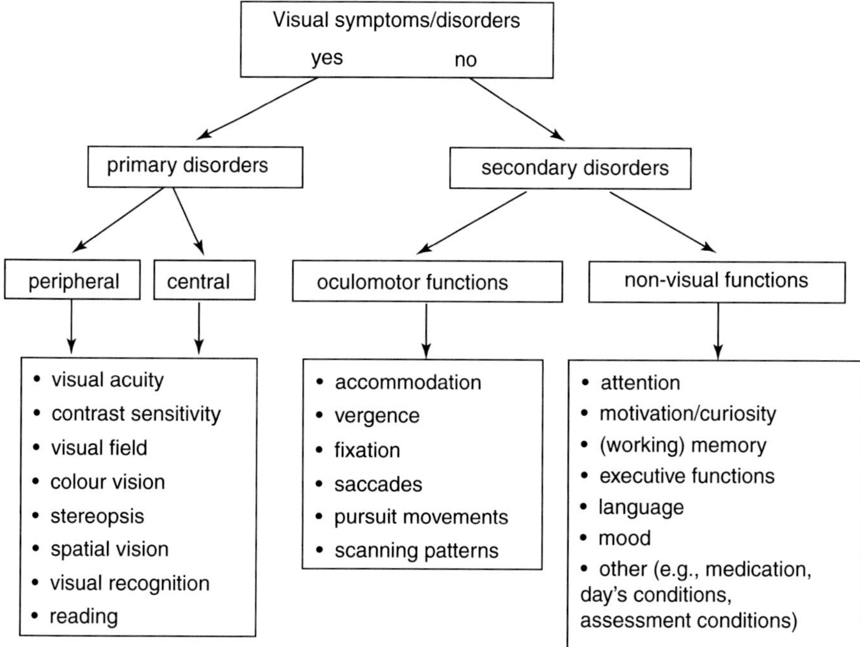

Fig. 6.1 Schematic diagram of diagnostic steps in children with suspected visual impairments of peripheral and central origin (so-called primary visual disorders) or due to oculomotor or nonvisual disorders (so-called secondary visual impairments)

Figure 6.1 shows the various diagnostic steps in the visual and oculomotor assessment in suspected CVI in a schematic diagram; the proposed diagnostic procedure is also intended to help with differentiating primary and secondary visual and oculomotor dysfunction.

6.4.1 History Taking to Assist Diagnosis and Guide Management of CVI

History taking comprising systematic questioning of parents or other reference persons (e.g. grandparents, mother's help, kindergarten teachers), who can give information about the child, concerning development, in general, and visual development, in particular, but also about habits, preferences, difficulties and avoidance responses, and conditions of occurrence, is the first phase of diagnostics. Visual history taking should include questions on the child's visually guided behaviour in everyday life situations and play behaviour but also visual curiosity, attention to visual (and other) stimuli, dealing with other children (social behaviour), etc. For the older child who can communicate well, history taking in the absence of parents is indicated. More valid and reliable information can be gained if a standardised questionnaire is used, which addresses visual performance and behaviour in

Table 6.2 The visual skills inventory of McCulloch et al. (2007)

Q1	Is your child aware of a spoonful or food coming towards his/her mouth?
Q2	Does your child reach for a small/large silent object?
Q3	Does your child's vision seem better vision in bright light/dim light?
Q4	Does your child reach for a drink bottle?
Q5	Does your child see a small/large silent object?
Q6	Does your child reach for a small/large noisy object?
Q7	Does your child react to you approaching him without sound clues?
Q8	Does your child follow your movements around a room when you have given him no sound clues?
Q9	Does your child return your smile when you smile without any sound?
Q10	Is your child aware of himself in a mirror; if yes: 6 ft (1.8 m), 4 ft (1.4 m), 2 ft (0.7 m), 1 ft (0.35 m) or less?
Q11	Does your child screw up his eyes when taken into bright sunlight?

Q question

everyday life conditions of the child. McCulloch et al. (2007) have used an inventory with 16 questions about visual skills and behaviour in familiar conditions to comprehensively assess 76 children (age, 7 months to 16 years) with marked neurological impairments. Visual skills and visual behaviour were rated by carers. In addition, structured clinical histories were taken, and visual acuity was measured using VEP acuity and acuity cards. Acuity ranged from mere light perception to normal and was positively associated with carer's responses and reports. Two independent factors were found, which were significantly correlated with the outcome of visual assessment. Factor 1 was visual recognition and was correlated with visual acuity; factor 2 was visually dependent social interactions. The authors eventually identified items with the highest validity for predicting visual skills and visual behaviour (see Table 6.2). Interestingly, overall correlations between item frequencies with acuity card measures were considerably higher than with VEP acuity. Ortibus et al. (2011) investigated the utility of a CVI questionnaire as a screening instrument in children with and without CVI (mean age, 6 years) who in addition underwent a detailed visual assessment including visual perceptual and visuomotor tests. The questionnaire consists of 46 items; covers visual attention, visual fixation, visual field and the influence of a familiar environment; and is filled out by parents. Sensitivity ranges from 33.3 to 76.7 % and specificity from 70.6 to 97.1 %; thus, the questionnaire has good predictive value for the identification of children with CVI. Ferziger et al. (2011) evaluated an interdisciplinary functional questionnaire for children with cerebral palsy and intellectual disability. The questionnaire proved valid and reliable information about daily visual performance and predicted visual function with respect to task-orientated visual function and basic visual skills and may be a useful instrument for visual assessment in children with CP. Although it appears obvious to ask parents and carers to fill out visual function questionnaires, because they can respond in a standardised form, it seems sensible to also question the children with CVI in a semi-standardised form to obtain more personal and individual information regarding their difficulties in various everyday life situations and how they cope with them, provided the child possesses sufficient linguistic and intellectual capability.

More detailed structured history taking using an inventory of questions, rather than a questionnaire, where clarification and more detail is sought as required for positive responses, can also be applied, particularly to move on from diagnosis to characterisation of the behavioural impact of the visual disability. One such recently validated inventory of 51 questions (Dutton et al. 2010; Macintyre-Béon et al. 2012) has proven effective in characterising the visual behaviours in children born prematurely (Macintyre-Béon et al. 2013).

The diagnosis of a number of visual conditions can only be made by *history taking*. Examples include the subjective symptoms of visual migraine (the fortification spectrum), amaurosis fugax (intermittent fleeting loss of vision) or Charles Bonnet syndrome (formed visual hallucinations as a sequel to loss of vision). Similarly, many of the adaptive and reactive behaviours seen in children with CVI can only be identified by taking a structured history, because they are features of everyday living, or they are no longer manifest but informative, or they comprise the older child's subjective experiences, none of which are evident on assessment.

This section describes history taking methods, using both open and closed question sets, designed to contribute to the dual objectives of working towards a diagnosis and optimally managing each child with CVI. History taking precedes and can thus be used to guide assessment for cooperative older children. However, assessment of vision needs the child's cooperation. For younger children, it is often best to 'capture the moment' and assess vision and eye movements before detailed history taking, which can then be carried out while the child is playing or being looked after.

6.4.1.1 Interview Method

Ideally the room for the interview is clean, tidy and uncluttered and has wheelchair access, space for a number of people and facilities for play. (Watching the child at play can be very informative.) The range of equipment and resources needed to fully assess vision in children of all ages ideally needs to be available.

The child and accompanying adults are welcomed and introductions made. The interviewer uses a calm voice, is kind and friendly and involves the child. The older child is made to feel important and is invited to contribute, on occasion without parents present for some of the time. Siblings and grandparents if present are also involved and can in many cases contribute useful information.

The way a question is asked can influence the answer. The question 'What are your concerns about John's vision?' is open and does not lead. The question 'What happens when you take John into a supermarket?' is a closed but non-leading question, while the question 'Does David become upset when you take him into a supermarket?' is both a closed and a leading question, as the expected answer is implied. Each type of question has its place. Open, non-leading questions are used to elicit the story for the first time and to contribute to the diagnosis. Closed, non-leading questions are used to find out more about issues raised. Closed, leading questions potentially providing expected answers can be helpful later in the interview, when working out how best to help the child once the diagnostic picture has been elicited using the open, non-leading approach. Closed leading questions can help parents recognise the behavioural features being sought, as it may not have occurred to them that behaviours they see each day are in any way unusual, meaning that this information may not otherwise be elicited. Such questions can lead to their realisation that behaviours that they deemed 'normal' are in fact reactions or adaptive strategies to circumvent visual disorders. (However, such leading questions must be used advisedly, and responses interpreted carefully, because a small minority of families can, in our experience, take on board and 'file' this information to use inappropriately at a later stage to potentially enhance the story for perceived gain. Such an outcome is of course counterproductive for all parties.)

The approach we recommend comprises:

Initial Administration

- Ascertaining the previous medical history from the referral letter and case notes.

Taking the History

- Seeking the story
- Clarifying the story
- Extending the story
- Asking open expert questions to seek diagnostic patterns of visual behaviour
- Using an open question inventory, if required, to seek the full range of the visual difficulties and their impact
- Selecting and employing supplementary question sets as required from a closed question inventory
- Finding out what the family has already been told and understands
- Understanding the wishes, agenda and aspirations of the child and family
- Finding out about the day-to-day practical and psychological impacts the visual difficulties are having upon the child and family (to work towards identifying and implementing ways of ameliorating any adverse impact)

Assimilating the Information

- Identifying typical clusters of features elicited to cross validate the responses and make sense of the information to contribute to the diagnosis and its pattern
- Assembling and documenting the story and drawing conclusions
- Using the information gathered by history taking and examination, to guide further tailored assessments if required
- Documenting all the features elicited to compile a prioritised tailored comprehensive list of interventional strategies to use at home, at school and elsewhere

- Communicating the Diagnosis and Management Plan
- Selecting the initial strategies to work on
- Writing a salient comprehensive report that all can understand and planning the approach to management

Initial Administration

Ascertaining the previous medical history from the referral letter and case notes. It is very helpful to have appraised and mastered all the available information before the child and accompanying adults enter the room. This gives the family confidence, and assists in guiding the strategies and pathway of history taking and assessment.

Taking the History

Seeking the story. For some children, the interview will be their first, and parents will want their observations of how their child behaves explained. For others, there may have been a number of previous encounters with a range of professionals who may have given different explanations of the findings and who may have provided a range of interpretations. Before giving any explanations, or making any plans, it is wise to ask the question 'What have you been told already?' followed by 'What do you understand about your child's vision?' The answers to these questions are crucial to knowing how to later go about explaining what has been identified and what needs to be done. If an explanation is given which is contrary to the parents'/caregivers' prior beliefs or explanations, this has the potential to cause difficulties.

The first question is open. For example, ask 'What would you like to get out of this interview?' and then listen without interruption. Parents may have a pre-planned agenda. They need to be given the opportunity to express it. If they are interrupted, this can break their train of thought, and useful information can be lost. (Parents can be invited in advance to prepare a list of questions if they wish, because material can otherwise be omitted when there is a lot to communicate.) A note is made of each key issue. Doing so in the form of a mind-map can prove helpful, as this can then be embellished as each issue is developed.

Clarifying the story. The initial history is clarified and developed in terms of 'time, place and person', as appropriate. For example, *John becomes distressed in busy shopping centres.*

Time

When did he first show this behaviour? *When he was a toddler.*

How often does it happen? *Whenever we go to the supermarket. We don't take him now.*

How long does it last for when it happens? *The whole time he's in the shop, and for a while after until he calms down.*

Has it happened recently? If so, what happened? *Yes, last month during Christmas shopping. He had to go back and sit quietly in the car with his dad.*

Place

Where does this happen? Can you give any examples? *Yes. He went to a party. We took him early when it was quiet, but as soon as the games began and the boys ran around, he hid in a corner and wouldn't come out.*

Person

What is his behaviour like? *It varies. Sometimes he becomes withdrawn like at the party; other times he can get distressed and angry.*

Is there anything that makes it better? *He's great when he is out walking in the countryside. We never see this behaviour then.*

Is there anything that makes it worse? *Additional noise. He will stand crying in the corner with his fingers in his ears.*

Does it upset David when it happens? *Yes. He's 7 years old. He doesn't want to be different, but he's beginning to understand that he is, and a child in his class is beginning to bully him.*

Extending the story. To comprehensively extend the history a number of key issues need to be remembered. These can be considered in the following sets of three.

Asking specific questions to seek patterns of visual behaviour. Visual behaviours due to cerebral visual impairment occur in recognisable patterns that tend to occur in the triplets outlined in the box below. When one element of the triplet is affected, then evidence of dysfunction of the other two needs to be sought by salient questioning. These features may need to be specifically sought by closed history taking as they may have been considered the child's 'normal' behaviour. They may, for example, have been attributed to inappropriate behaviour or to lack of intelligence and may not have been recognised as being related to disorders of vision. In some cases the visual behaviours may have been labelled as atypical autistic spectrum disorder, without recognition of the visual contribution.

Box: Issues to Consider

Each dysfunction can impact upon:
Access to information (both distant and near)
Social interaction
Visual guidance of movement of the arms, legs and body
Adaptations/reactions the child makes include:
Adaptive behaviours that make best use of intact vision
Reactive behaviours manifesting, for example, in anger or distress
Avoidance of difficult situations
Psychological impacts include:
Emotional: feelings, emotions, anxieties
Interpersonal: interaction with other children
Fatigue: due to the effort needed to utilise vision

Structured history taking considers the impact of how the measured visual functions such as visual acuity, contrast sensitivity and visual field predictably impact upon the three domains of social interaction, access to information and mobility. Additional question inventories act as a prompt to ensure full history taking, in which issues raised are clarified as required, and additional questions may be asked. This is essential for children with CVI as each child's condition is unique.

Using an open question inventory, if required, to seek the full range of the visual difficulties and their impact. Two question inventories are presented below. Table 6.3 presents a set of closed non-leading questions aimed at helping older children, parents and caregivers to describe behaviours that are commonly described (Ahmed and Dutton 1996; Dutton et al. 1996, 2004, 2006; Gillen and Dutton 2003; Drummond and Dutton 2007; Saidkasimova et al. 2007). It seeks evidence of typical adaptive and reactive behaviours seen in children with perceptual and cognitive visual dysfunction and addresses parents' perceptions of the child's emotional development, as well as their hopes and aspirations for their child's future.

Selecting and employing supplementary question sets as required, from a closed question inventory. Table 6.4 comprises a published set of closed leading questions (Dutton and Bax 2010) that was gradually assembled during a series of studies aimed at identifying and characterising visual behaviours in children with hydrocephalus (Houliston et al. 1999; Andersson et al. 2006) and those born prematurely (Macintyre-Béon et al. 2012, 2013), as well as seeking evidence of sets of such behaviours in a large longitudinal cohort study of children (Williams et al. 2011). In clinical practice, we recommend employing the non-leading questions described in Table 6.3 to move towards the diagnosis, proceeding to salient closed leading questions from Table 6.4 for issues that Table 6.3 questions have not clarified. Positive responses to these questions are clarified using the above technique of considering 'time, place and person' to gain as full an understanding as possible.

Finding out what the family has already been told and understands. The family may have seen other practitioners and have a range of knowledge. Sometimes information they have been given or their interpretation of it conflicts with the emerging results, and this needs to be taken into account and dealt with sensitively, constructively and without criticism.

Understanding the wishes, agenda and aspirations of the child and family. Knowledge of what the family understands about the child's condition and how this links in with their ambitions for the child is important.

Finding out about the impact the visual difficulties are having upon the child and the child's family (to later identify ways of ameliorating any adverse impact). The impact of profound visual impairment upon the child is usually well understood by the family, and appropriate action has commonly been taken. However, questions that seek whether there is evidence of visual processing disorders are asked.

When visual difficulties are less severe, and the child has adopted strategies to cope with them, such difficulties can easily be missed, and the behaviours attributed to specific behavioural disorders. The impact of less severe visual impairment can, therefore, be wide-ranging and profound. The questioning strategy seeks information about the following issues:

Table 6.3 An inventory of specific, targeted, non-leading questions that seek typical behaviours commonly seen in children with a diagnosis of CVI

Non-leading question	Anticipated answer	Possible explanation
Visual field/attentional impairment		
How well does your child...		
Clear food from his/her plate?	Food tends to be left on the right/left/near side of the plate	Food consistently left on the right, left or near side of the plate indicates possible visual inattention or visual field impairment in the area indicated
Cope with reading?	Tends to miss the start of a line. Tends to miss the next word. Misses text at the bottom of the page	Suggests left or right acquired hemianopia, or lower visual field impairment
Cross roads?	Misses traffic coming from the right/left	Suggests right or left hemianopia or inattention
Cope with going through doorways?	Consistently bumps into one side	Suggests right- or left-sided visual inattention. (left more common)
Does your child...		
Do anything to help ensure that food on the plate is not missed?	The plate is rotated to find food that has been missed	This is a strategy children often use to compensate for a visual field or attentional deficit
Sit at table in any particular way?	The body is rotated slightly	This suggests possible left- or right-sided inattention
Lower visual field impairment		
How does your child...		
Walk along with you?	Holds onto my clothes, or pocket or belt (pulling down)	Gains advance tactile guidance to ground height
Behave when a coffee table has been moved?	Can bump into it and become angry that the table has been moved	The table is inadequately seen in the lower visual field, and prior mapping of its location has been disturbed
Go down a slide?	Goes down on stomach	Wants to use the upper visual field to see down the slide
	Refuses to go down sitting	Absent lower visual field makes it frightening to go down while sitting
Find shoes?	Shoes on the ground cannot be found	Shoes not seen in absent lower visual field
Put on shoes?	Either lifts the foot up onto a step or lies on back with foot in the air	Foot has to be raised so as to see it
Jump off a wall or a bench?	Frightened to do so	Fear of landing because ground cannot be seen.
Jump into a swimming pool?	Frightened to do so	Fear of not knowing height to jump and possibly landing on someone
Go down stairs?	Going down by sitting on the steps or holding the banister with both hands	Cannot see the steps

Table 6.3 (continued)

Non-leading question	Anticipated answer	Possible explanation
Negotiate pavement kerbs?	Walks off steps by mistake. Trips over kerbs. Lifts foot too early/late, high/low	Kerbs may be incompletely seen or not seen at all
Deal with low obstacles?	Collision is frequent	Low obstacles are not seen
Go from one place to another?	Runs everywhere (and tends to trip often)	Most children with lower visual field impairment tend to run frequently, perhaps to get to the more distant visible ground ahead, while its location is registered
Go up and down slopes?	Slopes are much easier to walk up than down. The child can often 'get stuck' at the top	The ground ahead on downward slopes may not be visible unless the head it tipped down, but this can interfere with balance
Watch TV?	Lies on the floor watching it upside down	Using intact upper visual field
Cross floor boundaries?	Probes the floor boundary with the foot before crossing it	Floor boundaries and steps may be difficult to distinguish due to low contrast, low acuity or lower visual field impairment
Play with wheeled toys?	Wheeled toys are very popular and used all the time (by younger children)	Such toys give a tactile guide to the height of the ground ahead and (by bumping into them) the locations of obstacles
Cope with obstacles on the floor?	They are tripped over	Because they are not seen
Clear food from his/her plate?	Food is left on the near side of the plate	Because it is not seen, suggesting the potential for superadded inattention in the lower visual field
Fill a cup or glass with water?	This can be very difficult	Because it is in the lower visual field and of low contrast
Read?	The bottom of the page may be missed	Because it is not seen
Find toys that are low down and nearby?	These are easily missed	Because they are in an 'invisible area'
Left hemianopia/inattention		
How does your child…		
Sit at the dining table?	Tends to adopt a slight body turn to see both knife and fork	Body turn helps compensate for hemi-inattention, more so on the left side, which tends to be more severely affected than the right
Walk along?	Walks with a slight upper body turn to the left. Collides with obstacles on the left especially when distracted or tired	Body turn minimises collisions in those with left inattention, but concentration is needed, and lack of concentration accentuates features of lack of awareness on the left

(continued)

Table 6.3 (continued)

Non-leading question	Anticipated answer	Possible explanation
Choose to read?	Some children with acquired left hemianopia choose to read vertically upwards	Reading in this way becomes easier because the lack of vision occludes the material that has just been read and does not interfere with reading in the same way as horizontal reading
Right hemianopia/inattention		
How does your child…		
Draw pictures?	For some children the right side of the picture is consistently drawn poorly	Right-sided attentional dysfunction can interfere with artistic representation on the right
Choose to read?	Some children with acquired right hemianopia choose to read vertically downwards	Analogous explanation as above for left hemianopia
Impaired visual perception of movement		
How well does your child see…		
Moving traffic?	'He isn't allowed out on the road, because he doesn't see traffic'	Slow visual, attentional or intellectual visual processing. (Independent of whether risk is appreciated)
Fast moving animals like terriers?	These animals tend to startle and frighten	They may not be seen while moving and can be described as popping out from nowhere when they stop
Rapid or fleeting facial expressions?	Affected children can miss the nuances of rapid facial expression	Impaired movement perception, delayed attention or slow intellectual processing warrant consideration
Moving balls?	Children commonly say that a kicked ball vanishes until it slows down	Suggestive of impaired perception of fast movement
Does your child prefer…		
Slow or rapid film and TV?	Slow moving film and TV is preferred	Slow visual/attentional processing can preclude fast moving imagery from being seen
Pattern of 'dorsal stream dysfunction' – handling complex scenes		
How does your child…		
Find a toy in a toy box?	Strategies include: (1) empty the box and spread toys out, (2) ask an adult, (3) choose a different toy, and (4) don't bother	Impaired visual search is limited by overlap, or the number of items that can be seen at once, which in turn impairs search and attention
Find an object on a patterned background?	Commonly missed unless background pattern and/or clutter is eliminated	The amount of pattern or clutter reaches a threshold beyond which affected children cannot identify what is being sought
Pick out an item of clothing from a pile?	The clothes are spread out to find the item that is wanted	When garments are overlapped, the lower items that are partly covered cannot be distinguished

Table 6.3 (continued)

Non-leading question	Anticipated answer	Possible explanation
See a distant object?	This may take time and may not be possible	In most cases, the more distant the view, the more items to be seen, and items pointed out tend not to be seen
Find someone in a group of people?	Finding a friend on the playground or a parent at the school gate is very difficult	This visual search task is difficult. Parents tend to explain that they stand in a specific location at the school gate while wearing clothing that stands out
Choose to watch the television?	Affected children get very close to the TV and move their heads to see component parts of the imagery	They have difficulty embracing the whole visual scene
Find letters on a keyboard?	This is another visual search task…	…which becomes easier as the letter locations are learned and touch typing skills mastered
Maintain eye contact?	Eye contact during conversation tends to be impaired	The dual task of viewing and interpreting the face and facial expression is unattainable by many with 'dorsal stream dysfunction'
Find their way around in a busy place?	Disorientation is common but tends to be confined to crowded situations	Unlike the intrinsic egocentric disorientation of topographical agnosia, the disorientating factor appears to be scene complexity
Cope with team sports?	Considerable difficulty is commonly described	The combination of difficulties with visual search, and the commonly associated difficulty with movement vision, along with other factors renders team sport very difficult
Do arithmetical calculations?	School arithmetic books are often difficult to cope with	Text and image crowding, and jumbling of numbers in rows and columns, are often described as rendering arithmetic difficult
Know where you are calling from?	Inability to locate the source of a voice is commonly described	Sound source locations are likely mapped in the multimodal map of the surroundings created by posterior parietal function
React when disturbed when working?	Distraction while working can lead to angry outbursts	Schoolwork requires considerable focus. A behaviour of striking an adjacent distracting restless child is not uncommon. However, may also be caused by inability to divide attention
Behave in crowded places, e.g. shopping malls?	Crowded places are disliked and can cause discomfort, distress or anger	Crowded visual and auditory scenes can be overwhelming. However, may also be caused by inability to divide attention
Go about copying information?	Copying is difficult, slow, inaccurate and arduous	Impaired visual search is compounded because both the source and destination of copied information have to be repeatedly located

(continued)

Table 6.3 (continued)

Non-leading question	Anticipated answer	Possible explanation
Communicate verbally?	Affected children are commonly very fluent verbal communicators	Verbal communication tends to develop well and can substitute and compensate in part for the visual difficulties
Does your child...		
Always see big obvious items?	Large obvious items are intermittently missed	The nature of 'simultanagnostic' vision is that only a small number of items are parallel processed and perceived at once. If by chance items other than the big obvious one are being attended to, the big 'obvious' one may not be seen
Pattern of 'dorsal stream dysfunction' – guiding movement of the limbs		
How does your child...		
Reach out to pick something up	Reaching without looking is a commonly used approach	This commonly observed behaviour suggests that visual guidance of hand and arm movement is more easily performed in the peripheral visual field
Reach out to pick up an object from a table?	Items can be mis-reached for	Compensatory strategies used include: supplementary body or limb contact with the table, whole hand placement on the object and overreaching and gathering up
Put things down on a table?	Items may miss the table or be smashed down	Localisation of the vertical and horizontal dimensions of the table are inaccurate without tactile supplementation of visual guidance of movement
Walk over a floor boundary when looking at it?	Flat floor boundaries may be investigated by a probing foot or even hand	Steps and floor boundaries are not easily differentiated by visual means alone
Walk across a carpet with large patterns?	Some children walk around large patterns as if they are obstacles	Mapping of the surroundings for motor guidance is limited
Respond to pictorial decorations on a plate?	Some younger affected children reach out to grasp images as if they are 3D	Mapping of the image for motor guidance is deficient
Get into a bath?	Getting into a bath can be frightening	The depth of a bath can be difficult to estimate
Pattern of 'dorsal stream dysfunction' – impaired attention		
What happens when your child...		
Is walking along, and you start a conversation?	Obstacles are walked in to	Simultaneous dual processing is difficult. However, may also be caused by inability to divide attention
Is distracted while trying to do school work?	It can be very difficult to get back to what was being done	The apparently random nature of impaired parallel processing ('simultanagnostic vision') renders it difficult to reembrace the data set being worked on

Table 6.3 (continued)

Non-leading question	Anticipated answer	Possible explanation
Behave when there is an obstacle like a baby on the floor?	As a young child he/she walked straight over the baby without noticing	In some cases lower visual field impairment is accompanied by both an inability to estimate depth for motor activity and what appears to be a form of visual inattention
Pattern of 'ventral stream dysfunction'		
Does your child...[a]		
Recognise you and photographs of you?	Varied degrees of prosopagnosia can be described	Difficulty to select and use individual facial features to recognise persons based on face perception only
Respond appropriately to facial expressions?	Facial expressions may not convey meaning	Lack of language interpretation from facial expression can be part of the clinical picture
Maintain eye contact?	Eye contact may not be made nor maintained	Eye contact tends not to be maintained by those for whom the face fails to convey information
Recognise shapes and objects?	Shapes have to be colour coded to enable recognition	Impaired shape and object discrimination and/or identification and recognition, respectively, of variable degree can be part of the picture
Correctly identify left and right shoes?	This is a common problem	Impaired analysis of shape orientation may be evident
Navigate in well-known places?	Gets lost even around the home	Disorientation due to topographical agnosia is profound
Remember where things are normally kept?	Never seems to know where things go	Impaired visual localisation of objects. Topographical agnosia also affects localisation of possessions
How does your child handle...		
Strangers?	Strangers are greeted in the same way as friends and relatives	Prosopagnosia leads to strangers not being differentiated visually from those who are known
Telling the time from a clock?	Numbers may be inaccessible	Number symbols may be unintelligible
Reading?	Variants of alexia may be evident	Words may be unintelligible
Geometry?	Representational shapes and objects may be unintelligible	Difficulty envisioning shapes can render geometry difficult
The child's emotional development		
Is your child aware...		
Of his/her visual condition?	Yes, no or in part	Awareness of 'abnormal' vision and insight into its consequences depends crucially on child's corresponding experiences
Is your child...		
Affected emotionally by the visual difficulties?	Yes, no or in part	As they grow up, children become aware of their differences, particularly if they are teased or bullied

(continued)

Table 6.3 (continued)

Non-leading question	Anticipated answer	Possible explanation
Parental hopes and aspirations		
What are your hopes for...		
The outcome of this visit?	An aspirational description	The outcome is optimised if as many aspirations as possible are worked towards
Your child's future?	An expression of hopes and expectations	It is important to work towards the parents' and the child's aspirations

While the questions are formulated for parents and caregivers, they can be easily amended to ask affected children. A spontaneously volunteered history matching this table, for which there is no alternative explanation, is highly suggestive of CVI (this list is linked to the range of supportive strategies described in Table 6.4)

[a]These are more direct questions. If there is a need to do so, more indirect forms of questioning can be employed

Table 6.4 Inventory of direct questions to ask of parents/carers of children with cerebral visual impairment and acuities of 6/60 or better

	Never	Rarely	Sometimes	Often	Always	NA
Questions seeking evidence of visual field impairment or impaired visual attention on one or other side						
Does your child...						
1. Trip over toys and obstacles on the floor?						
2. Have difficulty walking down stairs?						
3. Trip at the edges of pavements going up?						
4. Trip at the edges of pavements going down?						
5. Appear to 'get stuck' at the top of a slide/hill?						
6. Look down when crossing floor boundaries, e.g. where lino meets carpet?						
7. Leave food on the near or far side of their plate?						
If so, on which side?	Near/		Far			
8. Leave food on the right or left side of their plate?						
If so, on which side?	Right/		Left			
Does your child...						
9. Have difficulty finding the beginning of a line when reading?						

Table 6.4 (continued)

	Never	Rarely	Sometimes	Often	Always	NA
10. Have difficulty finding the next word when reading?						
11. Walk out in front of traffic? If so, which side?	Right/	Left/	Both			
12. Bump into doorframes or partly open doors?						
If so, which side?	Right/	Left/	Both			
13. Miss pictures or words on one side of a page?						
If so, which side?	Right/	Left/	Both			
Questions seeking evidence of impaired perception of movement						
Does your child...						
14. Have difficulty seeing passing vehicles when they are in a moving car?						
15. Have difficulty seeing things which are moving quickly, such as small animals?						
16. Avoid watching fast moving TV?						
17. Choose to watch slow moving TV?						
18. Have difficulty catching a ball?						
Questions seeking evidence of difficulty handling the complexity of a visual scene						
Does your child...						
19. Have difficulty seeing something which is pointed out in the distance?						
20. Have difficulty finding a close friend or relative who is standing in a group?						
21. Have difficulty finding an item in a supermarket, e.g. finding the breakfast cereal they want?						
22. Get lost in places where there is a lot to see, e.g. a crowded shop?						
23. Get lost in places which are well known to them?						
24. Have difficulty locating an item of clothing in a pile of clothes?						
25. Have difficulty selecting a chosen toy in a toy box?						
26. Sit closer to the television than about 30 cm?						
27. Find copying words or drawings time consuming and difficult?						

(continued)

Table 6.4 (continued)

	Never	Rarely	Sometimes	Often	Always	NA
Questions seeking evidence impairment of visually guided movement of the body and further evidence of visual field impairment						
28. When walking, does your child hold onto your clothes, tugging down?						
29. Does your child find uneven ground difficult to walk over?						
30. Does your child bump into low furniture such as a coffee table?						
31. Is low furniture bumped in to if it is moved?						
32. Does your child get angry if furniture is moved?						
33. Does your child explore floor boundaries (e.g. lino/carpet) with their foot before crossing the boundary?						
34. Does your child find inside floor boundaries difficult to cross?						
34a. If so…, boundaries that are new to them?						
34b. Boundaries that are well known to them?						
Questions seeking evidence of impairment of visually guided movement of the upper limbs						
35. Does your child reach incorrectly for objects, that is, do they reach beyond or around the object?						
36. When picking up an object, does your child grasp incorrectly, that is, do they miss or knock the object over?						
Questions seeking evidence of impaired visual attention						
37. Does your child find it difficult to keep to task for more than 5 min?						
38. After being distracted does your child find it difficult to get back to what they were doing?						
39. Does your child bump into things when walking and having a conversation?						
40. Does your child miss objects which are obvious to you because they are different from their background and seem to 'pop out', e.g. a bright ball in the grass?						
Questions seeking evidence of behavioural difficulties associated with crowded environments						

Table 6.4 (continued)

	Never	Rarely	Sometimes	Often	Always	NA
41. Do rooms with a lot of clutter cause difficult behaviour?						
42. Do quiet places/open countryside cause difficult behaviour?						
43. Is behaviour in a busy supermarket or shopping centre difficult?						
44. Does your child react angrily when other restless children cause distraction?						
Questions evaluating the ability to recognise what is being looked at and to navigate						
Does your child…						
45. Have difficulty recognising close relatives in real life?						
46. Have difficulty recognising close relatives from photographs?						
47. Mistakenly identify strangers as people known to them?						
48. Have difficulty understanding the meaning of facial expressions?						
49. Have difficulty naming common colours?						
50. Have difficulty naming basic shapes such as squares, triangles and circles?						
51. Have difficulty recognising familiar objects such as the family car?						

For each of the items listed, the box which best describes the child's behaviour is ticked (Question 23 relates to the final category of questions, but is located where it fits conceptually with its position in the questioning strategy)
NA not applicable

The impact of the visual impairment on the child in relation to:

- Social interactions and relationships
- Education, with respect to:
  - Near (e.g. reading and writing)
  - Middle distance (e.g. reading music and seeing information conveyed by facial expression)
  - Distant (accessing information from the whiteboard and TV)

The impact of the visual impairment on the family – when appropriate:

- Social interactions and relations
- Work
- Income

As children with CVI grow up and come to realise that others can do things they cannot, this can impact upon self-esteem. The range of behaviours described can lead to misunderstanding (Freeman 2010). Teasing and bullying can contribute and have long-term adverse effects (Sourander et al. 2009). In cases where the CVI has not been diagnosed, criticism for poor performance can exacerbate the situation. It is therefore important to be aware of potential consequences for psychological health during long-term follow-up.

Assimilating the Information

Identifying typical clusters of features elicited, to cross validate the responses, make sense of the information and contribute to the diagnosis and its pattern. A comprehensive understanding of each child's CVI and its impact upon the child and family can be gained by considering them in terms of the clusters/patterns of behaviours described in Tables 6.3 and 6.4.

Assembling and documenting the story and drawing conclusions. The overall picture is assembled holistically and set in the context of the child's needs.

Using the information elicited at this stage to reach a preliminary diagnosis. During the process of eliciting the history, a typical pattern is likely to have emerged.

Using the information gathered by history taking and examination, to guide further tailored assessments if required. The information gathered may lead to suspicion of impaired perception of movement, or hitherto unsuspected visual field impairment of inattention, which in turn guides further assessments to complete the overall clinical picture.

Documenting all the features elicited and compiling a prioritised tailored comprehensive list of interventional strategies to use at home, at school and elsewhere. A range of interventional and adaptive strategies matched to the information elicited can be considered and recommended (see Sect. 7.6).

Communicating the Diagnosis and Management Plan

Selecting the initial strategies to work on. A wide range of management strategies can be considered, but families can usually only cope with and implement a limited number. One needs to ascertain the goals and ambitions of the family and tailor any recommendations made, to enable them to work towards these.

Writing a salient comprehensive report that all can understand, and plan the approach to management. The report that is assembled and written as a sequel to detailed examination and history taking needs to be written in clear, understandable nontechnical language so that everyone engaged in looking after the child can understand and implement the recommendations made.

In Table 6.5, a selection of the many approaches that parents and teachers have successfully applied for children with CVI is summarised.

Table 6.5 A selection of the many approaches that parents and teachers have successfully applied for children with cerebral visual impairment (assembled by the author GD from many case histories seen over 20 years)

Difficulty	Behaviour, adaptation and approaches taken	Possible explanation
Low corrected visual acuities for distance and/or near		
Unable to see facial expressions or recognise people, unless upclose	Families interact within the facial expression recognition distance, as do perceptive professionals. A black moustache, or dark lipstick, provide sufficient contrast for smiles to be seen	Low visual acuity leads to faces being blank and meaningless beyond a critical distance
Unable to see pictures and text	Getting close to gain geometric magnification, enlargement of text and images, optical magnification, CCTV and computing magnification are all used	Low acuity preclude access to subthreshold detail
Unable to see to navigate	Assisted by an accompanying sighted person. Mobility training is implemented early	Low acuity precludes identification of obstacles, hazards and landmarks
Unable to see in the distance	Many families with older affected children find that a mobile phone with a camera allows distant targets to be found, identified and enlarged on screen	Image crowding can be minimised In nystagmus, near acuity is often better
Unable to see when near	Enlargement of near materials to be within the limitations of functional visual acuity. Correction for even small degrees of hypermetropia can be helpful, as well as a near correction in some cases	Lenses for hypermetropia and correction for poor accommodation enlarge and bring into focus
Coping with spectacle wear		
Spectacles are uncomfortable	Glasses are removed. They may need adjustment for fit. Repeatedly, putting them on again in a gentle but firm manner usually proves successful	Some children with cerebral palsy appear to be more sensitive to touch
Spectacles for myopia interfere with near vision	Spectacles (that make the eyes look smaller) are removed and material is held very close to see	Myopia (without glasses) gives near magnification, with less crowding
Spectacles can be tiring to wear all day	Spectacles are removed when tired	Blurred vision can be more comfortable for children with visual crowding difficulties
Impaired perception of movement		
Small animals cause distress	Affected individuals startle and are upset by fast moving small animals	They seem to appear from nowhere due to dyskinetopsia, or slow visual attentional processing
Unable to move quickly	Moving quickly makes things disappear	Impaired movement perception

(continued)

Table 6.5 (continued)

Difficulty	Behaviour, adaptation and approaches taken	Possible explanation
Traffic is not seen	Cross at pedestrian crossings	Only slow traffic is seen
Fast movement not seen	Choose to watch TV and film with limited movement, and avoid fast moving films	Dyskinetopsia precludes perception of fast movement
Occasionally misses. Language within fast facial expression	Families and professionals need to use words to express their feelings and emotions, and give prolonged facial expressions to render them all visible	Fast facial expressions are not seen due to dyskinetopsia, but slow ones and expressions in photographs are seen and understood
Visual field defects and hemianopic lack of visual attention (recognising that many with hemianopia have good compensation and that the hemianopia may interfere less with daily living with time)		
Miss food on one side	Rotate the plate. Those lacking attention on one side find food if the plate is decentred to the sighted side, or chair is slightly rotated, 'better side' to table	Food on affected side is not seen or attended to
People not seen on affected side	Teachers, friends and family find they need to communicate from the side with best visual function. Child is seated in class with teacher to 'better side'	People are not seen and may not be attended to on affected side
Traffic missed on affected side	Mobile children may need to turn bodily to look to affected side because unilateral lack of attention, which may accompany hemianopia, relates to the body rather than the head and eyes	Inattention relates to the body schema and may not be compensated for by head and eye turn only
Toys and material in books not seen on affected side	Toys and books displaced off centre to the unaffected side for play and study, but placed at times on affected side to motivate search	Motivated search towards affected side may improve attention
Ventral stream dysfunction. (Isolated severe ventral stream dysfunction with good visual acuity is rare. Affected children are able to move around with their intact dorsal stream dysfunction and appear sighted, yet are unable to easily recognise what they are looking at. Ventral stream dysfunction is more commonly identified as an accompaniment to dorsal stream dysfunction)		
Lack of orientation within surrounding environment (topographical agnosia)	The child is easily lost, even in places that are known. Orientation in the class room can be assisted by colour-coded lines on the floor (in marked cases). Colour coding of doors in the home is used by some families. (The disorientation of ventral stream dysfunction is more marked than the clutter induced disorientation of dorsal stream dysfunction)	Temporal lobe damage can lead to severe impairment of recognising and navigating surroundings (topographical agnosia)

Table 6.5 (continued)

Difficulty	Behaviour, adaptation and approaches taken	Possible explanation
Difficulty or inability recognising people's faces (prosopagnosia), and the language of facial expression	A young child may turn her parent's head to look straight at her, to render it easier to recognise. Alternative identifiers such as colour of clothing, voice recognition and recognising the footfall may be so well substituted that the deficit may not be recognised for many years	Prosopagnosia accompanies damage to a structure called the fusiform gyrus in the temporal lobe, additional lack of ability to see language conveyed by facial expression is a common
	Family may go out together wearing clear identifiers such as bright coloured clothing	
	Affected children and adults may not look at people's faces when communicating	
Difficulty or inability to recognise animals	Four-legged animals may be indiscriminable, even when they are moving. Families may adapt by taking the child to children's farms where the animals can be experienced close to by the children	This problem occasionally accompanies prosopagnosia
Difficulty recognising objects (object agnosia)	The child may pick up one object after another before identifying and retrieving the chosen one by means of touch	Tactile recognition is being used instead of visual object recognition
Difficulty identifying family car in car park	Colour instead of shape tends to be used, so that it is easy to miss the car. Some families use a distinct identifier	Object agnosia results in alternative less robust recognition strategies
Lower visual field impairment and/or impaired visual guidance of the lower limbs due to dorsal stream dysfunction		
Learning to walk	May choose to lie on older sib's skateboard, pushing along with hands	Using upper visual field to see the ground ahead
Walking without tripping or bumping in to things	Wants to take a push-along wheeled toy wherever possible	Provides tactile guide to the height of the ground ahead and affords a mobile protective boundary
Unable to see ground immediately ahead	Paradoxically tends to run from place to place	May enable the child to get to the more distant seen ground before it is lost from memory
Jumping off a wall or a bench	Refuses to do so. Or is prepared to fall over, or may have already been taught how to do a commando roll	Cannot see the ground to land on
Jumping/diving into a swimming pool	Frightened of doing so	Cannot see or judge the height of the water

(continued)

Table 6.5 (continued)

Difficulty	Behaviour, adaptation and approaches taken	Possible explanation
Walking down slopes or over uneven ground	Finds it difficult. Holds onto clothing or belt of accompanying person while pulling down and walking slightly behind. Prefers not to hold a hand, unless it is consistently extended and held backwards. Older child may simply touch elbow of accompanying person	These strategies provide a tactile guide for the height of the ground ahead, with advance notice. (A 'loose' hand gives no such guidance unless it is extended and the elbow fixed to give a consistent tactile height guide)
	The mobile child may prefer to use a stick, walking stick or hiking poles on country walks	
Walking downstairs	Finds it difficult. Initially goes down step by step on backside. Later uses banister with both hands and goes down sideways. When older, may use heel to slide down each stair riser to judge height	Cannot see the stairs going down and has difficulty estimating their height
Going down slides	May refuse to go down a slide while sitting. May insist on going down head first	With a seated posture the slide below cannot be seen, but with a lying posture means that it can, in the upper visual field
Negotiating escalators	Avoids escalators and uses lift	Stepping on to a moving surface is very difficult
Difficulty crossing floor boundaries or walking over patterned floor, like tiles or carpet	Uses a foot to probe the height of ground ahead when there are floor boundaries or large patterns, especially in new places. Plain boundary free floor surfaces in the house may be needed	Those affected, look down and use central vision to inspect floor boundaries and pattern, yet still probe with the foot, suggestive of additional impaired visual guidance of movement of the feet
Cannot estimate height of the bottom of a bath	A coloured bath mat and handrail can help. Often the child prefers to use a shower	Lack of clearly visible contour renders the height of the bottom of the bath difficult to estimate
Misses the bottom of the TV screen	Chooses to lie on back on the ground or on sofa or chair, and to watch TV upside down. Or chooses to watch TV from below	Child prefers to use upper visual field to watch TV despite the picture being upside down, and habit persists
Putting shoes on	Lifts foot high onto step, or lies on back lifting the foot to do so	Cannot see feet well enough in lower visual field
Finding shoes on the floor	Allocate shoes in a specific location on floor or on a higher surface	Shoes and other possessions often lost when on the floor

Table 6.5 (continued)

Difficulty	Behaviour, adaptation and approaches taken	Possible explanation
Avoiding and negotiating low obstacles	Coffee tables are bumped in to especially when moved. The child can become angry if this happens. (Families have often removed them or have ensured that they are in a fixed location, and they involve the child in moving furniture)	Position of items in lower visual field is difficult to see and estimate
Wheelchair users cannot find items on their tray	Parents have found that tray needs to be elevated, and or moved further away, to become visible	Items need to be visible by being placed in area of intact visual field
Cannot see hand for a handshake	Avoids handshakes	The proffered hand may not be seen and this can cause embarrassment
Cannot see friends when looking down into a crowd	Family recognise this problem and wave and call out	Lower visual field impairment impairs search in lower visual field
Difficulty reaching for items	Automatically uses a wide finger gap, or an outstretched hand when reaching for an item. Or reaches beyond item and gathers it up	Variable combination of lower visual field impairment with dorsal stream dysfunction renders hand movement clumsy and the child compensates automatically
Difficulty seeing buttons	It is difficult to do up buttons, but this task may be found to be much easier in front of a full-length mirror	Buttons cannot be seen even when looking down if the visual field impairment involves the whole lower visual field, but they can be seen in a mirror
Difficulty putting items down	Items are often misplaced. Child may have already learned to use little finger as a tactile guide to locate and estimate height of surface	Visual guidance of movement needs to be supplemented by touch for putting items down (especially when tired)
Misses the lower part of a page	Prefers text to be held up high or placed on a book or music stand Text placed further away on desk allows lower part of page to be read more easily	Although one reads with the centre of the visual field, the lower visual field conducts gaze down the page
Impaired visual guidance of movement of the upper limbs. (Motor difficulties may mask aspects of impairment of visual guidance of movement, but for those with little or no motor difficulties, impaired visual guidance of movement (optic ataxia) may be evident as the principal problem)		

(continued)

Table 6.5 (continued)

Difficulty	Behaviour, adaptation and approaches taken	Possible explanation
Inaccuracy of reach	The in-flight movement of the hand is not matched to the spatial location. The gap between the finger and thumb is wide, or a whole hand is extended to grasp the target object. Or the object is gathered up. Some, with good control of movement, learn to extend a little finger, or the other hand, as a tactile guide to the location of the target surface can avoid misplacement of an object. Objects may need to be enlarged to facilitate grasp. Touching the table with part of the body can improve accuracy	The posterior parietal cortices are damaged leading to optic ataxia, commonly accompanied by simultanagnosia. (This may be misdiagnosed as dyspraxia or being motor in origin)
Disability giving attention to more than one issue at once		
Will not look at a face and listen at the same time	Looks away from people when listening to them	Disability giving attention to the face and the spoken word at the same time
Difficulty seeing and listening at the same time	Appears not to see when listening, in severe cases	Profound difficulty dividing attention between sight and sound
Great difficulty copying	Prolonged imperfect copying of information	Impairment of the dual task of visual search of source and target documents, while remembering the information
Cannot see all the information on TV screen	Chooses to watch material with slow presentation such as the weatherman. Gets very close to the TV, shifting the head and eyes to the elements that attract attention	The combined fast image movement and multiple details mean that it is easier to get very close to the TV to see it even if visual acuities are normal or near normal
Difficulties due to dorsal stream dysfunction		
Finding a relative or friend among a group of people	Parents learn to meet in specific locations, to wave, to call and to wear distinct clothing when meeting child from school, or when going out as a family. They 'know' this is 'normal' for their child	Impaired ability to identify a person in a group due to impaired visual search is a typical feature of dorsal stream dysfunction
	Older child may use a friend or sib as a guide, or stay at the side of the playground knowing it to be normal not to be able identify friends	
	Informed friends can adapt by 'adopting' and helping the child	

Table 6.5 (continued)

Difficulty	Behaviour, adaptation and approaches taken	Possible explanation
Easily gets lost in crowded places	Avoids crowded places, which can be distressing. Older child and adult know that it is normal to frequently ask for directions. Families have found that mobile phones are essential for older children, who can contact them if they get lost (Inability to locate where sounds are coming from can mean that calling out to the child may not help)	Crowded places with a lot of people and noise cause confusion
Easily gets lost in busy towns and shops	The young child can wander and get lost. Visits tend only made to known locations with limited distraction. Families have learned to visit places when quiet to learn the 'lie of the land' in advance	Town centres and shops can present too much visual input to analyse
Items pointed out in the distance cannot be seen	Some parents physically rotate the child towards the target and get them to look along a pointing arm. Digital cameras with a zoom facility can assist considerably	The further away one is, the more there is to see. (Except, e.g. for aircraft in the sky, which are more often seen)
Difficulty finding toys	The child tends to empty the toy box and spread toys out, line toys up, ask a parent/carer to find the toy, choose a random toy instead or not bother with toys. Sparse well-placed toys, in a plain uncluttered space overcome this difficulty	The 3D muddle of the contents of a toy box is difficult to cope with
Gets very close to the television	Watches separate elements of the television, shifting attention and gaze to items that attract attention	Impaired visual search limits how much can be seen
Does not watch cartoons and films with a lot of visual and auditory information	Either does not watch TV or watches the news reader or weatherman, or similar programmes with limited visual content. Films made before the invention of the zoom lens, where there is no zooming or panning may be preferred	Impaired visual search limits how much can be seen
Impaired reading of crowded text	Limit amount of text per page and limit background clutter	Impaired visual search can affect access to the written word. This can, in some, be overcome by minimising crowding with a typoscope or well-spaced text layout
	Some children learn to occlude surrounding text by using their fingers, a ruler or a self-made typoscope (an occluder with a slot cut out). A minority have already identified appropriate computer software (e.g. ACEreader)	

(continued)

Table 6.5 (continued)

Difficulty	Behaviour, adaptation and approaches taken	Possible explanation
Impaired ability to access numbers from the printed page	Some children find that this difficulty relates to an inability to access columns or rows of numbers accurately unless they are both presented and written on squared paper	Visual crowding can lead to numbers in columns and rows becoming jumbled
Inability to identify and find items of clothing from a pile	Clothes get spread out to find chosen item. This can cause conflict. Using small numbers of items of clothing placed in specific locations, or hung up as sets helps deal with the problem. Teaching the older more able child to iron and sort each item of clothing warrants consideration	A partially covered item of clothing can be difficult to identify
Problems finding items on school work station	The school workstation and tray easily becomes messy and disorganised. Strategies, such as a template of where to put things, can help deal with this difficulty	Overlap of objects can mean that they are not identified and found
Problems changing clothes at school	Items of clothes can get mixed up. Some children learn that a strategy of hanging up clothes sequentially as they are taken off can be reversed successfully, for getting dressed again. (Dressing apraxia may be an additional problem)	Overlap of clothing renders individual items difficult to find
Discomfort and anxiety related to dorsal stream dysfunction		
Shopping in supermarkets causes distress	Families learn to take child early or late when shop is quiet, or avoid doing so. The younger child likes to sit in the shopping trolley. The older child may like to push a small shopping trolley to feel safer (but this can be difficult to manage)	The visual and auditory noise, accompanied by inability to know whether shopping trolleys will collide into one, can be very distressing
	The child who gets lost is difficult to find and cannot identify where a calling voice is coming from. Older children can be given mobile phones to cater for this	
Tantrums in busy places	The distress caused by busy places can cause tantrums, which are difficult to manage. Families have learned to avoid these situations with the child	The visual and auditory 'noise' combined with inability to escape becomes overwhelming
	Retreating to a calm quiet environment can be effective	
Unable to go to family events and parties	Many families have adapted by going early, when quiet, and allowing the party to build up; taking the child away if distressed	Gradual build up of crowding is less distressing

Table 6.5 (continued)

Difficulty	Behaviour, adaptation and approaches taken	Possible explanation
Distress on car journeys	More profoundly impaired children can be distressed by the sensory input from car journeys. Parents may have found that window shields or dark glasses diminish the visual stimulation, while playing music through headphones can provide sufficient distraction	Engine noise and the moving scene can be distressing

6.4.2 Systematic Observation of Child's Behaviour

As mentioned in the preliminary notes to this chapter, systematic observation of behaviour may offer important information about visually guided activities in children with CVI. Table 6.6 contains a list of visual and oculomotor functions for systematic observation (see also Tables 2.14, 4.12, 6.1 and 6.2). Attention and curiosity should also be observed, because these two mental functions show intensive reciprocal interaction with vision; in addition, visual behaviour may be affected secondarily because of reduced/impaired curiosity.

6.4.3 Assessment of Visual Functions and Capacities

6.4.3.1 Visual Function and Functional Vision

The assessment of *visual function* evaluates peripheral vision, or visual field, and central vision, including acuity, contrast sensitivity and colour vision. The ability to see movement can also be evaluated. Such visual function tests measure the limits, or thresholds of visual capacity, which the child may have to struggle to reach, and contribute to diagnosis and follow-up of conditions causing visual impairment.

The assessment of *functional vision*, on the other hand, aims to ascertain the limitations of binocular vision during everyday life, for example, at school, under normal lighting conditions, when the child is tired in the afternoon. Arguably, once a diagnosis of a relatively static condition such as CVI has been established, assessment to determine binocular functional vision has the greater value, because this dictates the optimum environmental conditions (e.g. in terms of lighting and lack of clutter), and for educational materials (in terms of dimension, crowding and colour contrast), to render them easily accessible, at maximum speed without struggling, throughout the day (Lueck 2004). [In everyday life, colour and contrast are combined. Contrast sensitivity is the ability to discriminate shades of grey, whereas colour contrast perception is the ability to discriminate colours to which white or black have been added such as pink and brown, or navy blue and light blue.]

Table 6.6 List of items for systematic observation of behaviour of visual and oculomotor activities

Response to light (photophobia?)
Search for and maintenance of eye contact
Spontaneous gaze shifts in space (eye and head searching movements) with fixation of stimuli (visual exploration)
Fixation of a presented visual stimulus (e.g. light source, toy) in various directions of gaze (field of search/of attention, visual localisation in gaze direction)
Fixation of a presented stimulus outside the actual direction of gaze, i.e. in the peripheral visual field (visual field, visual localisation)
Grasping at an object (visual localisation and accuracy and character of reach)
Visual pursuit of a stimulus (movement vision, pursuit eye movements)
Following a visual stimulus (maintenance of fixation) when stimulus distance increases (distance vision)
Preference for coloured visual stimuli over uncoloured ones (visual perceptual preference, colour vision)
Preference of faces over other complex stimuli (visual perceptual preference)
Head position while fixating a stimulus
Visual behaviour during inspection of visual material (e.g. toys on a table, scenes on photographs)
Visual behaviour in rooms (spatial orientation and navigation)
Reidentifying (familiar) paths and places (visual-spatial navigation and memory)
Visually guided play behaviour (use of visual information for guidance of hands or for walking)
Behaviour during repeated presentations of a visual stimulus, for example, toys or faces (visual recognition)

As an analogy, the measurement of visual function is like measuring the feet, while the assessment of functional vision is like fitting shoes, the latter being more subjective by eliciting what suits the child best under everyday conditions.

6.4.3.2 Visual Acuity

Visual acuity in its simplest form refers to foveal spatial resolution of two dots or lines in close neighbourhood ('minimum separable'). As already mentioned, grating acuity is a different measure of acuity, which refers to a grating pattern; an acuity-equivalent value can, however, be calculated, by taking stimulus size and observer distance into account (stimulus distance in mm divided by stimulus size in mm × 0.00145).

For the assessment of visual acuity, standard conditions concerning lighting and optotype contrast are crucial. For children with CVI, higher contrasts and background illumination may be needed to obtain reliable responses. If children suffer, from additional visually impairing conditions such as impaired light adaptation causing photophobia, for example, children with albinism, atrophy of the optic nerve and after brain injury (see Sect. 4.5), testing conditions should be adapted to ameliorate visual discomfort. In this case, grating cards with low contrast symbols (Hyvarinen 2000) may cause less difficulty for the child (recognising that they are

Table 6.7 Assessment methods for measuring visual acuity in children

Months 1–12
Grating acuity test: patterns consisting of rectangular or sinusoidal contours with varying periods/frequencies (e.g. Teller acuity cards). PL, OR, OKN, VEP
Stycar rolling balls test: visual pursuit of rolling balls with varying size. OR (pursuit eye movements)
Nystagmus drum or band: striped pattern with varying periods/frequencies. OR (OKN)
Catford apparatus: drum with dot pattern with varying sizes. OKN
>1 year
In normal development, single optotypes (tumbling E's) or optotypes arranged in a line (>3 years) can be used to measure visual acuity. In children with CVI, the use of these acuity stimuli depends on their visual capacity and their cognitive development
Psychophysical tests (e.g. Cardiff Cards) can be used in CVI at closer distances taking into account the differing resolution measured

Modified after Hyvarinen (2000)
PL preferential looking, *OR* orienting responses, *OKN* optokinetic nystagmus, *VEP* pattern-evoked visual potentials

evaluating a somewhat different parameter). Grating acuity methods usually give a higher measure of visual acuity than optotypes (e.g. Landolt rings) (Stiers et al. 2004). The most commonly used method is the acuity card procedure (Teller et al. 1986; Mash and Dobson 2005). The method is described in the Teller Acuity Card manual available on the Internet. In brief this procedure requires the examiner to be masked to each acuity card being shown. A positive response is one where a clear head/eye movement is correctly and consistently made towards a picture or grating. The acuity is determined from the lowest spatial frequency that gives positive responses, taking the distance at which the grating is held from the child into account.

The Stycar rolling balls test consists of 10 white balls that differ in size; the smallest size, which elicits a reliable pursuit eye movement, has in the past been accepted as an acuity equivalent. However, as the balls are singular, this test only evaluates detection, or the ability to see a single target, but not resolution, and markedly overestimates central visual function. This procedure has therefore largely been replaced by other methods (Rydberg et al. 1999), but may be helpful in assessing functional vision in children with severe CVI. The visual interest particularly of younger children (2–7 years) when examining visual acuity can be improved by the use of animated objects on a screen. In this way, attention and accuracy and duration of fixation are enhanced, and false-negative responses can be reduced (Müller et al. 2009). For children with fixation difficulties because of congenital nystagmus and abnormal head posture, visual acuity should be assessed with their 'normal' head position, because acuity is best measured under this condition and acuity values may be higher compared with testing with a 'normal', but for them unusual head posture (Stevens and Hertle 2003). Depending on the child's age, different visual acuity testing tools are available (Table 6.7). It should be noted that PL methods yield lower spatial resolution values compared with orienting responses and VEP recordings

Table 6.8 Conversion table for measures of visual acuity

Measures that are independent of distance					Snellen notation measured at distances of				
LogMAR	Modified LogMAR	Decimal	Cycles per degree	Log cycles per degree	6 m	5 m	4 m	1 m	20 ft
−0.3	1.3	2.00	60	1.8	6/3	5/2.5	4/2	1/0.5	20/10
−0.2	1.2	1.60	48	1.7	6/4	5/3.2	4/2.5	1/0.6	20/12
−0.1	1.1	1.26	38	1.6	6/5	5/4	4/3.2	1/0.8	20/16
0.0	1.0	1.00	30	1.5	6/6	5/5	4/4	1/1	20/20
0.1	0.9	0.80	24	1.4	6/8	5/6	4/5	1/1.3	20/25
0.2	0.8	0.63	19	1.3	6/10	5/8	4/6	1/1.6	20/32
0.3	0.7	0.50	15	1.2	6/12	5/10	4/8	1/2	20/40
0.4	0.6	0.40	12	1.1	6/15	5/13	4/10	1/2.5	20/50
0.5	0.5	0.32	9.5	1.0	6/19	5/16	4/13	1/3.2	20/63
0.6	0.4	0.25	7.5	0.9	6/24	5/20	4/16	1/4	20/80
0.7	0.3	0.20	6.0	0.8	6/30	5/25	4/20	1/5	20/100
0.8	0.2	0.16	4.8	0.7	6/38	5/32	4/25	1/6	20/125
0.9	0.1	0.13	3.8	0.6	6/48	5/40	4/32	1/8	20/160
1.0	0.0	0.10	3.0	0.5	6/60	5/50	4/40	1/10	20/200
1.1	−0.1	0.08	2.4	0.4	6/76	5/63	4/50	1/13	20/250
1.2	−0.2	0.06	1.9	0.3	6/95	5/80	4/63	1/16	20/320
1.3	−0.3	0.05	1.5	0.2	6/120	5/100	4/80	1/20	20/400

(Katsumi et al. 1995, 1997; Mackie et al. 1995; Watson et al. 2009). This difference may be explained by the higher demand on cognitive performance, in particular, attention in PL; however, PL may also ‘produce’ more reliable results than VEP recordings (Bane and Birch 1992; Tinelli et al. 2008). Rydberg et al. (1999b) have found it useful to distinguish between ‘detection acuity’ and ‘resolution acuity’ and ‘recognition acuity’. For recognition acuity tests, the stimulus has to be recognised; examples include the BUST-D symbol test, the Sheridan-Gardiner (S-G) single letters test, the LH single symbol test, the HVOT test, the Kay picture test and the Glasgow acuity test (McGraw et al. 2000). Rydberg et al. (1999) conclude from the outcome of their study with 105 children with assumed normal vision or visual impairment due to ocular diseases or strabismus that reliable visual acuity measurements can only be obtained with a recognition test using linear letters or symbols.

As different measures of visual acuity are used, Table 6.8 contains a conversion table for measures of visual acuity. The primary measure for visual acuity, tested at maximum contrast and at specified levels of lighting, is the logarithm of the minimum angle of resolution (or LogMAR). The measure 0.0 equates with 1.00 decimal, and 6/6 or 20/20 Snellen. For this level of visual acuity, the component parts of the image are separated by an angle of 1/60 of a degree (or 1 min of arc) when viewed by the eye.

6.4.3.3 Visual Field

In the first years, the visual field is tested at the behavioural level. Binocular visual field testing is carried out in young children, when homonymous visual field defects are suspected, such that both eyes are affected similarly. A visual stimulus is initially moved slowly radially inwards along the bi-oblique meridians towards the centre of the visual fields. If the target is not responded to in one quadrant, or one hemifield, then the test is repeated moving the target from the blind to the sighted visual field towards the presumed boundary for a potential quadrantic, hemianopic or lower or upper visual field deficit. In this way the visual field boundaries are demarcated. This type of visual field assessment is similar to kinetic perimetry; accurate observation of the child's actual gaze direction when the stimulus is moved is important. Circular stimuli of sufficient size (e.g. 3° in diameter, or if vision is low, a size matched to acuity) and of sufficient contrast to the background are recommended. The visual field border is defined as the distance from the central gaze direction, where the child has first detected the stimulus (eccentricity). The examiner should pay attention that visual stimulus movement starts at about the same distance from the centre along both horizontal and vertical and the four bi-oblique meridians in random order and that each trial is repeated at least twice (but not successively) to obtain a sufficiently reliable measure for visual field size (see also Mash and Dobson 2005).

A simple method of standardised quantitative perimetric testing in young children has been developed by the Swiss low vision expert Rosemarie Nef-Landolt (so-called Nef perimeter; cited in Hyvarinen 2000). The 'perimeter' consists of a big transparent semicircular screen; the examiner sits behind this screen and slowly moves a light stimulus (e.g. a hand lamp) from the periphery to the centre while observing the child's fixation of the centre of the screen. Alternatively, stationary light stimuli may appear briefly at different distances and directions from the centre. In both instances, orientation responses (gaze shifts or pointing to the target when detected) are used as behavioural measures for light detection.

By means of a specific method of presentation (276 single diodes with yellow light 7.5° apart along both horizontal and vertical and the four bi-oblique meridians, and 4 red shining diodes in the centre of a hemisphere as fixation stimulus), Cummings et al. (1988) determined the monocular visual field in 12 healthy children between the ages of 2 and 5 years and in 5 adults (17–38 years). The distance between the fixation stimuli and the observer's eye was 33 cm; visual targets subtended a diameter of 42 s of arc; target luminance was 1.2 log cd/m^2, and background luminance was 0.2 cd/m^2. Behavioural responses comprised eye movements to fixate illuminated targets (saccadic eye movements). Subjects' fixation of the red stimuli in the centre of the screen, before the appearance of yellow visual targets in the periphery, was carefully monitored. Peripheral positions, at which subjects responded to the target stimuli, but beyond which did not, were taken as the visual field border. For comparison, the visual fields of 10 children older than 2 years and 9 months and 5 adults were also examined with the Goldmann perimeter (stimulus III_{4e}, 26 min of arc; luminance, 2.5 cd/m^2; background, 1.0 cd/m^2). At the age of 2 years, children showed visual field sizes similar to those of older children and adults; there were no significant differences between the two perimetric assessment methods. Furthermore, repetition of measurements in children revealed sufficient reliability. Other authors, who have also used a kind of kinetic perimetry, found that the size of the visual field shows a similar extent to adults at first at the age of 6 years (Hargadon et al. 2010), but development of attention (field of attention) may play a more significant role in younger than in older children or in adults when the visual field is determined (see also Sect. 2.3.1). In children, who possess only light-dark discrimination, the determination of the 'minimum area of light attractiveness', which is defined as the minimal intensity of a visual stimulus that elicits a reliable response, may be a helpful method for assessing light vision in general but also to roughly estimate visual field extent.

A novel method of visual field plotting designed for use in young children employs automatic detection of eye movements to look at any chosen targets on a computer screen. Saccades to each successive target are detected. Preliminary studies have shown that this method of oculokinetic perimetry (Damato 1985) provides visual field plots that match those of Humphrey visual field analysis in those who can be tested and gives convincing plots in very young children for whom other objective methodologies are not practicable (Murray et al. 2013).

6.4.3.4 Field of Gaze

A very useful method to reliably and quickly assess oculomotor compensation for homonymous visual field loss is the determination of the binocular field of gaze or visual search field (Zihl 2011). The field of gaze can be measured using a perimeter, but in contrast to visual field assessment which requires accurate fixation of a stimulus in the centre of the sphere, the subject is instructed to leave the fixation stimulus on command and to search for the light target as quickly as possible using saccadic shifts only (without head movements). The target is moved slowly (speed, ~1°/s) at the main meridians from the periphery towards the centre. Upon detecting the light target, the subject presses a buzzer key; the corresponding target positions serve as indicators for the field of gaze (Zihl 2011). Figure 6.2 shows schematically the normal extent of the field of gaze and its extent in the case of homonymous hemianopia. Of course, the field of gaze can also be qualitatively assessed using similar conditions to confrontation perimetry.

6.4.3.5 Spatial Contrast Sensitivity

Contrast sensitivity (CS) is a measure for spatial resolution capacity, combined with the capacity of the visual system to ostensibly discriminate shades of grey. Both measures depend on peripheral and central components of the visual system (see Sect. 2.3.3). Most methods of assessment of contrast vision comprise patterns with dark and light stripes varying in both resolutions, for example, LEA gratings

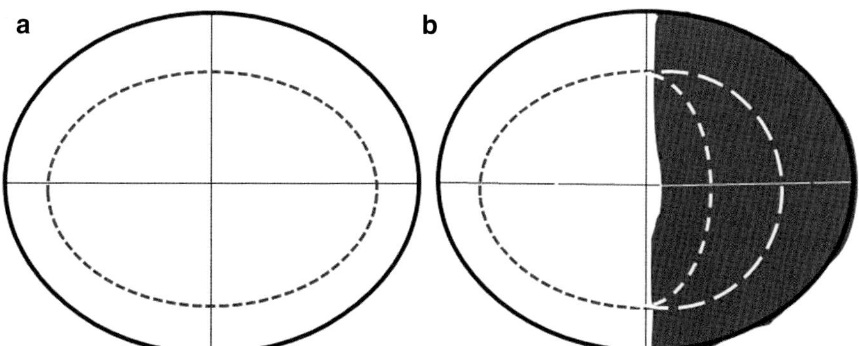

Fig. 6.2 Visual field and field of gaze. (**a**) Normal extension of binocular visual field (*solid line*) and of binocular field of gaze (*broken line*; range of eye motility). (**b**) Example of the size of the field of gaze (*broken lines*) in right-sided homonymous hemianopia (*dark area*) in a case of normal extension (**a**, full oculomotor compensation of hemianopia *longer dashes*) and a case with restricted field of gaze (**b**, incomplete oculomotor compensation *shorter dashes*)

(Hyvarinen 2000) or the Cambridge Low Contrast Grating test (e.g. Nielsen et al. 2007b). Children either indicate verbally (yes-no responses), whether they can see a grating pattern, or can discriminate grating orientation, or point to the pattern still visible to them and or to align their hand with the orientation of the perceived pattern. Nielsen et al. (2007b) have compared the outcome of the Cambridge Low contrast Gratings test in 99 normal healthy children (age 2–14 years) and in 146 children with developmental delay. Adult contrast sensitivity level was reached after the age of 10 years. The authors have found it a useful tool for assessing CS because of its simplicity. Larsson et al. (2006) have used the VISTECH 6500 test with five spatial frequencies (1.5–18 cycles/degree) to assess CS in 205 prematurely born children and in 215 children born at term. At the time of assessment, children were 10 years old. CS was significantly lower in children born preterm, indicating the diagnostic value of this test. However, the authors mention that the ecological validity of the reduced CS in daily life is unclear. Kvarnstrom and Jakobsson (2005) compared the LEA symbol chart and the Hooper Visual Organization Test (HVOT, LM) chart in a total of 478 children at the age of 3, and once more at the age of 4 years in 440 children. The rates of correspondence varied between 92 and 97 %. The difference in CS was less than 1/10th of a line. The authors conclude that at the age of 3 years, children can cooperate adequately with CS assessment, but examination time is a little longer, and the testability rate is about 10 % lower than for 4-year-olds.

Gratings can also be presented on a screen/monitor, while sensitivity is assessed using the method of PL (see Sect. 6.2). In early childhood, this may be the method of choice for the evaluation of contrast vision and also visual acuity ('grating acuity'). Essential prerequisites for this assessment are an intact central visual field, sufficient fixation accuracy and duration and sufficient concentration. As a rule, normally sighted young children no longer look at and fixate on gratings they can no longer perceive, because such gratings appear as a grey surface. By this

Table 6.9 Summary of some points relevant to assessment of contrast vision in children

Distance between the eye and grating pattern should be selected such that the entire pattern is within the field of search of the child
The test pattern should be presented within a visual field region, which is known to have the capacity to resolve the grating in a normally sighted child
The test pattern should be presented such that the child's attention is maximally captured
The child should possess sufficiently developed eye and head movements, so that he or she can look at the pattern and fixate it without difficulty, and the examiner can observe the child's fixation behaviour without difficulty
Before presenting a new pattern, the child should be asked to look straight ahead, while the examiner determines whether and when this is achieved by acoustic or tactile cues or by verbal instruction rather than vision
Paired patterns should be presented at the same distance from the child's line of sight (straight-ahead direction), such that the extent of gaze shift is about the same in both directions
Presenting paired patterns in a horizontal direction is preferable, but patterns can also be shown vertically or in any other axis if this represents a better testing condition, for example, in children with horizontal nystagmus, hemianopia or inattention to one side
In children with restricted horizontal gaze shifts, head shifts can be used as a behavioural response; however, it should be considered that head movements are slower and less accurate compared with saccadic movements
Very young children often use very small eye gaze shifts, but the direction of gaze shift can be observed with sufficient reliability. In such children, opening of the eyelids, increase in breathing frequency, uttering or grasping at the perceived pattern sometimes can be observed and used for spatial resolution estimation
When grating visual acuity is measured, many short breaks should be introduced, to avert habituation effects, and fatigue. Both effects can be avoided or at least minimised by presenting gratings with varying frequency and contrast in random order

Modified after Hyvarinen (2000)

procedure, difference thresholds for spatial frequency and for contrast can also be determined by stepwise approximation of the variable stimulus to the standard stimulus. The last discriminated difference can then as taken as the contrast threshold value.

A simple method for the assessment of CS and grating acuity is the use of a drum or a band with a grating pattern, which is moved in left and right directions, respectively, to elicit OKN (see Sect. 2.7.7). The pattern consists of vertical black-and-white stripes or grey contrast with varying width. To follow the moving drum or band with higher spatial frequencies of stripes (i.e. thinner stripes), a higher spatial resolution is needed to fixate the stripes. Thus, smooth pursuit eye movements can be used as a correlate of spatial resolution capacity. The highest spatial frequency followed is taken as an indicator for spatial resolution; however, this value cannot be used to calculate visual acuity for optotypes or symbols. It has been shown in children with myopia, hyperopia or astigmatism that no systematic correlation exists between the outcome of OKN grating acuity and visual acuity for optotypes (Cetinkaya et al. 2008). Table 6.9 summarises some points relevant for CS assessment. It should be mentioned that the use of tasks based on detection of raisins and puffed rice is not a reliable method for the assessment of CS, while the detection of black-and-white sugar strands against a white-and-black background may be a simple but sensitive subjective evaluation of CS at high contrast, although the outcome of this type of testing cannot be used as an indication of visual acuity (Rydberg and Han 1999). Furthermore, strabismus may secondarily affect CS (Rydberg and Han 1999).

Contrast sensitivity can also be evaluated without estimating spatial resolution. The Pelli-Robson test has the advantage of measuring the limit of contrast perception without a 'floor effect', in which children with normal vision can all see the lowest contrast target (Leat and Wegmann 2004), while the Cardiff contrast test employs preferential looking, so that it is applicable to the young and more disabled children.

6.4.3.6 Colour Vision

Examining colour hue discrimination should focus on foveal or central colour vision, because this portion of the visual field possesses the highest discrimination capacity. This does not mean that it may not be very useful to assess colour discrimination in more peripheral regions if central foveal vision is significantly impaired or absent (causing a relative or absolute central scotoma). Colour discrimination can be assessed in two different ways: discrimination between colours and greys, and discrimination between colours, that are close to one another with respect to their hue. In both conditions, stimulus pairs (colour-grey or colour-colour) are presented, whereby positioning (left-right, up-down) is at random, while the distance between stimuli is identical. Circles are usually used as the stimuli, but their size should not be too small, so as to avoid interference by low visual acuity. The colour stimuli should be identical with respect to saturation and greyscale (see, e.g. the PV-17 Colour Vision Test; Hyvarinen 2000). The background should be homogeneous (i.e. without texture) and uniform in colour, without blending effects; daylight conditions are recommended. As normal children by the age of 5 months find coloured stimuli more interesting than grey (see Sect. 2.3.4), it can be assumed that at this age a consistent preference for colours exists, which manifests itself by the child's orienting responses and longer fixation durations (Mercer et al. 1991; Catherwood et al. 1996). Apart from simple coloured forms (dots, circles, etc.), coloured patterns and scenes may also be used when required. For determination of difference thresholds, pairs of colours are shown, whereby one colour stimulus remains unchanged (standard stimulus), while the other colour stimulus (variable stimulus) is approximated in steps to the standard stimulus, until the child no longer shows any preference. This value can be taken as the difference threshold for the colour spectrum tested.

For children older than 3 years, the use of standardised colour vision tests is recommended, for example, the HRR Test, PACT, the M-R M Test, a children's version of the Ishihara Tests or the Colour Kid Test (see Shute and Westall 2000; Bailey et al. 2004). Children older than 5 years are able to perform a special version of the Farnsworth-Munsell 100 hue test (Farnsworth 1943; Ling and Stephen 2008) for which extensive normative values are available (Kinnear and Sahraie 2002). Concerning arrangement of grey hues in series, in the Lanthony New Colour test, children <12 years may find it difficult to apply the concept of arranging them in series properly, and artefacts may occur (Ling and Dain 2008; Dain and Ling 2009).

Processing of chromatic stimuli can also be assessed by means of VEP recording. By the age of 2–3 months, such potentials can be reliably recorded (Ruddock and Harding 1994). However, the limitations concerning VEP estimation of contrast vision and visual acuity (see Sect. 6.3) apply equally to VEP colour estimation.

6.4.3.7 Visual Space Perception

A distinction needs to be made between evaluation of the subjective appreciation of depth, the ability to guide limb and body movement through three-dimensional space and appreciation of one's location in the visual scene, for the purposes of navigation. Assessment therefore includes (1) measurement of appreciation of depth, or stereopsis; (2) observation of visual guidance of movement through depth (a 'dorsal stream function' which can in some individuals be abnormal despite intact stereopsis), along with subjective appreciation of orientation and dimension; and (3) topographical orientation, an ostensibly 'ventral stream function'.

Stereopsis can be assessed in 12-month-old children with the so-called random dot stereoacuity cards, using PL. Observation of whether the young child reaches out to grasp the wing of the Stereo Fly test provides behavioural evidence of stereopsis. Measured stereoacuity improves significantly until the end of the second year (Birch and Salomao 1998) and progressively thereafter between 4 and 5.5 years of age (Tomac and Altay 2000). For children ≥8 years, various stereo tests (e.g. Lang I and II, Titmus test, TNO test; Broadbent and Westall 1990) are available. However, these tests require a high level of cooperation of the child, including, for some, toleration of polarised or red/green glasses. Furthermore, amblyopia and disorders of eye alignment and accommodation may impair stereopsis secondarily (Ohlsson et al. 2001; Huynh et al. 2005).

Perception of visual space can be considered in a number of ways. The principal capacities of visual space perception are localisation of stimuli as a pictorial percept, and the perception of direction, distance, location, dimension and orientation, for the purpose of visual guidance of movement. Both capacities can be observed fairly well, with accuracy of fixation providing an index of the perception of direction, while reaching and grasping provide a useful indicator of the accuracy of localisation and distance/direction perception in the context of guiding upper limb movement through the visual scene. For the purposes of objective analysis, recordings of gaze shifts and grasping movements by means of video- or eye movement recording is recommended (Aring et al. 2007; Schmitt et al. 2007; Gredebäck et al. 2010; Pel et al. 2010). Gaze shifts and grasping can be used in children ≥5 months, with the accuracy being greater under binocular than monocular conditions (see Sect. 2.3.5). Reach and grasp of an item while a child is sitting at a desk can be graded, in our experience, with respect to the in-flight configuration of the hand and arm, and the adaptations the child makes for any inaccuracy. The in-flight pre-configured gap between the fingers and orientation of the reaching hand are assessed to determine whether they match the size and orientation of the target object. The child with optic ataxia tends to adopt one of three

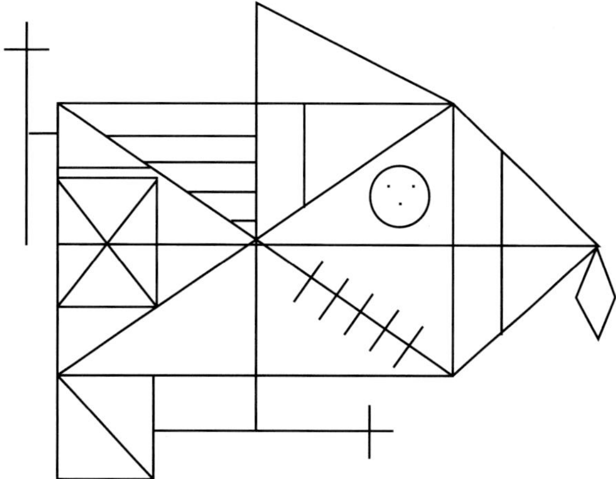

Fig. 6.3 Rey-Osterrieth Complex Figure (Osterrieth 1946)

strategies: (1) a wide finger to thumb gap is adopted; (2) the whole hand is extended and placed down upon the object, which is then grasped once the hand position has been adjusted; or (3) the hand reaches beyond the target object to gather it up. It is important to observe whether any part of the child's body is in contact with the desk during this exercise, because contact of the body or a leg with the desk provides tactile supplementation to the visual guidance, which manifestly improves in many cases. If this occurs observation and grading of movement with and without body contact with the desk is warranted. (The implications for habilitation being self-evident.)

For older children, who are already able to match positions, lengths and orientation of lines and spatial directions (axes), tests for adults can be used. The Visual Object and Space Perception Battery (VOSP) is a valid tool for the assessment of difficulties with objects and space perception in adults (Rapport et al. 1998). It includes four subtests that address visual space perception, dot counting, position discrimination, number location and cube analysis, and can also be used in children from 8 years onwards (Weber et al. 2004). Copying of spatial arrays and (complex) figures is another useful test; however, it is important to note that constructive abilities also contribute to the ability to copy three-dimensional arrays. A very popular figure used for the assessment of copying is the Rey-Osterrieth Complex Figure (Osterrieth 1946; Lezak et al. 2012; see Fig. 6.3). For this test, which can be applied from the age of 5 years onwards, normative data for children between 5 and 14 years are available (Waber and Holmes 1985; Anderson et al. 2001a). It is important to note that difficulties with copying of figures may be explained by impaired visual-spatial functions but also by visuo-constructive disorders.

Topographical orientation can be assessed by learning of new paths varying in difficulty, defined, for example, by the number of relevant land marks at intersections (Brunsdon et al. 2007).

6.4.3.8 Form Vision

Form discrimination can be assessed in newborns by means of PL because preference for particular complex imagery is already present. Form stimuli should differ only with respect to form, while size, contrast, etc. should be identical, suprathreshold and thereby visible. As with colour stimuli, form stimuli are presented in pairs, for example, form vs. grey surface, horizontal vs. vertical form elements (single lines, gratings), circular/oval vs. rectangular, etc. They are presented at random on the left or right side at the same distance from the midline. The frequency of any orienting responses (gaze shifts) and the duration of fixation are taken as indicators of preference.

Another approach to assess form vision is to determine the so-called differential sensitivity, by means of PL. Pairs of forms, e.g. square and circle or triangle and rectangle, of the same overall dimensions and contrast are used; the difference lying in the membership to a particular class of forms (e.g. round vs. rectangular). The difference between the form pairs is progressively decreased for successive presentations until no preference is shown, i.e. frequency of orienting responses and duration of fixations no longer show any bias in favour of the differing stimuli.

6.4.3.9 Object and Face Perception

For the assessment of *object perception*, real objects and objects in photographs taken in the fronto-parallel plane should in principle be shown because, particularly for young children, this perspective is easiest to interpret. Real objects usually elicit more reliable responses because of their 3D character; photographs possess only two dimensions (see Sects. 2.3.6 and 2.3.7). The assessment procedure is similar to that for colours and forms, including the determination of difference threshold between classes of objects. To avoid too great a demand on visual memory, the time between pair presentations should not be longer than 3–5 s. For children aged 8 years or older, the Visual Object and Space Perception Battery (VOSP) can be used as a valid and reliable measure (as long as all elements of the test fall within the limits of functional visual acuity; otherwise false-negative results are likely). The object part comprises 4 subtests: incomplete letters, silhouettes, object decision and progressive silhouettes (Weber et al. 2004). Of course, this test should not be applied to children who have difficulties with letter reading.

Face perception can be assessed for the following capacities: (1) discrimination (unfamiliar) face-non-face (e.g. complex object or figure); (2) discrimination of two (unfamiliar) faces, whereby similarity can be decreased to determine the difference threshold; (3) recognition of familiar faces (as well as employing new faces that are shown to the child repeatedly, i.e. face learning); and (4) discrimination and identification of facial expression (see below). To avoid false-positive results and misinterpretation, all testing materials need to be within the limits of the child's functional visual acuity. Already in the first month, infants prefer faces over non-faces and show longer fixation durations for faces by the age of 3 months. At 4 months of age, children can discriminate between familiar and non-familiar faces and can discriminate between different static facial expressions (see Sect. 2.3.8). For assessment of these capacities, PL can be used as described above (see Sect. 6.2). For testing facial discrimination, only faces that do not differ significantly with respect to non-facial features (e.g. hair, beard, glasses, facial expression) are used; otherwise the child can base his discrimination on these features and less so upon the face itself. Ideally, faces should have a nearly ‘neutral’ friendly facial expression. For testing face recognition, it is important to make sure that the child either has seen the face in question frequently in a similar context or has been shown a new face on a photograph frequently in the context of systematic visual learning. For the assessment of discrimination of facial expression, pairs of faces are used, which primarily differ with respect to facial expression, but not with regard to other facial features. Facial expressions used may include: happy, surprised and friendly (positive affective response) and sad, anxious and angry (negative affective response). Video clips may be very helpful for testing facial expressions, because the child can see the change in the facial expression from more neutral to the facial expression intended, and make use of the movement of face parts.

Interpretation of facial expression has temporal and spatial limitations, in our clinical experience. While clear static facial expressions can be differentiated and identified, the significance of more subtle and more rapid expressions can be missed by children with CVI. An approximate operator-dependent subjective clinical test that can provide useful information is the determination of the facial expression recognition distance (this is important to establish in school children who may not pick up the requisite language from their teachers). The examiner presents three expressions (e.g. happy, sad and angry) at a close distance and then asks for them to be repeatedly identified at progressively increasing distances. Children with low visual acuity manifest a consistent distance at which these expressions cannot be identified. The distance element makes no difference for those who cannot interpret facial expression. Modifications of this evaluation include making expressions of lesser amplitude, or for shorter durations. In this way, children who, for example, have periventricular leucomalacia causing impaired perception of movement can be assessed to provide an indicator for teachers and parents as to how long facial expressions need to be maintained to be recognised and reciprocated. No standardisations exist for this ‘rule-of-thumb’ approach.

6.4.4 **The Test Battery of** Atkinson et al. (2002b)

Atkinson et al. (2002b) have developed a comprehensive test battery for the assessment of functional vision and oculomotor functions in children from birth to the age of 3 years and have also collected normative data. The test battery comprises 22 visual tests; nine of them evaluate ‘core functions’ and can be used across the entire range of 36 months. They also describe ‘additional tests’ that can be used only at a particular age. These tests assess more complex visual, visual-cognitive, visual-spatial and visuomotor capacities. All tests should be administered at least three times to prove reliability and reproducibility of responses. Table 6.10

Table 6.10 Brief summary of test battery ABCDEFV

Tests	Age	Function/capacity assessed
Core functional tests		
Pupil response	0–36 months	Pupil function (response to light and accommodation)
Response to light	0–36 months	Visually elicited orienting response
Collateral gaze shifts	0–36 months	Horizontal saccadic and pursuit eye movements to visual stimuli
Peripheral refixation	0–36 months	Detection of visual stimuli in the peripheral visual field, visual attention
Corneal reflexes	0–36 months	Binocular direction of eyes (strabismus?)
Vergence movement to approaching stimulus	0–36 months	Binocular vision
Attention to far space stimuli	0–36 months	Sustained attention to distant visual stimuli (visual far acuity?)
Defensive response (blinking)	0–36 months	Visuomotor response to an approaching stimulus (distance vision?)
Visual fixation of a falling stimulus	0–36 months	Visual cognition: early form of object permanence
Optional		
OKN	0–36 months	'Reflexive' eye movements (saccades, pursuit eye movements)
Visual acuity cards	0–36 months	Visual acuity (spatial resolution)
Videorefraction	0–36 months	Accommodation, refraction[a]
Additional tests		
Lang test	2 years	Stereopsis
Grasping	4 months	Visuomotor development
Grasping of yarn	1 year	Visual control of fingers (scissors grip), (coarse) contrast vision
Searching for partially covered object	6 months	Visual cognition: object permanence
Searching for completely covered object	6 months	Visual cognition: object permanence
Placing forms	2 years	Form recognition, discovering and recognition of spatial relations, visual planning, visual control of fingers
Embedded figures	2 years	Figure-ground discrimination, form recognition
Building with blocks; free play	1 year	Discovering and recognising of spatial relations, visual control of action
Copying a figure with blocks	18 months	Discovering and recognising spatial relations, visual planning, visual control of hand and finger movements
Putting a letter into an envelope	2 years	Discovering/recognising spatial relations, visual planning, visual control of the hand (praxis)

Modified after Atkinson et al. (2002b)

m months, *Additional tests* minimum age, *OKN* optokinetic nystagmus, *object permanence* child knows that an object continues to exist when outside his field of vision (visual memory)

[a]Dynamic retinoscopy for accommodative range and basic retinoscopy for refractive error are recommended

summarises the various tests and the respective visual and gaze functions and capacities. Normative data are available for nine age groups (total, 318 children) between 0 and 6 weeks and 31–36 months (28–43 in each group). At least 85 % of all children passed each subtest at the corresponding age. This comprehensive test battery is easy to apply and does not require high cognitive demands on the child. Visual localisation, visual exploration/visual search, colour vision and object and face discrimination and recognition are not included and have to be added separately.

6.5 Oculomotor Functions

Like visual capacities, systematic expert observation techniques are very useful for the assessment of oculomotor functions. Eye movement recording methods, e.g. infrared and video recording, allow more accurate and reliable assessments of eye movements and fixation (Aring et al. 2007; Schmitt et al. 2007; Ayton et al. 2009; Gredebäck et al. 2010; Pel et al. 2010) and support further detailed analysis and diagnostic classification.

6.5.1 Convergence and Accommodation

A target visible to the child is moved towards the child's eyes to a distance of around 6 cm and then away again. The resulting converging and diverging movements of the eyes are observed. If the eyes stop converging (sometimes turning out) before 6–10 cm, convergence is deficient. Rarely there may be a lag in subsequent divergence, which if marked, warrants a neuro-ophthalmic opinion.

Accommodation, accompanied by constriction of the pupils, should occur in register with convergence as a synkinesis. If pupil constriction does not take place as a visible target (matched to the child's visual acuity) is moved towards the eyes, lack of accommodation is likely, and referral for refraction is required (Saunders et al. 2008).

6.5.2 Fixation

For diagnostic judgement of fixation accuracy, the following parameters are useful:

- Spontaneous fixation of particular visual stimuli such as small toys and pictures (of sufficient dimension matched to functional acuity). The more disabled children respond better to favourite toys and objects.
- Quality of fixation: intentional, coordinated, nystagmoid or drifting.
- Central vs. eccentric fixation, associated with abnormal head posture.
- Duration of fixation at an interesting visual stimulus.
- Position of the eyes: aligned or not, on cover and prism cover testing.

6.5.3 Saccadic Eye Movements

Shifts of eye position in response to interesting visual stimuli can be elicited in normally developed children by the age of 5 months. Spontaneous saccades are evaluated with respect to frequency, amplitude, direction and velocity.

Children with efficient compensation for homonymous visual field loss often show hypometric saccades (reduced amplitudes) with additional corrective saccades to the affected side (Mezey et al. 1998), but do not omit targets on this side; as a consequence, they may take more time for visual exploration and visual search. In contrast, children with less efficient compensation show fewer and more hypometric saccadic movements towards the affected size, but can shift their eye gaze without difficulty to more peripheral stimuli on command, or when pursuing a moving stimulus towards the far periphery. In the case of bilateral homonymous hemianopia, this applies to both sides. Children with visual neglect do not spontaneously use saccades towards the neglected side and cannot shift fixation to that side on command, at least in the acute phase of an acquired neglect. Children with Balint syndrome show this phenomenon to both sides of space as a form of apraxia of gaze.

6.5.4 Pursuit Eye Movements

As pursuit eye movements are much slower than saccadic movements, they can also be observed more reliably. In children with CVI, latencies may be increased, and pursuit may be possible only for low stimulus speeds. Absent, delayed or jerky pursuit eye movements towards one side may be indicative of homonymous visual field loss affecting also the macular region, and of visual neglect. Paradoxically however, rarely, extensive pathology causing hemianopia can also lead to a supranuclear gaze palsy impairing pursuit in the direction of the sighted side (Choi et al. 2012). Loss of fixation in pursuing a moving stimulus may also be explained by a relative or absolute central scotoma.

6.5.5 Visual Exploration and Visual Search

Oculomotor scanning patterns involved in visual exploration and visual search should be examined under two conditions: (1) spontaneous exploration of a scene, without defined instruction concerning what to search for (free exploration or search), and (2) exploration of a scene or searching for targets with prior defined instruction concerning what the task is, for example, to search for defined targets visual functioning permitted (Fig. 6.4). The child may either point to targets or may cancel targets with a pencil. The first condition primarily focuses on visual curiosity and spontaneous scanning of the scene (or even the surrounding area), while the second condition implies visual-spatial organisation of scanning and efficient interplay between global and local processing. However, both conditions are useful in detecting or omitting stimuli in one (hemianopia, visual neglect) or both hemifields (tunnel vision, Balint syndrome).

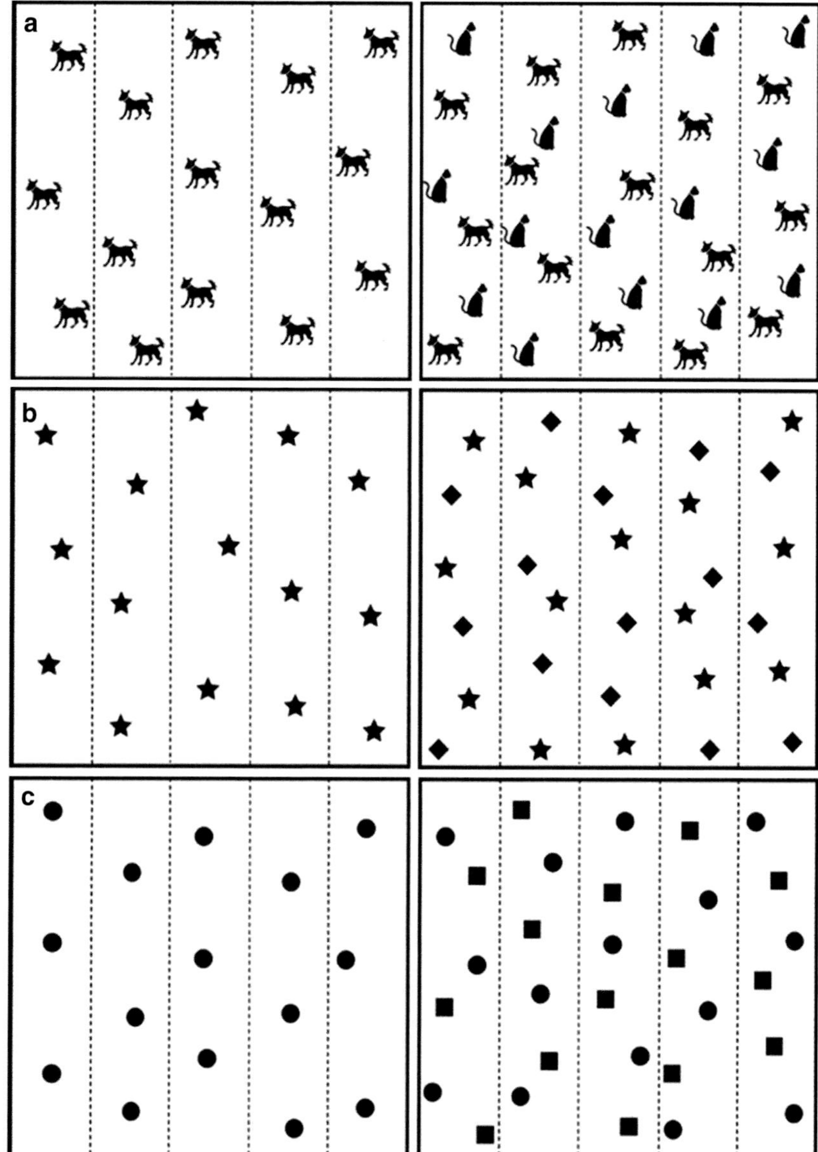

Fig. 6.4 Stimulus arrays for cancellation/visual search with different task demands. Left-sided figures in (**a–c**) cancellation of all stimuli (*dogs, stars, dots*), right-sided figures: cancellation of targets (*dogs, stars, dots*) distributed among non-targets (*cats, diamonds, squares*). *Broken grey lines*: sectors for performance analysis. Task parameters: speed (total search/cancellation times) and accuracy (number of omissions). Stimulus arrays should cover at least 30×20 cm at reading distance

Visual scanning and visual attention in space can be quantitatively assessed using the Teddy Bear Cancellation Test (Laurent-Vannier et al. 2006). Fifteen targets and 60 distractors are distributed proportionately in a pseudorandom array in five columns on a A4 sheet of white paper (see Fig. 6.5). The number of omissions is used as the performance index; analysis of performance can be carried out for the

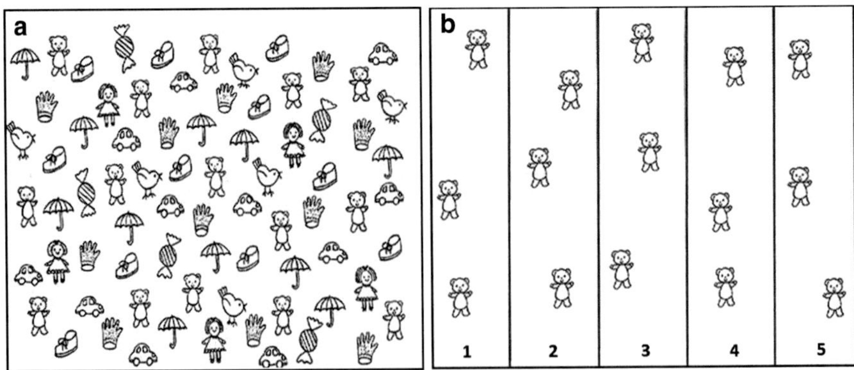

Fig. 6.5 Teddy bear cancellation test (Laurent-Vannier et al. 2006. © Wiley reprinted with permission). (**a**) Test form, (**b**) location of targets in five columns for assessment of cancellation performance

entire scene, or for the left and right hemispaces. For use in children, it has to be recognised that children under 6 years show a higher number of omissions. The time required to perform the task can be used as an indicator of visual scanning performance.

An experimental method that allows a more accurate, quantitative assessment of information processing in space is the *visual search paradigm*. This paradigm allows the measurement of visual search performance in conditions with an increasing number of stimuli (so-called set size). A target is embedded among non-targets (distractors), which differ clearly from the target with respect to colour, form, size, orientation, etc. This stimulus condition allows the observer to grasp the target at once, irrespective of the number of distractors; i.e. the observer does not need more time to detect the target when the number of distractors is increased. This mode of stimulus processing is called parallel visual search (Duncan and Humphreys 1989; Eckstein 2011). Figure 6.6 shows examples of stimulus conditions for parallel visual feature search. The subject is asked to fixate a stimulus in the centre of an empty screen, which is followed by the presentation of a stimulus array consisting of several stimuli. Typically, in 50 % of the trials, a target is present; in 50 %, it is absent. Upon appearance of this stimulus field, the subject is asked to search for a defined target among distractors (i.e. a red circle among green circles, or a circle among triangles) and to press a button when the target has been detected. Usually, subjects are instructed to respond differentially to the presence and absence of a target by pressing different response buttons. It is important that the subject is instructed that accuracy goes before speed of response. Search performance can be assessed by using the search accuracy (hits/misses) and by search speed (response times). The visual search paradigm has been proven useful in the assessment and rehabilitation of visual information processing deficits in adults with cerebral visual disorders (Zihl 2011) as well as children with CVI (see Chap. 9).

The *useful field of view (UFOV)* investigation is a valid indicator for overview, distribution and shift of attention in visual space, and also parallel processing of visual stimuli in space. To determine the UFOV, eye movements or pointing movements may be used. Children may touch the targets, shift their gaze to detect and

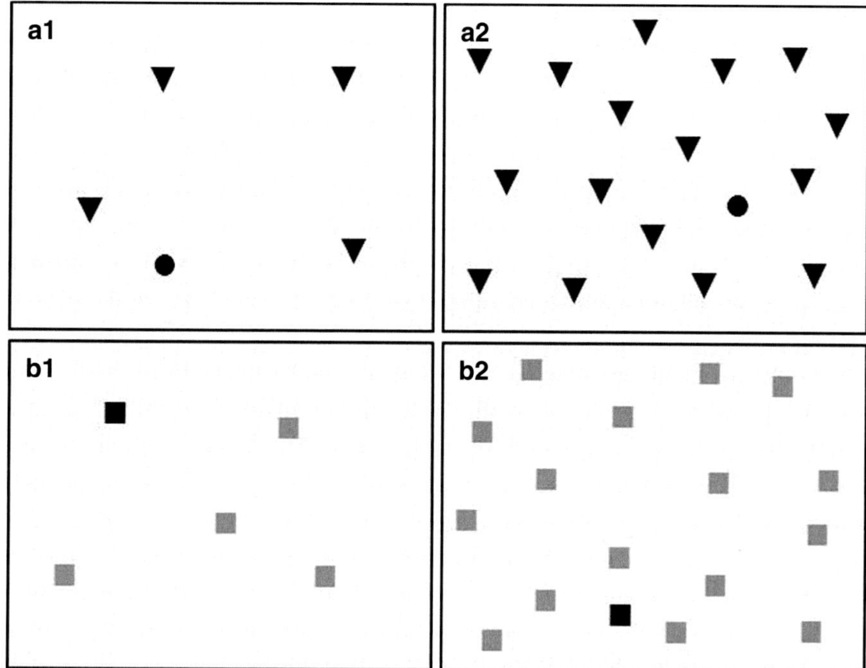

Fig. 6.6 Stimulus arrays for the assessment of parallel visual search performance using a form (**a**, *black circle*) as target among other forms (*triangles*, non-targets) or a colour (**b**, e.g. red or yellow square, indicated in *black*) as target among other colours (e.g. green or blue squares, non-targets, indicated in *grey*). *A1* and *B1* comprise a set size (total number of stimuli shown) of 5, and in *A2* and *B2* the set size is 17

recognise complex visual stimuli presented in the peripheral visual field and/or detect targets in the presence of distractors. Bennet et al. (2009) have used a simple software-based UFOV to assess the three components mentioned to determine the UFOV in 135 healthy children and young adults (age range, 5–22 years). They found a monotonic improvement of UFOV performance in all performance parameters (processing speed, selective attention, divided attention); by the age of 14 years, UFOV scores had reached adult levels. The UFOV test described has the advantage of being objective, standardised, simple and valid for the assessment of the UFOV and thus of attention and visual information processing in space.

6.6 Writing a Report

Reports on the outcome of visual functions/dysfunctions, cognitive functions and emotional/social behaviour can be written for a variety of recipients; usually they are prepared for the paediatric neurologist, the ophthalmologist, the practitioner or the neuropsychologist ('experts'). In addition, parents and other responsible persons (e.g. teachers) should also know and understand the outcome of such assessments to support the child with CVI. Of course, official reports read differently from more informal reports. Therefore, we provide the reader with examples for formal and less formal reports. The advantage of writing them for parents is that the material is naturally written in a form of language that they and others serving the child can understand. This is essential if the intensive work entailed is to optimally benefit the child.

6.6.1 Example of a Report to Experts

The report to experts consists of a concise although complete description of the outcome of diagnostic assessment of a child with CVI; its interpretation in the context of the cognitive, speech, motor, emotional and social context; and, if appropriate, a proposal for interventional measures. The following report serves as an example.

6.6.1.1 Neuropsychological Assessment

Case history: This 11-year-old boy J. was referred to a neuropsychological assessment because of 'vague' visual difficulties in school, particularly with reading but also 'holistic' perception.

History taking: J. reports that he has difficulty with seeing several children, objects or even letters at once; he finds that it takes a lot of effort to look at one after another and then to 'make an overall picture' out of it.

Neurological diagnosis: Preterm birth. Normal motor, speech and social development. An MRI scan 6 weeks ago did not reveal any pathological signs.

Ophthalmological diagnosis: Normal visual acuity. Visual field not tested. Accommodation and vergence, fixation and saccadic and pursuit eye movements are unremarkable.

Visual field: Concentric homonymous constriction; visual field extent is 30° in both hemifields. No indication for psychogenic field constriction.

Field of gaze: Normal size in all directions; prompt saccadic responses to peripheral light stimuli.

Visual localisation: Correct, without difficulties.

Visual search: Failure in parallel search; stimuli (targets and non-targets) are identified in a purely serial fashion. J. omits several stimuli particularly in peripheral space.

Visual scene perception: Characterised by serial processing mode. J. reports many details, but finds it difficult to put these details together. J. needs a considerable amount of time to gather the important features. When asked to first gain a more global impression and then to look for the details, he performs immediately much better and can report the main significance of the scene.

Visual object perception: No evidence for visual agnosia for single objects.

Visual face perception: No evidence for difficulties with familiar faces.

Text processing/reading: Mainly serial processing of letters and digits (letter-by-letter reading), higher performance for shorter words (2–3 letters).

Assessment of cognitive capacities: Normal performance levels in attention, verbal memory and executive function, apart from a slightly reduced cognitive flexibility.

Summary: Severe impairment in parallel processing of visual stimuli, causing difficulties with global perception of scenes, larger and complex objects, and with text processing. This impairment cannot be explained by the concentric visual field restriction, but can be understood as a fundamental difficulty with parallel visual information processing. There is, however, no indication of any visual agnostic disorders. The neuropsychological outcome is compatible with the diagnosis of CVI. At the moment it is unclear, whether developmental dyslexia is also present.

Proposal for intervention: Systematic practice with parallel processing of simple and more and more complex scenes, and with text processing.

6.6.2 Example of a Report to Parents

The advantage of writing reports for parents is that the material is naturally written in a form of language that they and others serving the child can understand. This is essential if the intensive work entailed is to optimally benefit the child.

Dear 'Parents',

When we met your 5-year-old daughter with you this week, we discussed a number of issues concerning her vision and the way she sees and understands the world around her.

1. History
   You explained that 1 year ago your daughter sustained a head injury after a fall from a height. This resulted in bleeding inside the head, which required neurosurgical treatment. As a sequel to this injury, she has sustained significant impairment in her vision.
2. Visual history
   Since her injury, her vision, which was initially limited to perception of form and movement, has progressively improved. You explained that she has now become fully mobile and is able to move freely through her visual world. She copes well with stairs and pavements. She does not bump into people. She is able to reach out and grasp objects accurately.
   She has difficulty finding objects that she is looking for. This appears to be related more to difficulties with object recognition than with visual search.
   In particular, your daughter is unable to recognise faces. She cannot recognise objects, and she is unable to recognise shapes through vision. However, she is able to recognise shapes and objects very efficiently through touch. This means that she has impaired clarity of vision compounded by a specific difficulty in shape, object and face visual recognition, known as visual agnosia, as well as inability to recognise language conveyed by facial expression.

3. Assessment of visual function
   The visual acuity is a measure of how clearly one can see. We found that the most effective way of testing your daughter's visual acuity at this stage was with Cardiff cards. Your daughter was able to identify the location of the targets on the cards (whether they were at the top or bottom of the card) despite being unable to recognise them, at a distance of 20 cm but not beyond. The measure, which was obtained at this distance, equates with that of 1.0 logMAR (or 6/60) for near. The results were however variable and subject to fatigue.
   Contrast was assessed using Cardiff contrast cards. Your daughter was able to identify the location of the images (but not their identity) down to a contrast level of 12 %.
   The visual field is an assessment of the area over which one can see. Your daughter was able to locate a moving target within her left visual field but not within her right, while being tested with both eyes open. This means that she has lack of conscious vision on the right side otherwise known as right hemianopia. She does not however bump into anything on her right side and may therefore have significant retention of subconscious right-sided visual function for the purposes of visual guidance of movement.
   Colour vision for primary colours was assessed. Your daughter is able to identify the primary colours when shown large objects greater than 3 cm across, but is unable to do so for smaller objects. She identifies the colours with more accuracy if the targets are moving than if they are static. In our experience, these are features of cerebral impairment of the ability to perceive colour.
   Your daughter was unable to identify the shapes on the Cardiff cards. She did not know whether she was looking at a house or a fish or a car. Although she was unable to identify basic shapes using vision, when she used her finger to trace shapes, she accurately identified a circle, a triangle, a square and capital letters which she already knew, by recognising the shape conveyed to her mind by the trajectory of the finger.
   Your daughter was asked to find, identify and pick up a coin when placed on a distant large plain playmat. She was able to do this easily. She was then asked to pick up a coin from among other items. To do this, she had to pick up and touch each item in turn to find out what it was in order to correctly pick up the coin; she did so accurately once she had been able to feel it in order to identify it. This indicates that your daughter is unable to differentiate one object from another simply through vision.
4. Explanation, opinion and recommendations
   Your daughter is known to have sustained a severe injury to the back of the brain or the occipital lobes. This is the part of the brain responsible for conscious visual processing. The result of this is that she has profound visual difficulties with respect to seeing and recognising what she is looking at. She also has difficulty identifying information in her right visual field. This is consistent with the reported MRI scan findings. Notwithstanding, she has excellent visual guidance of movement and is able to move through the visual world without difficulty.

She has a reduced visual acuity, and all information presented visually needs to be checked to make sure it is visible. She has an intact ability to see movement, and can guide her movement through the visual world.

She has loss of visual perception to her right. Information that is presented visually is worth presenting off centre to the left, to find out if this enhances her ability to access it. In the classroom, she will be able to give more attention to events taking place on her left side, so she is best placed so that her teacher tends to be more often on her left side as well. When her teacher or classroom assistant works with her, they are best seated on her left side too. The same applies to sitting with relatives and friends and reading stories. You want to be on the side she can attend to best.

We discussed a number of strategies that are worth considering helping your daughter to both make sense of her visual world and develop further the visual skills she has already regained.

We use vision for mobility. This is a function that is well retained for your daughter, but there may be times when she needs assistance, particularly when she is tired.

We use vision for access to information. As explained above, she is unable to recognise what she is looking at despite having a variable near visual acuity of between 1.0 logMAR (6/60).

Despite this impaired visual recognition your daughter is able to use her finger to trace over shapes and letters, which she already knows from her schooling before the time of her accident, and to recognise them through her knowledge of the movement she has made. This is known as 'pantomiming'. From our experience and from the literature, it is known that pantomiming in this way can be practised so that eventually the person who is using it becomes able to imagine the pantomiming action without actually doing it, by which time it becomes possible to recognise the shape or letter that she is looking at. This is therefore a useful strategy to employ repeatedly as it provides a potential means of gradually gaining an alternative form of visual perception. She can currently identify upper-case letters in this way. It will be worthwhile experimenting with moving onto writing in large script with a marker pen, to write joined up lower-case script to determine whether she can eventually learn to access lower-case letters by imagined pantomiming and to write them in the same way.

It is planned that your daughter will be taught Braille next term. This is entirely appropriate. It could well be worthwhile providing Braille letters next to text letters which are big enough to pantomime as well (about 5 cm) as this will provide the dual training model of both tactile and pantomiming recognition.

We use vision for social interaction, and your daughter cannot recognise people nor understand their facial expressions. We discussed verbal communication. I explained that it is very helpful to have the concept of being a 'radio parent'. Close your eyes and listen to the television. It does not make sense. Close your eyes and listen to the radio and it does make sense. One therefore needs to communicate as if one is on the radio. This technique of verbal communication is always used when teaching those who cannot see. I also explained that there are a number of scenarios in which it can prove helpful:

- In normal conversation;
- To enhance her visual experiences as they happen;
- To explain your emotions at the same time as giving facial expressions, in order to link the expressions to her understanding of the emotions as conveyed by language.

We discussed further her inability to recognise facial expressions and to recognise people. These interfere with social interaction. Everyone needs to know that she is unable to recognise people's faces and unable to see the language within facial expression. It can help if friends wear coloured identifiers so that she can recognise one from another visually. It also helps if all her friends know that they need to let her know who they are, so that she does not miss out by missing them, in the playground, for example. When going out and about with the family, it helps considerably if everyone wears clothes, which are bright, coloured and easily identified, so that they can be seen and identified from any direction even in the distance.

In the context of your daughter's on-going education, it is important that all the teachers understand and recognise the paradoxes of her visual behaviour. By watching her motor performance, it appears that she is the same as any other girl and has no visual problems. It is therefore difficult to believe that she has profound visual impairment in terms of the ability to recognise what she is looking at. This therefore requires the use of all the well-known methodologies of teaching somebody who is unable to see.

Prognosis

It is difficult to predict the long-term outcome. It is our experience that people with this specific type visual disorder continue to develop a range of compensatory strategies over a period of many years. A positive approach, which fully understands and recognises the nature of her visual deficits and strives to circumvent them along the lines described in this report, is likely to reap dividends. It is now known that the visual system, like other parts of the brain, can be developed through practice, and this is known as neuroplasticity. By providing your daughter with approaches that she finds fun and motivating, she is very likely to progressively improve in her capacity to understand the world around her. In terms of the curriculum, the principal means of accessing and processing information will need to employ blind methodologies and will need to focus on auditory and tactile approaches. However, simultaneous presentation of clear simple matching imagery also needs to be employed wherever this is practicable and appropriate in order to associate the visual images as she sees them, with the parallel information provided by the other senses. This is likely to enhance further recovery of her capacity to recognise what she is looking at over the next decade or so and progressively lead to her on-going rehabilitation.

With kind regards

Addendum

Follow-up information provided by the parents a year later explained that this child made considerable improvements. The pantomiming methodology allowed her to recognise letters and interpret short words. She is still using Braille as this remains faster. She is progressively gaining an ability to identify and select objects and to recognise language in facial expressions. She is a happy confident and popular girl. Her school classmates have all been taught about her visual condition and accept and accommodate it well.

Conclusion

Many families and children who have been followed up long term have fed back to the authors that the outcome of the approach outlined in this chapter has had a number of benefits.

- An immediate beneficial effect of providing families with an in-depth understanding of the nature of a child's CVI and its impact upon performance and behaviour is that those children who had been criticised for 'clumsiness', lack of giving attention, inability to see things that are just in front of them or not looking at someone who is talking to them, are no longer criticised but are understood.
- The analysis and explanation of the impact of CVI on the child's everyday life, results in family, friends and acquaintances being given an explanation of the child's behaviours and actions to take to ameliorate any difficulties.
- The specific strategies recommended facilitate development.
- Most children managed in this way gain considerable benefits from both improved home and school conditions, and the enhanced understanding that the information gives to the child and family.

7 Intervention

7.1 Some Introductory Remarks

Brain developmental disorders and those occurring in early childhood give rise to a variety of functional impairments. This does not however necessarily mean that these impairments, and their consequences for everyday life activities, are immutable, that the developmental processes and functional capacities of the (very) young brain are persistently affected or that the capacity of adaptation to these functional consequences in terms of learning will be irreversibly reduced or lost. Thus, specific and systematic intervention measures are needed as early as possible after brain injury, or the onset of brain dysfunction.

The principal aim of all early intervention measures is to minimise the degree of disability to facilitate self-reliance and independent daily life activities, with better participation in social and school activities and programmes, leading eventually to a higher quality of life. In essence, the child with visual impairment learns from life, for life.

All our knowledge, creativity and willingness are needed to develop tailor-made and problem-oriented solutions for intervention. Assessment of children with CVI to characterise the nature of each child's condition for the purpose of planned intervention needs close cooperation by all disciplines involved. Intervention measures first of all aim to ameliorate the degree of visual disability in everyday life and reduce and minimise social disadvantage. This can be achieved by first eliciting and quantifying the limits of each visual capacity and working within these thresholds, when catering for each of the child's needs. Approaches aimed at improving the affected visual capacity, for example, visual acuity, as well as efficient compensation strategies to overcome each visual dysfunction, e.g. visual field defects by gaze shifts; the use of technical aids, e.g. magnifying glasses; modified parenting strategies; and environmental modification in the home, are all considered. Often a combination of functional improvement and compensation techniques is the optimal strategy. Substitution for impaired or lost visual capacity is, at least in adults, the most frequently employed measure, because recovery of visual function after acquired brain injury appears the

J. Zihl, G. Dutton, *Cerebral Visual Impairment in Children: Visuoperceptive and Visuocognitive Disorders*, DOI 10.1007/978-3-7091-1815-3_7

exception rather than the rule (Zihl 2011). For children with CVI, research results concerning substitution for impaired visual capacities are still somewhat sparse compared with adults. It appears that (spontaneous) recovery and adaptation to visual dysfunction in children occurs more often, provided that other functional systems particularly involved in vision are sufficiently spared and can develop normally. Attention, learning, memory and executive function, as well as motivation to learn more about the visual world are crucial prerequisites for flexible adaptation and the use of (spared) visual capacities in an optimal way. However, as Hoyt (2003) has shown, just living in a natural environment is not sufficient to elicit improvements in vision.

In principle, the following approaches aimed at minimising cerebral visual disability are possible:

- Ensure that environmental conditions and all communication and materials used are accessible to and matched to the developing needs of the child, by being supra-threshold for each of the child's measured/estimated perceptual limitations.
- Return/recovery of impaired visual capacities, spontaneously or after systematic training.
- Development of efficient strategies for using impaired visual capacities (improvement of residual visual capacities).
- Substitution of impaired or lost visual capacities by other functions or capacities (substitution by functional compensation).
- Substitution of impaired or lost visual capacities by technical aids.

Parents and caregivers need to be closely involved in all habilitational efforts, so that they can be shown how to help their child, and encouraged to integrate and appropriately extend any successful outcomes of intervention into their child's activities of everyday living.

7.2 Spontaneous Recovery and Spontaneous Adaptation in Children with CVI

In adults with acquired CVI, spontaneous recovery has been reported for nearly all visual capacities; however, the degree of recovery is rarely complete (Zihl 2011). Children with severe CVI may develop some useful vision (Duchowny et al. 1974; Kaye and Herskowitz 1986; Lambert et al. 1987). The temporal course of recovery from cerebral blindness follows a typical pattern. In the first phase, children are able to detect moving and flickering light stimuli. Perception of (very) bright colours, contours and simple forms follows. Some children eventually develop contrast vision and visual acuity, which allow perception and identification of forms, objects, faces, scenes, etc. However, improvement can come to an end at each stage and for each visual capacity. Remarkable visual capacities (detection and discrimination of visual stimuli, movement vision) and visually guided behaviour (fixation, tracking, reaching) have been reported in single cases with congenital absence of normal occipital cortex or early bilateral occipital injury (e.g. Dubowitz et al. 1986;

Summers and MacDonald 1990; Giaschi et al. 2003) indicating that development of vision may in part also be mediated by subcortical and/or extrastriate visual structures. Bova et al. (2008) reported the case of a boy with bilateral occipital lobe infarction at the age of 2.5 years. Complete cerebral blindness lasted a few weeks, then perception of movement returned, followed by progressive recovery of visual acuity, visual field and oculomotor functions. At the age of 6 years and 8 months, the boy had developed normal acuity (10/10), but still showed incomplete bilateral upper hemianopia (the pathway of the optic radiations serving the upper visual fields runs through the temporal lobe) and difficulties with complex visual form perception (e.g. overlapping figures) and complex visual-spatial tasks (e.g. Block design, Rey's figure). Similar patterns of recovery have been reported by Innocenti et al. (1999), Werth (2007) and Muckli et al. (2009). These reports also illustrate that spontaneous recovery from cerebral blindness may take place over a number of years. Furthermore, the degree of recovery after brain injury early in life may not always be greater than later in adulthood, i.e. plasticity in childhood may also be limited, indicating that 'young is not always better' because vulnerability in the developing brain may be more crucial with respect to signal transmission and neuronal connectivity (Anderson 2003; Giza and Prins 2006). On the other hand, as Cioni et al. (2011) have pointed out, some mechanisms underlying brain plasticity may no longer be available at a later stage of maturation, in particular in the visual, sensorimotor and language systems.

As with adults, children with complete cerebral blindness are not always aware of their blindness (Barnet et al. 1970). In the course of recovery from cerebral blindness, visual perceptions without external stimuli (visual hallucinations) may occur (White and Jan 1992), which can be incorrectly taken to be real, and thus may impede awareness of blindness, or correct interpretation of any vision present, or improvement of vision. Many children with complete cerebral blindness also manifest cognitive dysfunction, which may impair awareness, as well as impeding visual assessment and intervention (Barnet et al. 1970; Jan et al. 1977; see also Matsuba and Jan 2006). Interestingly, Guzzetta et al. (2010) have found stronger awareness for visual stimuli in terms of 'conscious feelings' in subjects with cerebral blindness after early brain injury compared with subjects who have suffered brain injury later in life. Unfortunately, the use of electrophysiological correlates of vision may yield equivocal results because children with cerebral blindness may sometimes show preserved pattern-generated VEP (Frank and Torres 1979), but for many children with CVI, there is a good correlation between VEP and preferential looking methodologies (Mackie et al. 1995) showing that results warrant interpretation in the context of the whole clinical picture.

Partial recovery of vision has been reported in children with homonymous hemianopia, impaired visual acuity and contrast sensitivity (Groenendaal and van Hof-van Duin 1990; Porro et al. 1998), with a time of recovery that may take several years. Kedar et al. (2006) have reported spontaneous recovery of vision in about 40 % of 31 children with homonymous visual field defects. Matsuba and Jan (2006) found spontaneous improvement of visual acuity over two or more years in 97 of 194 children (50 %). Seventy-five of the children (38.7 %) did not show any change in acuity, while the remainder deteriorated (18, or 9.3 %); in 4 children, acuity could not be assessed properly. Children with better visual acuity values at follow-up also showed better cognitive outcomes. Furthermore, independent mobility was associated with higher visual acuity, indicating a favourable effect of vision on motor outcome. Similar observations had been previously reported by van Hof-van Duin et al. (1998) who found that visual outcome in children with CVI could be predicted by grating acuity at the age of 12–24 months in 27 out of 39 children (69.2 %). Watson et al. (2007) reported improvement of visual acuity in 49 % of 34 children and of contrast vision in 47 % of 39 children, but no relation was found between improvement in visual acuity and the aetiology of CVI.

Surprisingly, children with early more or less total bilateral occipital lobe injury in the first year of life may show recovery/preservation of 'low' vision in the central portion of their visual field, which allows them to detect a visual stimulus in motion, to fixate a stimulus or to follow a stimulus with eye and head movements (Werth 2006, 2007). An even more surprising picture emerges after loss of one occipital lobe, because – in contrast to adults – children may exhibit a nearly full visual field, at least for perception of light. This preservation of visual field contralateral to occipital injury may be explained by morphological reorganisation of retinal afferent pathways to the striate cortex and thus of transformation of cortical visual field representation (Muckli et al. 2009). Alternatively, light perception may also be mediated by subcortical structures, which are known to receive afferent signals from the retina and project to the striate cortex (Werth 2008). The latter hypothesis is supported by a study in 23 children with uni- or bilateral homonymous visual field defects with spared perception of moving visual stimuli in affected visual field regions (Boyle et al. 2005). Children can also recover from visual neglect; in contrast to adulthood, it seems that this disorder tends not to become chronic in children (Ferro et al. 1984; Trauner 2003; Kleinman et al. 2010).

De Haan and Campbell (1991) presented a 15-year follow-up of a 27-year-old female patient with developmental prosopagnosia with relatively preserved basic visuo-sensory functions which were largely intact and relatively well-preserved discrimination of a face and a 'non-face'. In contrast, recognition of familiar faces was severely impaired, and facial expression recognition was difficult, so that the patient may not have been able to learn representations of faces. Joy and Brunsdon (2002) reported spontaneous improvement of visual face discrimination and identification and recognition in a 7-year-old boy with congenital prosopagnosia, who was assessed for the first time at the age of 4 years. In contrast, impaired visual recognition of familiar faces may not show any change (see also Ariel and Sadeh 1996; Sect. 4.3.8).

A particularly impressive example of spontaneous adaptation by highly efficient compensation strategies has been reported by Lê et al. (2002). The authors assessed in detail a 30-year-old man (SB), who suffered from bilateral posterior brain injury because of meningoencephalitis at the age of 3 years. Injury affected both ventral (occipito-temporal) pathways and the right dorsal (occipito-parietal) route, as verified by MRI. From his 6th to 16th year, SB had been in an institution for visually disabled children and young adults; during the ensuing 4 years, he followed a professional training. As acquisition of visual reading ability was not possible, he learned the Braille system, which he mastered fluently. He was unable to visually recognise stimuli, but had no difficulties with tactile recognition of the same items. What was remarkable with SB was the discrepancy between his severe CVI and his visually guided activities in everyday life, including sport activities; because of this mismatch, some teachers questioned his severe visual disability. He showed more or less normal visual-spatial orientation and navigation, learned how to ride a motorcycle and played as goalkeeper in an amateur football team. There were no impairments in cognition, language or motor functions. Detailed visual assessment revealed complete left-sided homonymous hemianopia without visual neglect, the distance binocular visual acuity for forms at a distance of 5 m was estimated 0.6. He showed impaired contrast sensitivity for middle and high spatial frequencies, cerebral achromatopsia and impaired form vision. Foveal light sensitivity was normal, and stereopsis was not impaired. Visual identification and recognition were severely impaired; SB could, however, 'guess' real objects with the help of characteristic (individual) features and properties. A similar outcome was found for faces. Although SB could correctly discriminate faces as identical or different in pairwise presentation, he was absolutely unable to visually recognise 'familiar' faces and also had difficulties identifying facial expressions. Reading was impossible, because SB also showed visual agnosia for letters (pure alexia). His visual imagination of colours was completely absent, while for other visual categories (objects, animals, faces), it was rudimentary. In sharp contrast to SB's profoundly impaired visual identification and recognition, were his capacities in topographical orientation and navigation and in visually guided grasping. Sparing of just one (i.e. the left) dorsal visual processing route and the intensive spontaneous use of spared visual capacity (and possibly residual visual capacities belonging to the ventral routes) in everyday life had ensured that visual perceptual learning became sufficient to acquire remarkable visual-spatial skills. In situations, which primarily demanded visual-spatial capacities, SB behaved like a sighted person, while in situations that demanded visual identification and recognition, he behaved like a person who had become blind. Interestingly, SB never chose to be registered as visually impaired. SB's visuospatial capacities in some ways resemble that of case DF, the patient who inspired the dual-route processing model of Milner and Goodale (2006). However, as Schenk (2006) has convincingly argued, spared visuomotor capacities in bilateral ventral route injury can alternatively be explained by redundancy of visuomotor control (see also Schenk and McIntosh 2010). Apart from the sparing and further development of visual-spatial and possibly also visual-cognitive skills, the case of SB tells us that visual development and adaptation to everyday life visual challenges require preserved (visual) learning capacity, including visual memory, attention and executive function, and a high level of motivation for visual information (visual curiosity). Thus, an optimal combination of functional brain plasticity, adequate (visual) environment and intensive practice of visuomotor actions and activities may explain SB's significant improvements in useful vision and thus provide an excellent example of environmental- and practice-dependent plasticity of the visual system (see Chap. 1). Visuomotor experience over several years can manifestly enhance spontaneous adaptation to early CVI.

A positive interaction between vision and motor activities has also been reported by Pavlova et al. (2007), who examined the association between visual-spatial navigation and paresis in the upper and lower limb extremities in 14 preterm children with PVL at the age of 13–16 years. Children with upper limb paresis showed higher performance in a maze task than children with lower limb paresis. The authors concluded that children with intact lower limbs, i.e. with normal walking, also showed better visual navigation. This observation is underlined by Evenson et al. (2009) who found that reduced visual acuity accords a higher risk of motor problems in preterm children but not in term children small for gestational age.

In conclusion, despite many positive examples of spontaneous recovery of visual capacities and spontaneous adaptation, many children with CVI may exhibit persistent visual impairment (see Hoyt 2003), which may cause disability well into, if not during adulthood: in addition, persistent CVI may further affect overall health, self-perception, educational attainment, job choices and social interactions (Davidson and Quinn 2011). Thus, intervention measures are required as early as possible, to reduce the degree of visual handicap; to support an optimal visual, cognitive and social development of children with CVI; and to guarantee the best options possible for later life.

In the following sections, intervention strategies in children with CVI are described and discussed. Because scientifically proven programmes of intervention in children with CVI are not available, the strategies proposed represent recommendations of intervention. Of course, intervention in children with CVI should also be based on general principles of rehabilitation. Therefore, it seems helpful to first outline some fundamental issues that are relevant for visual rehabilitation in general, and for the rehabilitation in children with CVI in particular. The proposed intervention measures and strategies are exemplified by single-case reports in Chap. 9.

7.3 Methodical Considerations in Visual Rehabilitation and Special Early Education in Children with CVI

7.3.1 Functional Visual Assessment

A crucial prerequisite for adequate intervention and special early education are assessment methods that comprise all important domains of development and fulfil the criteria of validity, reliability and objectivity (see Chap. 6) in the context of ensuring that every element of every test is easily visible to the child being assessed. These assessment methods should also possess ecological validity, i.e. should provide relevant information about the quality and quantity of individual visual disability (so-called assessment of functional vision; see, e.g. Colenbrander 2009, Boot et al. 2010; cf. Sect. 6.1). To gain such information, standardised methods for the comprehensive assessment of visual capacities should be combined with systematic observation in everyday life conditions and feedback from the child and his parents, family members and other significant persons. A further significance of

Table 7.1 Summary of tasks of functional diagnostics

Assessing *specific* visual impairment(s) and determining all functional binocular, spectacle corrected visual capacities in the context of everyday performance (evaluating positive and negative pictures of performance)
Assessing the *degree of severity* of visual impairment(s)
Identifying skills abilities and strengths
Deciding upon and recommending interventions, matched to the capacity of the child/family/professionals to implement them
Assessing outcome of interventions
Continuing the cycle

functional visual assessment is the valid and reliable measurement of the effects of intervention in terms of reduction of severity of visual disability in both the clinical and the child's own settings (Table 7.1).

For children with CVI, functional assessment should comprise evaluation of all visual functions and capacities (e.g. contrast vision and visual acuity for form vision), particularly in relation to the higher-level visual perceptual components that they serve. For example, the diagnosis 'homonymous concentric restriction of the visual field' does not communicate how wide the child's overview might be or whether the child efficiently uses compensatory gaze shifts, for example. The same argument applies for 'impaired spatial contrast sensitivity'. This description does not contain valid information concerning whether form vision and object and face perception are impaired, and to what degree, or not impaired at all. In essence, measures of functional vision need to be evaluated, explained and set in the context of education and everyday living.

The amount of light required for optimum visual performance needs to be considered for each child with low vision, because the ability to discriminate elements of an image starts to diminish below a critical level of background or ambient lighting, in the same way as it does for those with normal vision, but not infrequently at a higher level of lighting. On the other hand, there is a group of children with profound visual impairment due to CVI whose vision is paradoxically enhanced when light levels are reduced (Good and Hou 2006), and functional vision in this group needs to be evaluated in mesopic conditions of lighting, to determine whether performance improves.

Functional visual assessment differs from the assessment of visual function in a number of ways. Visual function assessments, such as visual acuity, contrast sensitivity, visual fields and stereopsis, are determinations of threshold levels of vision. In particular, visual acuity is measured to determine the resolution of the visual system with each eye in turn, tested at maximum contrast ideally under specified bright lighting conditions in defined standard conditions. In contrast, assessment of functional vision is carried out under ambient lighting conditions, with both eyes open with optimal spectacle correction if required, with the aim of determining what can be reliably, consistently and comfortably seen and appreciated in daily life, ideally both when wide awake in the morning and when tired later in the day (recognising the increased fatiguability of the visual system in many children with CVI). *The functional visual acuity*, for example, tends to be two- to threefold larger than the measured visual acuity, which for everyone, sighted and visually impaired alike, denotes the lower limit of visual function. (Fully sighted people do not choose to read text at their level of binocular visual acuity; they prefer text which is two- to threefold larger, reflecting their functional visual acuity; Lueck 2004.) It is clearly very important that threshold acuity measures are not communicated as those to be used by families and professionals working with children with CVI, as all visual information presented needs to be well within the perceptual limitations of the child. Visual acuity specifies the minimum perceptible line thickness and minimum perceptible gap thickness between lines found in text or imagery, whereas the functional visual acuity specifies the measure that ensures that all elements are visible during everyday viewing in ambient lighting.

Similarly, *functional contrast sensitivity* assessment is carried out to ensure that all adjacent greyscale elements of all images presented are perceptible, as contrast sensitivity can be diminished in children with CVI (Good et al. 2012). Greyscale black-and-white images as seen in black-and-white photography are now not commonly shown to children. Colour contrast also needs to be considered. For example, light blue is blue to which white has been added, and navy blue is blue to which black has been added. The ability to differentiate these two colours is thus an evaluation of contrast sensitivity in the context of a blue background. This conceptual model applies to all colours and needs to be born in mind by all those investigating, looking after and teaching children with low vision.

Colour vision in its own right is also evaluated from a functional standpoint, by evaluating which adjacent colours, at which degrees of saturation can be differentiated, and by determining which coloured objects are identified or missed against which backgrounds.

The functional visual field embraces a number of concepts. Apart from eye movement detection methods, which show considerable promise in evaluating attentional visual fields in children (Murray et al. 2009), the visual field is commonly assessed with the head and eyes looking in a single direction. On the other hand, functional visual field evaluation assesses whether there is lack of visual function in any area of the visual field, during everyday living. It takes into account the visual field per se, visual attention throughout the visual field, any reflex vision that brings about saccadic eye movement to peripheral targets and any divergent strabismus compensating for hemianopia, as well as detrimental features such as tonic eye movements that limit visual access in the direction opposite to the deviation.

The peripheral lower visual field is needed for walking and running. Thus, the functional lower visual field is evaluated with both eyes open while looking straight ahead. The subject is given support, if needed, while elevating a straight leg until the foot is seen, for each leg in turn. Functional peripheral lower visual field impairment is evident if the foot has to be elevated to a degree that would encompass more than two paces ahead (more than 20°). (Standard visual field testing employs targets that do not evaluate this peripheral area of the visual field, so that peripheral lower visual field impairment interfering with walking may not be identified using standard measures.)

Evidence of impaired parallel visual processing and its degree are elicited in children for whom prior history taking reveals impaired visual search. The number of items that can be simultaneously perceived is elicited, and the degrees to which background pattern and surrounding clutter interfere with this process during everyday living are evaluated.

The accuracy of visual guidance of movement of the arms and hands, and the legs and feet, in the context of everyday living, is sought by both history taking and assessment.

Key issues to consider include:

1. Comprehensive evaluation of the day-to-day consequences of dysfunction of the central visual system and its effects on behaviour and individual experiences of the child.
2. Functional visual assessment to cover the quality (type) and quantity (degree of severity) of the child's visual impairments in a valid and reliable way, in relation to the child's developmental age.
3. Evaluation and communication of the spared visual capacities (providing both 'positive' and 'negative' pictures of development and performance).
4. In children with CVI, developmental stages of cognition, motor functions and activities, as well as language, motivation, emotion and social behaviour, are also assessed, and the results of visual assessment are interpreted in this context. This form of interpretation is important, because it potentially allows differentiation between primary and secondary visual impairments (e.g. due to attentional dysfunction) and informs the need for intervention measures and specialist early education (impairments in these functional domains should of course be treated separately and specifically, when required).
5. The effects of intervention and special early education should be strictly monitored; this helps avoid inappropriate or suboptimal application of intervention measures and can be used to change treatment or education programmes as required. All experts in this field, who are responsible for the child's further development, are primarily responsible for proper assessment and intervention, ideally based on scientifically proven or at least face-value evidence.
6. Although intervention and the effects of special early education are assessed using appropriate measures, the main outcome measure is *useful vision*. Of course, one is on the right track, if after intervention the child shows improved visual acuity, but the crucial test of efficacy is ecological validity, i.e. whether the child benefits from improved acuity in visual localisation, spatial orientation and navigation, form vision, object and face perception and visual recognition.
7. The results of visual assessment, the conclusions reached and recommended actions to be taken need to be communicated to all interested parties in easily understood language. Specific advice on care and parenting includes information about how not to criticise behaviours due to CVI but instead to support the child, along with description of specific targeted strategies that the child, caregivers and family can all implement on a day-to-day basis (Sect. 7.4).

7.3.2 Requirements of Intervention Measures

Successful adaptation to the challenge of brain dysfunction particularly during development depends on two main prerequisites: enriched environments and systematic experience (van Praag et al. 2000; Nithianantharajah and Hannan 2006; Kolb et al. 2011; Eckert and Abraham 2013). In addition, the availability of learning capacity, including cognitive (perception, attention, memory, executive function) and motor functions involved in learning, also appears crucial, because in the absence of the critical minimum of learning capacity, interactions between enriched environment and systematic experience cannot take place, i.e. environment- and experience-dependent plasticity cannot operate. In children with CVI, the enriched environment may be understood as stimulus conditions, which on the one hand support the child's endeavours and on the other make sufficient demands on a child's visual and cognitive equipment at a given time of individual development, but do not over expend the child's capacities. Thus, adequate visual sensory enrichment is optimally adapted to the child's visual-cognitive capacities, which also includes controlled intervention conditions. On the other hand, experience-dependent plasticity implies that systematic practice is required for visual perceptual and visual-cognitive learning to lead to improvement of vision in the context of action and thus behaviour. Systematic practice should, therefore, consist of a fair balance between given (and assumed) visual, cognitive and motor capacity of a child and tailor-made task demands that are essential for successful intervention measures. Both enriched environments and systematic practice with the use of such environments in the behavioural context are known to modulate neuronal efficacy and thus functional brain capacity (van Praag et al. 2000; Berlucchi 2011; Eckert and Abraham 2013).

For children with CVI, the concept of enrichment includes the need for all training to be administered in an environment free from clutter and noise and in a creative way by skilled individuals, in a form of motivational play that is interesting, challenging, varied, rewarding and fun. Children with CVI have to work hard to 'see' and are easily fatigued, which can manifest as lack of engagement and sometimes distress. This needs to be recognised and positively catered for. Children need to be happy and wide awake to actively participate and learn.

As already mentioned in the introduction to this chapter, adequate application of interventional measures in children with CVI requires professional diagnostic assessment with mastery of the methods of intervention and early special education, which are tailor-made and individually adapted to the complexity of the child's individual challenges.

Intervention procedures may be non-specific or specific and systematic or nonsystematic.

Non-specific intervention aims at general (i.e. non-specific) activation of visual functions. They are indicated whenever a child shows little spontaneous activity, because of global or specific (visual curiosity) motivation difficulties, or insufficient attention (alertness, sustained attention, mental processing, concentration). Non-specific methods are, however, unsuitable for specific treatment of visual impairments where their application may even prove inappropriate.

Specific intervention allows tailor-made treatment of visual impairment, i.e. intervention is adapted to the individual type and severity of defined visual impairment. Thereby it is ensured that improvement of the visual impairment in question is the focus of intervention and of main therapeutic activities. However, it should be recognised that the higher the specificity of the method of intervention, the higher the demands for the child. If the requisite (cognition, motivation, etc.) requirements are not available, the degree of specificity can be diminished, or, in the extreme case, the child can initially be afforded adequate non-specific intervention, followed later by specific intervention.

Nonsystematic intervention comprises inconsistent performance in relation to stimulus and/or task conditions, instruction, duration (including breaks) and time of intervention, type of mediation of learning strategies and time and form of feedback. This 'form' of intervention has limited application and should therefore be avoided, because both the child and the therapist cannot develop a clear structured approach to intervention. Furthermore, no valid framework for the assessment of the outcome of such intervention can be established.

Systematic intervention, in contrast, is based on standardised rules concerning stimulus and task conditions and instructions; defined duration of intervention phases, including time points, length of breaks and time of intervention (i.e. excluding unfavourable times of the day); and regular and unequivocal feedback, which is focused on specific aspects of intervention that can be easily grasped, mastered and willingly implemented by the child. Systematic conditions of intervention also imply that the child can become sufficiently familiar with the intervention procedure and thus gain certainty, which supports self-confidence and enhances motivation and attention and guarantees compliance. Of course, systematic intervention should not be understood and applied in too stringent a form, for example, concerning time structure. If, for example, a chosen treatment poses excessive demands on a child, then the structure is simplified; this clearly poses more demands on the teacher or therapist, but it also renders intervention more interesting and effective.

Developing a sensible, systematic and comprehensive plan of intervention in a 'holistic' context requires a stepwise procedure. The definition and monitoring of intermediate goals of intervention and the flexible adaptation of the process of intervention to its principal aims but also to the personal needs of the child in the context of individual demands in everyday life are a complex challenge. This challenge is best guided by evidence-based knowledge, personal experience and (professional) empathy. The plan of intervention is based on the negative and positive pictures of visual capacity, on existing proven procedures and means of intervention and on ecological validity. Close cooperation between all professional disciplines engaged in the intervention for children with CVI is, therefore, essential for the success of the intervention and early special education and, of course, for the child and his or her family. Regular exchange of information and individual experiences facilitates a flexible response to individual adaptation of intervention measures and also guarantees early identification and modification of unsuccessful training procedures or training conditions. Furthermore, visual stimulus materials used for practice should always also include affective components (e.g. colours) or an affectively potent context that uplifts mood, because task-irrelevant affective information is known to negatively influence visual cortical activity (Damaraju et al. 2009).

7.3.3 Perceptual Learning and the Requisite Cognitive Capacities

Improvement of vision in children with CVI is mainly based on perceptual learning, ensuring that materials used fall within each child's level of functional vision. The most basic form of visual perceptual learning is same-different discrimination, in which the number of stimulus features increases. More complex forms require acquisition of visual constancy and categorisation and ultimately identification and recognition (Goldstone 1998). Perceptual learning is based on brain plasticity (Fiorentini and Berardi 1997; Gilbert et al. 2009) and constitutes a fundamental type of learning in the pre-semantic period of child development, which however involves already attained complex cognitive capacities, e.g. problem solving (Coldren and Colombo 1994).

Perceptual learning has been shown to be efficient in children (and adults) with perceptual disorders with and without associated cognitive dysfunction (Greenfield 1985; Serna et al. 1997; Huurneman et al. 2013). An important factor in perceptual learning is the form of feedback. It has been shown that disabled children in particular learn to discriminate stimuli faster and with greater reliability, when errors are prevented straight away (so-called errorless learning; Sidman and Stoddard 1967). For example, in a typical visual discrimination paradigm, a child is shown a pair of stimuli of the same dimension, brightness, form or colour. Initial stimuli clearly differ, but differences are decreased stepwise, so that the child learns to detect increasingly fine differences in the respective stimulus dimensions, and the child's sensitivity for the stimulus dimensions improves. Feedback concerning correct and incorrect discrimination, respectively, is given immediately after each response; this procedure enhances sensitivity and prevents unfavourable discrimination criteria being learned. According to the level of discrimination performance and ability, feedback can be progressively diminished. Children who understand and use verbal instruction can respond verbally; if this is not the case, fixation, pointing or grasping at the correct stimulus, possibly associated with head shaking ('yes'-'no'), can be used as alternative behavioural responses. Video-based recordings of the child's responses may be helpful for later analysis of responses in the various discrimination conditions; in addition, the child benefits from the therapist's overt interest in his responses and his attention to the stimuli during practice (joint attention).

As mentioned earlier, cognition is a crucial prerequisite for perceptual learning. In the following section, cognitive capacities required for perceptual learning in children with CVI are briefly summarised and commented upon. A wide range of issues need to be considered with respect to age and level of visual, intellectual and motor function.

7.3.3.1 Attention

The following attentional capacities need to be considered:

- Sufficient alertness;
- Sufficient sustained attention with respect to intensity and duration;
- Sufficient concentration (focusing attention to a particular stimulus and reduction/prevention of distractibility);
- Capacity for dividing attention (paying of attention to two or more stimuli in the visual and/or other modalities in parallel).

In this context, distractions including discomfort, extraneous sound and visual stimuli and social distraction are identified and minimised as appropriate.

The interplay between attention and complexity of the visual task should be considered when planning visual perceptual practice; the more complex the task, the more attentional resources are required to perform it. Regular changes in the visual material and in task conditions (e.g. detection vs. discrimination) can enhance maintenance of attention (Fantz 1964). During early special education, stimuli with high attentional value, e.g. glittering stimuli and moving simple (unicoloured balls) and complex stimuli (travelling little cars, self-moving dolls, mobiles, etc.), presented against a contrasting plain background have been found very useful as a means of catching and maintaining attention in children with low vision (e.g. Hyvarinen 2000).

7.3.3.2 Learning and Memory

Optimal conditions for learning through intervention can be achieved by:

- Favourable conditions for attention/concentration and motivation;
- A good relationship with the therapist;
- Establishing a positive mood (frame of mind) for learning (interest in visual material and joy with practice tasks);
- Avoiding taxing and insufficient demands (mental over or under load);
- Regular affirmatory social signals to the child rewarding the performance despite an evident low level of performance.

For shaping practice conditions, the following considerations can prove helpful:

- Transparent organisation of the amount of information, with clearly limited packages of information belonging together;
- Pre-structuring of information: to (a) render tasks unambiguous to bring about an expected ‘performance’, (b) bring about global before detailed (local) processing and (c) accord recognisable significance to the stimuli;

- Transfer to other task/environmental conditions: regular repetition of tasks initially under equal and then later under changing context conditions;
- Confirming/rewarding: affirming, establishing and reinforcing the processes of self-monitoring of learning strategies (by giving unequivocal positive feedback; see above);
- Ecological validity: establishing the concrete relevance of the tasks to everyday life situations (so that the child understands what the purpose of learning is).

7.3.3.3 Executive Functions

When considering the cognitive and developmental level and the importance of integration of the perceptual learning into broader concepts of knowledge combined with a coherent framework of guidance and training in behaviour, the following issues can prove helpful:

- Visual perceptual tasks should be simple and concrete as far as possible;
- The complexity of tasks should be increased in steps, taking the child's mental processing into account, i.e. building associations between stimuli (colours, forms, objects), discovering logical connections between stimuli, predicting what may happen when …, etc.;
- Support of realistic self-assessment of visual capacities and visual performance as a solid basis for developing self-control.

7.3.3.4 Visuomotor Skills

Children with posterior parietal damage or dysfunction ranging in severity from dorsal stream dysfunction to Balint syndrome can manifest a range of disorders of visual guidance of movement (optic ataxia) that may compound cerebral palsy or may occur in the context of otherwise normal motor function. Accurate visual guidance of movement is predicated upon intact visual function, visual attention and the dorsal stream-mediated capacity to create an accurate internal emulation of the surroundings, to inform the motor cortex to bring about limb or body movement with accurate visual guidance (Milner and Goodale 2006).

7.3.4 Children with CVI Without Additional Cognitive Impairments

In children with CVI, but spared cognition, intervention can be primarily focused on improvement of vision, although the developmental cognitive stage should always be taken into account. Intervention may be arranged such that visual stimulus complexity and task demands are increased stepwise with regard to the defined (intermediate) goals of systematic practice. Table 7.2 summarises various aspects of both components.

Table 7.2 Classification of visual stimulus dimensions, of stimulus complexity and of visual perceptual performance

Visual stimuli can be classified according to individual or combined features and context:
Stimulus features
Brightness
Size
Colour
Form
Combination of features
Number, type of combination; level of complexity
Context conditions
e.g. same or different context; figure-ground relations
Complexity of a task can be qualified in terms of:
Detecting stimuli (type and number),
Comparing stimuli (same-different; new-familiar; smaller-larger, etc.),
Classifying (based on stimulus features; increase in number of features),
Identifying (based on stimulus features; increase in number of features),
Recognising (based on characteristic stimulus features; number of features; short- vs. long-term storing),
Manipulating (acting with objects based on particular object features),
Naming of visual stimuli (forms, colours, objects, faces),
Gaining knowledge (about context, functional aspects, 'history' of an individual object or person, personal experiences with a particular object/person, factual knowledge; visual semantic and episodic memory)

Important

- Successive levels of task difficulty should not be implemented before the child has reached the level of visual performance required for each level.
- The requisite cognitive and (fine) motor functions need to be considered for each task and must fall within each of the thresholds and capabilities of the child.

7.3.5 Children with CVI with Additional Cognitive Impairments

Some recommendations are given below concerning intervention methods to use for children with CVI with additional impairments of attention and learning/memory.

7.3.5.1 Insufficient Attentional Capacities

1. Establishing an adequate span of attention (sustained attention for at least 5–10 min) by using visual material and task conditions that do not pose particular difficulties for the child. Distracting stimuli including background pattern and clutter should be avoided. Other modalities (audition, touch) may be included to supplement but not substitute for vision.

2. Increase the span of attention to about 10–15 min by using complementary visual material and task conditions. Visual material should be diversified to enhance and maintain concentration and interest.
3. Increase in (visual) attentional task demands concerning material and task condition.
4. Practice with directing attention at particular visual stimuli or stimulus (object) features while 'neglecting' unessential features.
5. Extension of orientation of attention from one visual stimulus (object) to several stimuli (or objects) (aimed at developing the capacity to shift and divide attention and to carry out parallel processing).
6. Combinations of (1)–(5) to further increase the span of attention (30 min) and the capacity to handle diversity.
7. Practice of sustained attention/concentration and mental load under 'natural' conditions.

Important

- At the beginning of any intervention, the stimulus and task conditions should avoid all forms of distraction.
- Intervention procedures should be planned such that the child possesses the requisite vision and attention/capacity to perform the task.
- Successive levels of task difficulty should not be implemented until the child has gained the requisite attentional performance.

7.3.5.2 Insufficient Learning and Memory Capacities

The capacity to learn is the principal resource underpinning intervention, involving the acquisition of visual skills and the differentiation of visual perceptual capacities. Learning is needed when a very young child intends to fixate, observe and inspect a (complex) visual stimulus or to discriminate visual stimuli on the basis of different features. The outcome of such learning is stored in visual memory. Thus, even acquisition of 'lower' visual perceptual capacities requires learning and memory. Children with CVI commonly need to learn how to see, by developing activities and strategies to accurately process visual stimuli, or they may need to relearn such activities and strategies. Consideration of some main principles of learning may thus be useful in the context of intervention.

Development of learning strategies and learning habits is the crucial basis for:

- The acquisition and successful use of (individual) visual experiences and factual visual knowledge;
- The selection of executive activities (stored in episodic and semantic memory) and actions (stored in procedural memory) for the visual guidance of behaviour in diverse life situations (skills), including previous (planning) and later control (feedback) of the outcome of intentional behaviour;
- The development of long-term visual experiences and resulting routines and habits, which can be used as (successful) routines in the future;
- The development of optimal visual guidance of movement of both upper and lower limbs.

Table 7.3 Some components of intervention in children with CVI and impaired learning/memory

1. *Practising single and simple visually guided activities*: bringing about sufficient accuracy and duration of fixation without additional visual-perceptual demands
2. *Practising of successive visually guided activities*: e.g. fixation shifts between two or more stimuli without additional visual-perceptual demands, and guidance of limb movements with methods of tactile supplementation of the visual guidance of movement
3. *Practising (learning) of*:
Detection
Discrimination
Identification
Recognition
Association with personal experience
Association with (semantic) knowledge (including naming)

The development of visual routines and habits is a life-long process in healthy individuals also and includes flexible adaptation whenever needed, to cope successfully with the visual world and its demands. Table 7.3 summarises components of intervention in children with CVI and impaired learning/memory.

Important

- Action supports learning – perceptual learning entails action (gaze; pointing and grasping; drawing and constructing).
- Learning should always occur under conditions that are as error-free as possible. Immediate supportive feedback about the child's correct/incorrect approaches is important and facilitates faster and safer learning.
- Feedback should be simple, correct and unequivocal. Otherwise, the child with CVI may be put in a condition of excessive demand or may be overloaded with too much unclear information, which is useless and cannot (and should not!) be remembered.
- The child finds it difficult to understand why his or her responses are correct or incorrect.

7.4 Direct Interventions for the Visual Impairments of CVI

Direct intervention for specific visual impairments in children with CVI aims to ameliorate impaired visual capacities and compensate for irreversible visual impairments. For the individual child, it depends whether there is sufficient visual capacity in evidence, to work towards direct improvement, or whether compensation strategies will be sufficient. There is limited evidence for efficacy for direct intervention to improve vision in children with CVI (Williams et al. 2014), but lack of evidence for efficacy does not constitute evidence of lack of efficacy, and further systematic investigation in this area is required.

A good example is the work of Malkowicz et al. (2006) who showed that children with CVI can significantly benefit from systematic practice with discrimination and identification of visual stimuli.

The functional organisation of visual perception in the brain is based on parallel and serial processing and coding, organised within a form of hierarchy, in the sense that more complex ('higher') visual capacities depend, at least in part, on less complex, i.e. 'lower' visual capacities (see Chap. 2). For specific interventions, a sequence of steps emerges from the following functional organisation of the visual brain:

- Visual exploration and visual search processes
- Visual localisation, essential for accurate fixation and grasping
- Visual contrast sensitivity and visual acuity
- Visual space perception, in particular visual-spatial orientation and navigation
- Visual guidance of movement of the limbs and body
- Discrimination and classification of colours and forms
- Discrimination, classification and identification/recognition of complex stimuli, e.g. figures, objects, faces
- Visual memory (visual experience)

7.4.1 Visual Field and Field of Attention, Visual Exploration and Visual Search

The close association between detection of stimuli in the visual field and attention forms a useful basis for treating children with impaired detection in parts of the visual field.

7.4.1.1 Visual Field

It is unclear whether and to what extent vision can be restored by systematic training in adults with homonymous visual field loss (see Zihl 2011). A similar picture emerges for children with homonymous visual field defects; in single cases, recovery of vision has been reported after systematic practice with detection of slowly moving light targets along the visual field border requiring fixation and pursuit of the target, while no visual field changes were observed in the group without such practice (Werth and Moehrenschlager 1999; Werth and Seelos 2005). Based on fMRI outcome, the authors interpreted recovery of visual field as training-enhanced activity in spared striate and extrastriate visual cortices. In adults, the method of visual field restitution is still questioned, because only few patients have been reported to benefit from restitution training and the degree of visual field enlargement is usually fairly small. Moreover, restitution training is very demanding and time consuming, and evidence of (ecological) validity of this method has yet to be sufficiently proven (see Zihl 2011). In children, visual field restitution in single cases after systematic practice is a similarly interesting phenomenon, but empirical evidence with respect to the efficacy and efficiency of this treatment measure is as limited as it is for adults.

In visual field regions with depressed visual function (so-called cerebral amblyopia), visual performance (detection and localisation) may be improved by combined focusing of attention to the particular visual region to facilitate detection and localisation of the stimulus used. As a result, children may learn to spontaneously direct attention to affected visual field regions, leading to benefits in everyday life due to being more reliably able to detect both obstacles, and items that are being sought (Mezey et al. 1998). For this type of training, large moving uncoloured stimuli (black on white background or white on black background) and high-contrast coloured stimuli are used, which are initially presented in the centre (straight-ahead direction of gaze) and then at increasingly greater distances from the centre towards the periphery of the visual field. This stimulus condition facilitates stimulus detection and guides attention to where stimuli will appear. The session starts by seeking responses from the centre of the stimulus array, which is indicated by a big red light spot. Positive responses to target appearance comprise searching and orienting gaze shifts (eyes and head, later eyes only) or, if possible, additional verbal responses (yes-no). The positioning of stimulus appearance initially follows a systematic approach, but is later varied in a random way. This procedure establishes an expectation of stimulus appearance at variable positions in space and enhances the distribution of the child's anticipatory attention throughout the visual field. When the child's detection rate is at the level defined in the plan of treatment for a particular stimulus condition (e.g. 75–90 % correct responses), smaller stimuli and stimuli with lower contrast can be used to improve visual sensitivity. Initially, the stimulus presentation time should be as long as needed for reliable detection, but it is then successively reduced to speed up the process of visual search. A diminishing latency and an increasing accuracy of response indicate improvement in performance. Registration of eye movements and/or of pointing and grasping movements to targets by means of video- or infrared-recording techniques allows a more detailed analysis of speed and accuracy of detection and the gaze shifts involved. This approach can also be used for follow-up and longitudinal assessments (see also Sect. 6.2).

7.4.1.2 Field of Attention, Visual Exploration and Visual Search

The consistent association between directed visual attention, detection of a visual stimulus and subsequent localisation by gaze shifts can be used for the development or optimisation of oculomotor scanning strategies, which the child can, for example, also use to compensate for his or her visual field loss. The procedure is the same as described in the last section ('visual field'). The principal difference lies in the sequence of stimulus presentation. The stimulus is first presented in the spared visual field, then along the visual field border and finally outside the visual field. By this procedure, the field of visual search and thus of attention are systematically enlarged towards the periphery. After the child has developed systematic and reliable searching movements, stimuli are presented at random positions in both hemifields within and outside the spared visual field. After this phase, scenes (pictures, photographs, defined visual search arrays, possibly presented using an LCD screen), with a big red light spot in the centre (or in the LCD frame appearing before scene presentation) as standard reference position before scanning, are very useful to ensure the same starting point. The scene should extend at least 30° to the left and right and 15–20° upwards and downwards (total diameter, 60 × 30–40°). Set size (number of stimuli) can be increased stepwise, so that the child learns to search for

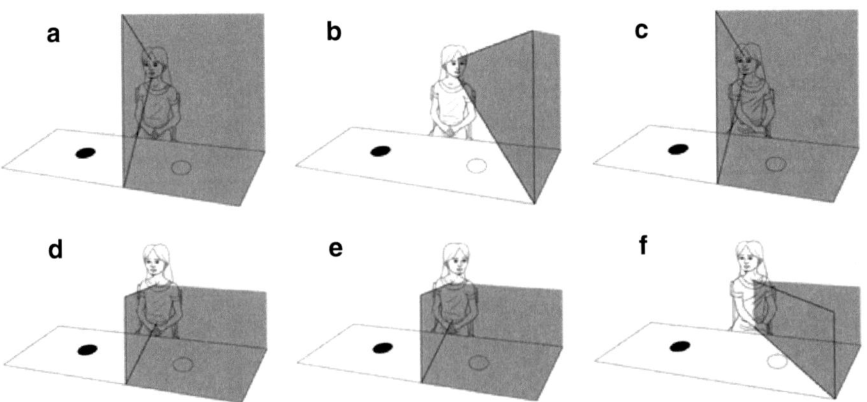

Fig. 7.1 Diagram showing left hemianopia due to right occipital pathology (**a**, **b** and **c**) and left hemi-inattention due to right focal posterior parietal pathology (**d**–**f**). For left hemianopia: (**a**) Looking straight ahead, the white disc is not seen. (**b**) Turning the head to the left, the white disc is revealed, but (**c**) by turning the body it is not. For left inattention: (**d**) Looking straight ahead, the white disc is not seen. (**e**) Turning the head to the left does not reveal the white disc, but (**f**) by turning the body it is revealed

more than one stimulus. At the final level of difficulty, a combination of targets and distractors may be used; however, distractors should differ clearly from targets (e.g. in size, form, colour), and the child should know the target(s), before the search is started. The use of the left hand for reaching for stimuli in left hemispace and externally alerting stimulation by sounds may be helpful in reducing left-sided visual neglect (Dobler et al. 2003). As the right posterior parietal lobe maps the surroundings with respect to the body, left-sided neglect relates to the body (Ting et al. 2011) and tends not compensated for by movement of the head and eyes. Instead, rotation of the body to the left, allows the midline of the body schema to point to the left side widening the field of visual attention to include more of the left side. Affected children commonly sit at table in this way, and when they do, food is no longer left on the left side of the plate. A slight rotation of the torso to the left when walking can also be seen as a probable adaptive response in some affected children, who commonly have an additional left hemiplegia (see Fig. 7.1).

7.4.2 Contrast Vision and Visual Acuity

For improving spatial contrast sensitivity and visual acuity, several procedures, which have been developed for treatment of childhood amblyopia, are available. It is, however, still unclear whether these procedures are also effective in children with CVI. It seems essential that, whatever procedure is used, active perceptual learning is involved, because 'passive' procedures (e.g. covering the eye with the better acuity and contrast sensitivity) alone are less efficient, at least for distant vision (Levi and Li 2009; Polat et al. 2009). Huurneman et al. (2013) used a perceptual learning paradigm (form and letter search and discrimination using PL) to improve near visual acuity in 45 children with visual impairment. Training included 12 sessions, 30 min each (two sessions weekly in 6 weeks). After practice, children showed significant improvements in near visual acuity. Binocular paradigms, where the child is actively engaged in a 'game' in which each eye is independently presented with separate elements of the task with the clarity of image presented to the better eye degraded to match the vision of the better eye, are showing promise (Knox et al. 2012).

7.4.3 Visual Space Perception and Spatial Orientation

7.4.3.1 Visual Localisation

Visual localisation of stimuli can be practised by employing tasks in which this visual capacity plays the most prominent role, e.g. fixation or, pointing to and grasping at simple visual stimuli or objects. It is important that any compounding effects of oculomotor deficiency (e.g. eye muscle paresis) (Weir et al. 2000) or motor dysfunction of both the upper extremities are recognised and taken into account. In the first phase of intervention, a visual stimulus (e.g. a small white or black ball with sufficient contrast attached to a thin rod) is presented in front of the child. The size of the stimulus is, of course, chosen to fall within the child's functional visual acuity. The child is asked to look at (fixate) the stimulus and to reach for and grasp it. Children with biparietal pathology commonly manifest impaired visual guidance of movement (optic ataxia) of the upper limbs that may occur in isolation or may be integral with the features of cerebral palsy. In this context, the opportunity needs to be given to supplement visual guidance of movement with tactile guidance. Potential approaches include:

- Encouraging the child to move a hand along a table to reach out for a target.
- Ensuring that part of the table is in contact with part of the body, to enhance feedback concerning the location of the target in three-dimensional space, through tactile means.
- Providing a tactile guide. This may be the arm and hand of the trainer. The child learns to reach out along the arm and hand and through this comes to know that reaching out will not cause injury.

Once the child has begun to master this visuomotor action, the stimulus is shown to the left and right of the mid position. At the beginning of intervention, stimulus position is varied systematically, i.e. predictive; later on, stimulus position is randomly varied. For enhancing directing of attention, salient (e.g. coloured) stimuli can be used. Gaze direction should always be straight ahead before the presentation of the next stimulus, so that the child learns to acquire the spatial reference. The lateral distance of the stimulus from the straight-ahead direction of gaze is also varied (e.g. between 5 and 30 deg eccentricity) as is distance, comfortably within the child's arm length (when training fixation, the distance can be larger). Fast and accurate fixation, pointing, reaching out and grasping are the goals of therapy.

Replacement of items requires visual guidance of vertical movement. For those who have difficulty estimating the vertical vector and can bang things down, or whose reach is short of the table surface, extension of the little finger as a supplementary tactile probe can be taught.

7.4.3.2 Distance Perception

If the child already possesses verbal competence and can give verbal responses, a stimulus array can be used to improve subjective discrimination of spatial distances. Identical stimuli (e.g. small white or black balls with sufficient contrast) are presented pairwise at either the same distance or at different distances, but within the same direction of gaze. For the simplest condition, the child has to decide, whether both stimuli are at the same distance or not (yes-no responses); at the next task level, the child indicates, which stimulus is nearer or further away to one or other side. Alternatively, three stimuli can be used; two are shown at the same distance, while the third differs in distance, i.e. either nearer or further away. The child has to identify, which stimulus differs with respect to distance ('take-the-odd-one-out' paradigm; Torgrud and Holborn 1989; Boelens 1992). Clearly when grasping is being trained within the programme, all targets need to be within easy reach.

7.4.3.3 Visual Orientation

Intervention for impaired visual orientation related to impaired search, often related to bilateral posterior parietal pathology, involves the development of a spatial reference system within the scene (the stimulus array comprising an array of different forms, or a natural scene shown as a picture, or presented on a TV screen) and in space. In the first phase of intervention, a scene or stimulus array with several visual stimuli (objects, e.g. toys or forms), shown at a table or a picture or using TV or LED screens, is used. The child is asked to search for a particular visual stimulus (object, form) among other stimuli; the background should provide good stimulus contrast. The child is informed about the targets and is asked to either point or grasp at stimuli or to indicate target position using a pointer when a TV or LCD screen is used for presentation. In the second phase, several different targets can be used for searching, and the number of distractors (set size) can be increased. Systematic practice aims at improving visual search performance in terms of accuracy and speed; the combination of both parameters is indicative of a coherent scanning strategy that is based on reliable visual orientation. Coherent visual search also implies updating of fixation position in visual-spatial working memory ('Where have I been already?') contingent upon intact posterior parietal ('dorsal') and fronto-parietal pathway function. It is recommended that the child first of all gains a complete overview over the scene or stimulus array (global perception) before local visual search and thus local processing is started and performed. Therefore, it may be helpful to use a small (15–20° in diameter) scene stimulus array before extending visual search to the full field of vision (~60° horizontally and 45° vertically). Set size can accordingly be increased from 3 to 15 (1 target, 2–14 distractors); the number of targets can also be increased from 1 to 8 in the largest stimulus display (as dictated initially by the set size that the child can simultaneously appraise).

Once the child has reached the targeted level of performance at the highest level of task difficulty for that child, the third phase of intervention, visual orientation, can be practised in everyday life conditions, i.e. in rooms and smaller places. In addition, learning of new paths with increasing number of landmarks in a smaller than a larger room is recommended. After a child has learned a fixed path through the room/place and can eventually successfully find a toy, the number of objects in the room/place (e.g. furniture) can be increased and the path can be made longer to increase task difficulty. It is, however, important that the child always starts from a fixed position in space, for example, the entrance door.

Impaired orientation related to temporal lobe damage, which is often accompanied by visual agnosia, is rare and more severe and commonly is associated with impaired face and object recognition. Brunsdon et al. (2007) have developed an intervention programme for the improvement of spatial orientation in a 6-year-old boy (CA) with topographical agnosia, who had suffered brain haemorrhage a few days after birth. Before entering school, CA received intensive intervention to improve motor, language and cognitive development. At the age of 5 years, CA was examined in detail for the first time by a neuropsychologist. Concerning language capacities, CA performed well although somewhat lower than age-matched normal children. In the vision modality, he exhibited left-sided homonymous hemianopia and a good functional visual acuity and had marked difficulties in figure-ground tasks, object constancy, visual localisation and visual-spatial working memory. In topographical orientation, his performance was worse. CA was unable to learn the position of landmarks; after 10 practice trials, he still had considerable difficulties remembering them (4 % correct responses; healthy age-matched children, 92 % correct responses). Furthermore, CA was unable to learn a path, which had been indicated by circle marks and arrows. Based on these test results, the following goals of intervention were defined: (1) improvement of visual identification of landmarks in the (familiar) surroundings of his school and of describing them verbally, when shown pictures of them; (2) improvement of navigating frequently used paths in the area surrounding his school (natural condition); and (3) design of strategies to aid successful learning of new paths in familiar as well as unfamiliar surroundings; these strategies were communicated to his parents and teachers. The entire period of intervention had two phases. In phase 1 (3 weeks), the focus of systematic practice was visual identification and recognition of landmarks and buildings (28 pictures) in familiar school surroundings. Phase 2 consisted of learning 10 new paths of increasing length, which CA had to remember. Before intervention, CA could correctly recognise only 17 out of 28 pictures (landmarks, ~ 60 %; normal children, 100 %); after phase 1, CA was able to correctly recognise all landmarks and buildings including their spatial location. Before phase 2, CA could correctly 'reproduce' only 3 out of 10 paths (30 %); after this training phase, CA was able to 'reproduce' double the number (60 %); in addition, CA required much less time to 'reproduce' paths. In the follow-up assessment, CA could correctly recognise all paths and could also use them correctly. The authors emphasise the importance of the ecological validity of their intervention procedure, which was as close as possible to everyday life. In addition, close collaboration of parents and teachers, who kept exactly to the intervention programme, was a highly supportive factor. That congenital topographical disorientation can still be remediated later in life has been reported by Incoccia et al. (2009). These authors trained navigational skills in several steps to a young woman with severe selective topographical disorientation: (1) exploring the surroundings systematically and carefully, (2) orienting in these surroundings and (3) moving in the surroundings using a language-based strategy. At the end of practice, she was able to navigate in her familiar environment by using various cognitive strategies. At follow-up after 1 year, she used these strategies as navigation routines and could successfully apply them in unfamiliar environments as well.

Supportive strategies devised by parents and successfully used for children seen by one author (GD), include colour coding of doors within the home, for a child with topographical agnosia due to temporal lobe damage, and composing songs as a verbal cue to route finding. A verse of one such song, written and sung by a 12-year-old girl with topographical agnosia, to independently make her way to school successfully for the first time was:

I go to lamp-post number three.
And then I go to the big green tree.

The song was sung in reverse to guide the return route. Within a few weeks, the strategy was no longer required.

7.4.4 Colour and Form Vision

Several measures of intervention exist for the improvement of colour and form vision. A very simple method of training, which can be used early in childhood, is preferential looking (PL; see Sect. 6.2). Pairs of colours or forms are presented, which at the lowest level of difficulty differ clearly. One stimulus serves as the standard and the other as the variable stimulus. Differences between paired stimuli are decreased stepwise by progressively approximating the colour hue or form of the variable stimulus to that of the standard stimulus in order to create increasing levels of difficulty. The child's 'task' is to match the two stimuli regarding same-different (yes-no responses). When the two stimuli look more or less the same, the child will no longer fixate the standard, which meanwhile is familiar, but now has 'lost' its familiar value, or the variable stimulus, which has 'lost' its saliency because of undetectable differences in colour hue or form. At the beginning of the intervention, stimuli may be taken from different visual categories. For colour discrimination, red vs. green or yellow vs. blue stimuli may be used at lower levels of difficulty; at higher levels, yellow vs. red and green vs. blue may be appropriate pairings. For form vision, comparable stimuli may be circle vs. square and circle vs. triangle, and circle vs. ellipse and square vs. rectangle. Using this procedure, the so-called difference threshold can be determined by repeated presentation; the lowest distinguishable difference indicates the discrimination sensitivity and can be used as a performance parameter (see also Sect. 6.2). Alternatively, the take-the-odd-one-out paradigm can be used (Torgrud and Holborn 1989; Boelens 1992;

see also Section on distance perception above). Three stimuli, colours or forms, are presented to the child; two of them are identical (standard stimuli), while the third one is different (variable stimulus). The child's task is to find the odd stimulus, which does not match with the two other stimuli; 'finding' is understood as fixation of the odd stimulus, pointing to it or grasping it or naming it. Feedback should be given immediately (errorless learning) to prevent children from laborious trial-and-error learning and to enhance correct perceptual learning. Differences between the odd stimuli and the two standard stimuli are decreased stepwise; therefore, increasing visual sensitivity is required for discrimination of more and more subtle stimulus differences. Stimulus positions should be varied at random, so that position is not the critical variable, but colours or forms are. Both paradigms, PL and take the odd one out, can be used separately but also in combination; thereby more variation in stimulus and task conditions is possible. This enhances attention and motivation of the child, without discontinuing the fundamental principle of treatment. Furthermore, the level of difficulty can easily be adapted to the level of individual performance (provided, adequate assessment has been carried out before the beginning of intervention). Table 7.4 summarises some visual stimulus classes and variations in practice with discrimination.

Table 7.4 Some classes of visual features for discrimination learning and forms of practice with stimulus dimensions

One-dimensional discrimination
Colour
Discrimination between colour categories (e.g. red, green, blue, yellow; black, white)
Discrimination within colour categories (e.g. between different red- or grey hues)
Form
Discrimination between form categories (e.g. circular vs. angular)
Discrimination within form categories (e.g. circular-oval, square-rectangle, rectangle-triangle, triangle-star)
Size
Discrimination of different sizes of the same form (e.g. circles with differing diameter)
Discrimination of different sizes of different forms (e.g. circle vs. square differing in size)
Multiple dimensional discriminations (constancy)
Colour constancy
Different forms (e.g. circles, squares or stars) paired with same or different colours (abstraction of colour from form)
Size constancy
Different forms (e.g. circles, squares or stars) paired with same or different sizes (abstraction of size from form)
Form constancy
Different colours (e.g. red, yellow, black) paired with same or different forms (abstraction of form from colour)
Different sizes paired with same or different forms (abstraction of form from size)
Different colours and sizes paired with different forms (abstraction of form from colour *and* size)

For some children, inability to name colours can be misinterpreted as impaired ability to discriminate colour, and for others pathological inability to name colour may be evident or even acquired after brain injury (colour anomia). A management technique that has repeatedly proved effective in one author's service (GD) has been to recognise that colour names are abstract concepts and that linkage of these words to real entities by repeatedly using terms, such as sky blue and grass green, leads to acquisition of colour naming skills in most affected children, even after the noun component has been relinquished a few weeks later.

7.4.5 Object and Face Perception

Intervention for improving object and face discrimination and identification and recognition, respectively, can be performed in the same way as for improving form and colour perception; instead of colour and form stimuli, objects and faces are used. It is important to note that therapists should clearly distinguish between discrimination, identification and recognition, respectively. Before beginning with training of the components mentioned, attention should be paid to whether the child possesses all prerequisites crucial for object and face perception, at least to a sufficient degree. These include visual acuity and contrast sensitivity, size and form vision and visual fixation and scanning. As very young children prefer complex visual stimuli over more simple ones (see Sects. 2.3.6 and 2.3.8), complex visual stimuli can also be used for intervention. Nevertheless, the use of less complex objects with very characteristic features is recommended for the beginning of the intervention, i.e. at the lowest level of task difficulty, increasing complexity with progressive levels of difficulty.

In the first phase of intervention, discrimination of *objects* is practised by using PL and take-the-odd-one-out paradigms (see Sect. 7.4.4). As objects, familiar toys and objects (e.g. fruit) are suitable, these are presented in pairs (standard and variable stimulus). Stimulus position is varied at random to prevent spatial position being the critical variable and to improve object constancy and visual recognition, because the standard stimulus becomes the invariant stimulus. Children should be given sufficient inspection (and decision) time; this also enables children with attentional dysfunction or delayed responses to engage in this type of practice. Gaze shifts, duration of fixation, pointing and grasping movements and verbal answers can be used as responses. At higher levels of difficulty, object features can be graduated, and the number of features can be increased. Also pictures and stimulus cards (e.g. memory cards) can now be used, provided real objects are shown in clear and unequivocal quality and in familiar perspective. Perspective may be varied at the highest level of visual object discrimination and identification levels, both between (different objects) and within object categories (same objects). Recognition of objects, using the same or similar object stimuli, is trained to the highest level of difficulty that the child can attain. Sufficient trials should be carried out, and recognition performance established (between 75 and 90 %) before starting this progressive element of the training. Feedback should be given immediately after responding (errorless learning) to enhance the child's perceptual learning strategy.

The intervention programme strategy for improving *face perception* is identical to that for improving object perception. Pairs of faces are presented, which differ clearly from each other; with increasing levels of difficulty, differences between faces are reduced to improve sensitivity for faces. Faces should possess 'neutral' facial expressions to avoid intermingling with facial expression discrimination. Face stimuli can include faces of younger and older children and younger and older adults, and are presented as (coloured) pictures or using a LCD screen. In the second phase, the child learns to discriminate between faces, which have already been presented, and new faces. For this, the standard face is paired with another face stimulus that changes with every trial. Of course, pictures also showing parents, sisters and brothers, etc. can be used. The child's task is to indicate which one of the two faces is the new one. In the third phase, recognition of faces is specifically practised, i.e. one or two (later 3 or 4) faces are shown repeatedly at different positions (left or right from the child's mid position), unless the child can indicate that this one face has already been presented before and has now become the familiar one. Response types are the same as for colour and form vision (Sect. 7.4.4); feedback is given in the same way as described for the treatment of object vision.

As a final phase of intervention, discrimination and identification of *facial expressions* are trained, if required. The procedure is the same as for face perception and identification, except that facial expression is varied for the variable face stimulus. At the next level of difficulty, pairs of faces with same/different facial expressions are used to improve overall recognition of both face identity and facial expression. Tables 7.5 and 7.6 summarise object and face stimulus and task conditions for improving object and face perception, respectively.

For the assessment of the outcome of perceptual learning and recognition performance for objects and faces, the following response types and response parameters can be used in accordance with the child's stage of development: (1) fixation and fixation duration, (2) pointing and grasping movements and (3) verbal responses. The moment a child has learned to visually recognise an object or face, he or she may show signs of surprise and joy; in the case of facial expression, imitation of the recognised expression may also be observed, particularly when the child deals with a positive expression. In the case of a negative facial expression, e.g. sadness or anger, the child may also imitate the facial expression, but may also respond by using avoidance behaviour or even by crying.

Of course, clear instructions are very important so that the child knows exactly what the perceptual task is, i.e. what the therapist expects as the response, and thus of the perceptual performance. Real objects should be given to the child after (not before!) correct visual recognition, for subsequent tactile exploration; this procedure supports and enhances building of intermodal associations.

Brunsdon et al. (2006) and Schmalzl et al. (2008) have published single-case studies on intervention in two 4-year-old children with developmental prosopagnosia. Training was mainly focused on the use of characteristic individual facial features for better discrimination and recognition of faces. The following phases and goals of intervention were defined: (1) improvement of visual discrimination and identification of features of unfamiliar faces; (2) improvement of visual identification of

Table 7.5 Some object stimulus and task conditions for improving object perception

1. Discrimination of objects
One-dimensional object features: colour, size, form
Value: degree of difference or similarity
Complexity: number and combination of features, which may also differ with respect to their degree of value (i.e. different colours in one object or colour and form elements in the same object)
Multidimensional object features: natural objects vs. object pictures
Familiar condition of perception: presentation of the same object in its most frequent and thus most familiar condition (i.e. familiar perspective)
Unfamiliar condition(s) of perception: presentation of the same object in various sizes, colours and perspectives
Forms of presentations and response categories
Parallel presentation of pairs of object stimuli, but with alternating position: same-different
Parallel presentation of two identical and one differing object (alternating positions): finding the differing object
2. Identification and recognition of objects
Identification/recognition of one object when two objects are presented in parallel, and one object is varied; position is alternated
Identification/recognition of one object under varying stimulus conditions (object constancy): presentation of a particular object with varying object features (form detail, colour, size, perspective)
Forms of presentations and response categories
Parallel presentation of pairs of object stimuli, but one object stimulus is varied; recognition of permanent object stimulus (position alternating)
Successive presentation (increasing time interval: 2–10 s) of one identical and one (or more) differing objects: recognising (remembering) the permanent object
(Motivation is driven by presenting these tasks in the context of enjoyable games with rewards.)

familiar faces shown on pictures on the basis of individual characteristic facial features; and (3) transfer of improved visual discrimination and recognition performance, acquired in phases (1) and (2), to new (i.e. unfamiliar) faces. Pictures of faces were presented on a screen; hair was removed from all pictures. Perceptual learning of faces consisted of several steps: identification of age (child vs. adult), gender (female vs. male) and specific facial features (e.g. bushy eyebrows, large nose, blubber lips). Training for both children lasted about 4 weeks and comprised 14 and 18 single sessions, respectively. Both children showed significant improvement in reliably discriminating facial features and faces of familiar people, independent of whether hair was present or not. Thus, both children successfully learned to use 'natural' facial features for individual identification and recognition. Improvement in selective processing has also been mirrored in scanning patterns of faces (Schmalzl et al. 2008). The improvements remained stable; however, generalisation of identification and recognition capacity to new faces was only observed a few weeks later, indicating that intensive and regular visual experience with new faces is required for successful application of learned processing and

Table 7.6 Some face stimulus and task conditions for improving face perception

1. **Discrimination of faces**
Learning to discriminate identity: same–different with respect to (global) form, age and facial details
Learning to discriminate facial expression: same face (person)-different facial expressions
Forms of presentations and response categories
Parallel presentation of pairs of face stimuli, but with alternating position: same-different
Parallel presentation of two identical and one differing face (alternating positions): finding the differing face
2. **Identification and recognition of faces**
Identification/recognition of one face when two faces are presented in parallel, and one face is varied; position is alternated
Identification/recognition of one face under varying stimulus conditions (face constancy): presentation of a particular face with varying facial features (form details, coloured or black-white, size, perspective)
Identification/recognition of varying facial expressions in the same person: pictures of the same face is shown, but facial expression is varied; particular facial expressions (e.g., 'neutral', 'friendly', 'happy', 'surprised') are shown repeatedly
Identification/recognition of the same facial expression in different people: pictures of different faces with the same (similar) facial expression are shown
Forms of presentation and response categories
Parallel presentation of pairs of face stimuli, but one face stimulus or a particular facial expression is varied; recognition of permanent face stimulus or facial expression (position alternating)
Successive presentation (increasing time interval: 2–10 s) of one identical and one (or more) differing faces or facial expression: recognising (remembering) the permanent face and facial expression, respectively
(Motivation is driven by presenting these tasks in the context of enjoyable games with rewards.)

identification strategies. The authors of both studies emphasise the necessity of systematic and specific treatment procedures at home as well, to support the training programme; in the study by Schmalzl et al. (2008), most of the training was carried out at home by the child's mother. DeGutis et al. (2011) found improved discrimination and recognition of faces after systematic practice using part-whole tasks in five subjects with developmental prosopagnosia. This improvement showed transfer to faces of other races too, indicating that visual recognition of faces can be successfully learned and generalised by improving discrimination of small facial differences even at a much later stage of development.

7.4.6 Text Processing and Reading

Developmental visual dyslexia can be caused by various visual deficits that impair text processing, e.g. low visual acuity, difficulties with discrimination of symbols and letters presented in a line (Pike et al. 1994), impaired ability to cope with visual crowding (Callens et al. 2013) or impaired organisation and guidance of eye movements in text processing (Lanzi et al. 1998; see also Sect. 4.3.9), which could be linked to the degree of crowding of text. Furthermore, learning to process text and thus to read also depends on attentional and executive capacities and on verbal memory (Fellenius et al. 2001; Sireteanu et al. 2006; Menghini et al. 2010; Vidyasagar and Pammer 2010). Thus, successful acquisition of text processing and reading requires visual, oculomotor, cognitive and linguistic capacities and their mutual interactions (Solan et al. 2001; Mackeben et al. 2004). Consequently, intervention measures aimed at improving text processing and reading should integrate all functions involved in reading (Menghini et al. 2010) and should also be tailor-made for the subtype of developmental visual dyslexia (Lorusso et al. 2011; Di Filippo and Zoccolotti 2012) and for the individual patterns of visual, oculomotor and cognitive functions.

A first step in improving text processing is to give children practice with form and letter discrimination, including coping with crowding effects (Martelli et al. 2009; Huurneman et al. 2013). The observation that systematic practice with non-reading functions, in particular controlled guidance of visual attention (and the requisite eye movement control) in terms of the spatial span of processing, spatial shifts of attention and inhibition of attention, may induce a greater improvement in reading performance compared with a training focused on reading, only highlights the importance of the role of cognitive prerequisites (Lorusso et al. 2006).

Practising faster text processing with imposed time constraint can considerably enhance reading speed and thus also improve text comprehension, because a minimal speed of text processing is crucial for fluent reading and text comprehension (Facoetti et al. 2003; Breznitz et al. 2013). Rapid processing of text material may also enhance letter-string association, whereby processing of longer words is more difficult (De Luca et al. 2010) and may thus require further practice with processing. In addition, for rapid processing of longer words and strings of words, regular fixation shifts that precede the text processing in time are required. Practising such 'oculomotor readiness' can considerably improve reading performance in dyslexic subjects (Solan et al. 2001); similarly this can benefit adult patients with hemianopic dyslexia (Zihl 2011). It is important to note, however, that limited horizontal eye movements per se may not always impair reading performance (Hodgetts et al. 1998).

Summarising the observations on intervention effects in developmental visual dyslexia, the following steps are recommended:

- Establishing the crucial visual (spatial resolution, form/letter discrimination), oculomotor (systematic successive fixation shifts in time and accuracy in the direction of text processing before text processing, which can be simply observed by watching the child's eyes while reading text printed on transparent material (Hyvarinen and Jacob 2011)), and cognitive prerequisites for

visual text processing (attention, in particular controlled spatial guidance of attention, visual and verbal working memory, executive function for monitoring of text processing operations);
- Learning of rapid processing of letters and of letter strings of increasing length (letter integration);
- Building accurate visual representations of letters and words;
- Practice with transfer of processing of words to processing of short and longer sentences, with consideration of semantics;
- Practice with comprehension of visually processed text material (single words of varying length, sentences of varying length).

As with other forms of systematic visual practice and experience, intensive, regular practice is associated with a better chance of acquiring efficient text processing skills in time, which appears to be an essential prerequisite, not only for text processing to become a routine but also to establish pleasure from reading, which eventually manifests itself in the ability of the dyslexic child to comprehend the content of an interesting story with sufficient ease.

Children with bilateral posterior parietal pathology causing difficulties with simultaneous/parallel processing of visual stimuli may only be able to access a very small number of words at once. In this context, a typoscope (comprising a slot in a sheet of black cardboard, or plastic matched to the print size used) can prove remarkably effective in facilitating reading. One young lady seen by the author GD over a number of years, who has periventricular white matter pathology also causing spastic diplegia, reads fluently, but only by reading through the 'slot' that she chooses to create with her fingers.

7.5 Special Intervention Measures in Children with Severe CVI

In children with severe cerebral visual impairment, often a further phase of intervention is required to guarantee that children can reliably use any improved visual capacities that they have gained, under conditions of everyday life through:

- Practice with independence in visually guided everyday life activities based on existing visual capacities;
- Learning strategies for spatial orientation and navigation based on the use of existing visual capacities;
- Learning to discriminate and identify simple objects;
- Improvement in cognitive domains of attention, memory (including imagery) and executive function and in language and in guidance of movement through vision and supplementary tactile means;
- Improvement of social perception and social behaviour with consideration of visual capacities.

7.6 Adaptive Strategies for the Child and Family for Home, School and Community

7.6.1 Adapting to the Needs of the Child

Cerebral visual impairment in children ranges widely in character and extent, yet an approach is needed that affords all affected children the best chance to develop in a way not disadvantaged by their different vision. Parents/caregivers and teachers have a fundamental part to play. Each needs to understand the specific limitations and strengths of the child with CVI to help him or her make best use of all their abilities. They need to enable and empower their child to explore and learn, by creating a world that stretches each of the child's perceptual and intellectual limits, by being within these limits and by being informative, captivating and motivating, ideally where possible, within an ambience of loving support, encouragement, affirmation and fun. They also need the knowledge, confidence and ability to communicate this information to others.

7.6.2 A Practical Model to Explain the Perceptual Limitations Caused by CVI

The commonest way of thinking about the vision of others is to assume that everyone sees in the same way as oneself, but this approach cannot be applied in the case of those with low vision. For them a correctly imagined and accurately conceived allocentric model of thought is needed, founded on a well-informed understanding of how their child sees. This enables living and schooling environments, toys, possessions, books and educational materials to be rendered accessible, enriched, attention grabbing and motivational and ready for exploration and learning. All need to understand that material that cannot be fully seen due to impaired vision has no meaning, cannot be attended to, does not motivate and cannot be learned from. Verbal communication referring to what the speaker can see, but the child cannot, has no value. It is also counterproductive because it teaches the child that it is normal for people to speak language with no meaning, arguably predisposing to the development of echolalia.

The specific limitations that CVI potentially causes on visual function are considered in the context of the actions that must be taken to ensure that they impact least upon the three principal requirements of vision:

- *Access to information*, whether it is near (e.g. playing with toys, looking at pictures or reading) or in the distance (e.g. a shop or a tree)
- *Social interaction*, whether this involves seeing and greeting someone in a group or recognising and responding to facial expressions or gesture
- *Visual guidance of mobility* of the upper and lower limbs and body

As explained in Chap. 1, learning cannot be inflicted. It is brought about by motivated exploration that culminates in neuroplastic development. Children can only explore what they perceive, and when vision in any of its characteristics is limited, early implementation of adaptive, compensatory and training strategies, all designed to comprehensively fall within each child's perceptual, attentional and intellectual limitations (or thresholds), reaps dividends. The approach that is needed for low vision is to provide the child with the means to live and learn comfortably within their limits of visual perception, with supplementation by alternative means, when the limits to access to information through vision would otherwise be unavoidably exceeded.

7.6.3 Explaining Cerebral Visual Impairment to Parents, Caregivers and Teachers

A clear basic model of how the brain sees and how this process is disturbed for the affected child is required, recognising that vision is not an 'outside-to-in' process, but that it ostensibly comprises a virtual mental representation of the surroundings, which for each child with CVI has specific limitations that commonly diminish as the child grows up. The importance of regularly ascertaining, knowing and working within these limits, and mastering ways of attaining this aim, must be fully recognised and understood.

An explanation needs to be given that an image of the outside world is not somehow transferred into the brain. Instead, the image data are reconstructed within the mind. (Studies of how optical illusions are perceived show that consciously processed visual imagery is ostensibly a reconstructed hypothetical virtual model of the surroundings, which is compellingly presented to consciousness as the actuality of the surroundings. The conscious mind ascribes the imagery to the outside world, despite it being a virtual representation.) When it is understood that the 'picture' of what we see is inside the brain, it can then be understood that the disordered image processing in the mind of a child with CVI is equally compellingly created as an alternative construct of the external world. It is this altered external construct that the child 'knows' to be their surrounding environment. This construct may have impaired clarity, contrast or colour, areas missing or anomalous matching and recognition, yet still conveys information, the nature of which needs to be understood so that it can be employed to maximum advantage, by ensuring that both the background scene and foreground materials are perceptible and afford interest, motivation and meaning.

As previously discussed, much image processing is implicit (unconscious) in nature, particularly in relation to visual guidance of movement of the limbs and body. The moment-to-moment consecutive acquisition of streaming incoming image data is temporarily stored and processed (then relinquished) in the form of a moving three-dimensional image construct, through which we are able to navigate without collision, because it matches the 'reality' of the 'outside world'. A multiplicity of elements of the surroundings are constantly being mapped with respect to shape and form, while the body's movement is guided through this virtual unconscious construct, with an innate subconscious automatic acceptance that it represents an accurate visual and auditory three-dimensional (3D) map of the surroundings, upon which the image data, discussed in the above paragraph, are superimposed. For the child, whose CVI is impairing this process, this virtual multimodal moving map of external space, is degraded. It holds less data. In a sense it has fewer but larger voxels than the typical child and leads to inaccuracy of movement or optic ataxia that is seen as clumsiness and is often exacerbated by fatigue. The degraded 3D map also holds fewer entities, so that fewer can be seen (impaired parallel processing) and fewer can be looked at (apraxia of gaze). When explaining the specific nature of the vision of a child with CVI, whose visual limitations and abilities have been elicited, this model of thinking can be conveyed in clear simple language that highlights and explains both visual abilities and visual limitations. Parents who have been keen observers of their child's behaviour are often able to identify with this model of thinking as it immediately explains all their observations, and what previously was a puzzle falls into place.

7.6.4 Approaches to Adopt for Day-to-Day Living at Home, at School and Out and About

Implementation of a plan, which takes all the issues described above into account and which is reviewed at appropriate intervals, is the fundamental approach that needs to be adopted for all children with CVI.

7.6.4.1 Generic Approaches

Affording Insight into the Difficulty with Vision. Children with CVI who are in mainstream school tend to start becoming aware of their visual disabilities when they come to recognise that they are unable to do things that others can do. At this stage, an approach that highlights how and why the vision that is normal to them differs from others needs to be carefully introduced, in a way that highlights their strengths and abilities. (In a sense, parents too may have had their form of 'anosognosia' or unawareness for their child's visual difficulties annulled by good explanation.)

Averting Criticism Through Knowledge and Understanding. When parents, relatives, friends, teachers and classmates have all been well taught about a child's CVI, the child's behaviours all become explicable and handled appropriately and kindly, rather than being the subject of criticism. Children under our care, who have had a late diagnosis, have given feedback that this approach became a 'turning point' for them. They were no longer being criticised for being unable to find things and being clumsy, for example. Instead appropriate measures were put in place. This can have a remarkably positive impact on the child's self-esteem and learning, as prior anxieties are eclipsed by a new sense of confidence.

Not Inflicting a Sighted Agenda That Becomes Inaccessible. Alertness is required, particularly at school, to ensure that there is no drift towards expecting the child who is doing well on account of appropriate provisions, to move on to a more 'normal-sighted agenda'. School textbooks empirically become progressively more crowded with smaller print for older children, and this can pass the threshold of the child's ability to cope with it. Print crowding can be problematic, and any child with CVI who has initially learned to read well, who starts to fall behind at the age of 7 or 8 years, needs to be assessed with respect to how they handle crowding of print. Appropriate measures of ensuring optimal sans serif font, as well as optimal print size, and line and word separation may be needed. The same applies to arithmetic for which textbook pages can be particularly crowded. The ability of children to handle columns and rows of numbers may need to be evaluated, while determining whether benefit accrues from both presenting and writing sums on squared paper that they can easily see.

Communication: Working Comfortably Within the Thresholds for Language Perception and Comprehension. Children with CVI may have specific language needs. As previously discussed, all language needs to be comprehensible and should not link to visual frames of reference to what the child is unable to see. Succinct verbal supplementation of what the child is currently experiencing helps to enhance acquisition of language.

Many children with CVI have additional developmental disorders that may impair acquisition of meaning and language, and those caring for and teaching affected children need to be taught how to match their use of language to the child's attention, speed of processing, age, intellect and prior knowledge while sensitively stretching the limits of the child's comprehension.

Low visual acuities, visual field deficits, impaired parallel processing, impaired oculomotor scanning, prosopagnosia and impaired interpretation of facial expression need all to be recognised as contributors to impaired social engagement. For children who manifest such difficulties, the strategies of language use need to accord with the principles of teaching children with autistic spectrum disorder, by being clear, meaningful and explicit about feelings and emotions.

7.6.4.2 Day-to-Day Approaches Matched to Typical Behaviours

Table 7.7 links with the structured history taking Table 6.4 in Chap. 6 and describes ideas that have proven helpful for some (but not all) children with each of the scenarios described. Most of the ideas suggested can be progressively and inconspicuously incorporated into everyday living and implemented in such a way that they empower the child to become progressively more independent. Gradually, many of the practical strategies are relinquished, as children develop and gain requisite skills.

Families are rarely able to cope with a long list of recommendations, matched to the needs of their child, and often benefit most, if the ideas are prioritised and suggested sequentially at the time of successive appointments. This of course requires a planned approach, by the professional with this responsibility. Table 7.7 is not a comprehensive list, and practitioners are recommended to amend it and add new items that have been identified as helping children under their care.

Table 7.7 Adaptive approaches to daily living that children with CVI, and their parents have described as being helpful (after McKillop et al. 2006; McKillop and Dutton 2008)

1. **Frequently walks or trips over obstacles on the ground**
Have good storage at home, nursery and school to help ensure the floor space is clear
Consider having plain, non-patterned floor surfaces
Give verbal reminders, when needed, to compensate for visual field impairment e.g., look down, look left, look right
Provide toys such as a pram or a wheeled toy for the younger child to push, to give guidance for the height of the ground ahead
Encourage the child to hold an arm, belt or clothing of an accompanying person, or to touch a nearby wall when needed
When walking and holding hands, assist the young child by holding one's arm straight, and slightly back when approaching uneven ground, kerbs or steps. This gives advance tactile information about the height of the ground ahead
Give tactile reminders e.g., a tap on the shoulder can mean 'there is a hazard ahead'
Train the child in a strategy of "slow, look, check, go" when moving around, and when out and about
2. **Has difficulty walking down steps or stairs**
Provide handrails at the correct height, on both sides if possible (for going up and down), and/or hold on to an adult or responsible older child for tactile guidance
Give additional verbal reminders to slow down and hold on to handrails
Use plain stair coverings, such as plain carpets, laminate or wood because pattern can cause distraction and appear like obstacles to some children
Minimise wall decorations and patterned paper as these can cause discomfort and distract
Give a warning sound, a touch or a verbal instruction when approaching the stairs
Use spotlighting on the stairs, especially at the top, bottom and landing, to create shadows and an enhanced sense of depth
Train in the ability to rub the heels successively down each stair riser, to give supplementary tactile guidance of step height
Allow the child to be first or last when using the stairs, especially if crowded. e.g. At school, make it routine for the child to leave early or late from class to avoid crowds on the stairs
3. **Trips or is unaware of the edge of pavements going up and/or going down.**
Use methods from section 1 above
Give additional verbal reminders e.g., "there's a kerb coming up in 3 steps"
Use locations where kerbs are lower (e.g. pedestrian crossings)
4. **Appears to get stuck at the top of a slide, or hill. (Related to impairment of the lower visual field.)**
Give verbal reminders to look down
Allow your child to go down slides head-first so as to use the intact upper visual field
Give help to get down when needed
Teach how to go down a hill sideways, advancing one foot at a time and drawing the other foot down to it
5. **Looks down or trips when crossing floor boundaries, for example where linoleum meets carpet?**
Use the same non-patterned floor covering throughout the house
Give additional verbal reminders and prompts e.g., the carpet finishes in three steps
Mark floor boundaries clearly

Table 7.7 (continued)

Use plain carpets and plain floor surfaces, using contrasting colours to highlight boundaries
Ensure good lighting at floor boundaries
Use additional physical support e.g., arm, rail, wall
Arrive early at new places to practice and help reinforce memories of where surfaces change
6. **Leaves food on the plate on the near or far side**
Position favourite foods on the place where it is usually missed to stimulate exploration
Develop a routine for the child to rotate the plate to look for food
Use plain plates with no pattern, and a colour chosen to contrast well with the food
Place food items on different plates, or place them one at a time onto the plate
Ensure good colour contrast between food and plate
Avoid gravy and sauces that can merge the appearance of the food
7. **Leaves food on their plate on the left or the right**
Consider ideas from Sect. 7.6
Displace the place setting towards the intact visual field
Rotate the child's chair slightly so that the functioning visual field faces the table
8. **Has difficulty stepping into the bath, which is not related to balance**
Apply coloured stickers along the edge of the bath and use a plain coloured mat at the bottom, to highlight the location and depth of the bath
9. **Has difficulty finding the beginning of a line or the next word when reading, or misses pictures or words on one side of a page (features suggesting hemianopia or hemi-inattention)**
Rotate the child's chair slightly so that the 'better side' is closest to the desk/table
Move text so that the page being read is to the right or left of the midline, as appropriate
Teach finger pointing at successive words for right hemianopia or inattention, and using a tactile guide such as a ruler on the left to help redirect gaze to the left side for left hemianopia or inattention
Some children with acquired hemianopia can rapidly master vertical downward reading for acquired right hemianopia and vertical upward reading for acquired left hemianopia
10. **Walks out in front of traffic (from the left/right/or both directions)**
Give additional verbal reminders. For example "Let's check it's safe to cross."
Teach to cross roads at pedestrian crossings
Encourage the child to listen for cars
Encourage the child to turn their whole body when they look for cars in each direction. (This can be assisted by parents doing the same thing to set an example.)
11. **Bumps into doorframes or partly open doors (left/right/both) due to hemianopia or hemi-inattention**
Strategies to consider
A bright coloured marker at eye level, placed on the unattended side can help the child to pass through the centre of the doorway
12. **Has difficulty seeing scenery from a moving vehicle**
Strategies to consider
Give advance verbal information and guidance, e.g. "There is a church coming up on your left"
Use wrap-around sunglasses with polaroid lenses to diminish visual distraction and reflections

(continued)

Table 7.7 (continued)

Take video recordings to review later
Let the older child sit in the front seat as approaching scenery is easier to see owing to less relative movement
13. **Has difficulty seeing things that are moving quickly, such as a friend in the playground**
Give additional verbal information, e.g. "Jenny is at the gate in a pink jacket"
Teach the child to use voice recognition to identify friends and family
Teach friends and teachers to introduce themselves when in moving groups of people
Give additional help to find friends/family in busy places such as the playground
Encourage the child to use a mobile phone to call or text the person they want to find
Use pre-arranged meeting points
14. **Finds it hard to see moving water e.g. to fill a cup**
Try using a clear plastic cup marked with nail polish to indicate the full level
Use a small cup that can be looked directly into
Use a fluid indicator. (A device that hangs over the rim of the cup and emits a sound when the liquid touches it.)
Learn by using coloured liquid (e.g. orange squash) and a contrasting cup (e.g. white)
Teach the older child to listen to the pitch as the cup/glass is filled. (A vessel as it fills emits a reproducible sound with progressively rising pitch, particularly when filled quickly.)
15. **Finds it hard to follow the cursor on a computer screen**
Use a large high contrasting cursor with a slow movement setting
16. **Avoids watching fast moving TV programmes and prefers to watch slow moving TV programmes**
Choose size of the screen to suit the child's scanning capacity
Sit close to the TV to view single elements and minimise other distractions
Minimise visual distractions around TV (eg. photos, pictures, patterned wall coverings)
Ensure class teacher is aware that many instructional TV programmes may be unsuitable, due to the speed and content complexity
Identify and show programs where the presenter sits or stands still
Choose films that have the least movement
17. Has difficulty seeing and catching a moving ball
Practice catching skills using a balloon that moves more slowly
Practice using large, brightly coloured beach balls
Use balls with sound or light effects
18. **Finds uneven ground difficult to walk on**
Refer for mobility tuition, with long cane training if appropriate
Give additional physical support e.g. hand rails/banisters as required
Hold onto adult's arm pulling down, adult should have a straight arm extended back and downwards when approaching uneven ground
Give additional verbal reminders and instructions- "you'll need to lift your feet higher here as the ground is bumpy"
Teach how to 'toe walk', placing the toes down before the heel, to probe then weight bear on uneven ground
Give additional reminders to look down when needed

Table 7.7 (continued)

Learn to use adjustable spring loaded telescopic hiking poles. (Other family members may wish to do so also.)
Make own walking stick to act as a guide, for example a stick picked up in the park
Minimise height variations on floor surfaces
Try white trainers to increase visibility of feet
19. **Bumps into low furniture, such as a small table**
Give additional verbal reminders e.g. "the coffee table is just in front of you"
Avoid moving furniture and involve child in helping when necessary
Minimise the amount of furniture in each room thus maximising the space available for free movement
Use plain carpet and wall coverings to reduce the amount of visual information being presented
Consider the style and shape of furniture to maximise the floor space
Enhance the colour contrast between furniture and the floor
20. **Collides with furniture and becomes angry, if it has been moved**
Avoid moving furniture, or involve the child in helping to do so
21. **Reaches incorrectly for objects, i.e. reaching beyond or around the object or when picking it up uses a wide incorrect reach and grasp, sometimes missing or knocking it over**
For the younger child and infant who is not reaching out nor engaging, provide a moving adult hand as a tactile guide, to reach out along, to interesting toys and targets, made to match functional acuity. (Having eliminated pattern and clutter – making a prior assumption of potential Balint syndrome.)
Use larger items that contrast in colour with the surface unit
Touching the surface that the object is on, with part of the body, helps to locate and envision the location of the surface, in height and distance, and improves accuracy of reach
Use the non-dominant hand to reach out along the surface unit to provide a tactile guide to locate the object in order to supplement visual guidance of movement through touch
Practice with games and toys (matched in visibility to functional visual acuity), that require targeting and controlled dexterity
22. **Has difficulty seeing something that is pointed out in the distance**
Share a digital camera to zoom in to item of interest. Record the scene to talk about it later. Help your child learn to do this
Give clear directions. e.g., "Your friend is just next to the nearest lamp post"
Play "I spy" games. Encourage your child to choose a distant object and give clues about it so that others have to find and identify it. (Consider using a digital camera with a zoom facility)
Encourage your child to regularly look at the view. Ask them to describe what they see and talk about it together
Give your child the requisite time to take in what they are seeing. Try not to rush them on to the next thing too quickly
If you spot something your child would enjoy, take them to it to learn from it close up
23. **Has difficulty finding a close friend or relative who is standing in a group, such as a parent at the school gate, or a friend in the playground**
Give additional verbal cues. Call out your child's name to allow voice recognition to assist with visual search (some children have difficulty working out where a voice is coming from and an additional wave to cue where to look may be needed)

(continued)

Table 7.7 (continued)

Wear a brightly coloured item of clothing which "pops out" from the background and is visible from all angles. (e.g. a bright jumper, luminous jacket or coloured hat showing your child in advance which item will be worn)
Let the child choose a pre-determined meeting point
Encourage child to use their voice to call out for the person they are looking for
Let the child have a mobile phone (which they have been taught how to use) to contact the person they are looking for
Teach the child's class about the child's vision, so they can understand and help compensate on the playground
24. **Has difficulty playing team games with many people moving**
Ensure school physical education staff are aware of this potential difficulty, as failure can affect confidence and self esteem
Choose individual sporting activities involving fewer people (e.g. Athletics and swimming)
25. **Has difficulty finding an item if there is too much visual information e.g. a tin of soup or cereal on a shelf**
Use linear storage systems to facilitate one-dimensional search (as in books in a library)
Give each item a specific location
Let the child sort and put away, organising items so that adjacent ones contrast with each other
26. **Has difficulty locating an item of clothing in a pile of clothes, drawers, wardrobe, or shoes in a pile**
Minimise the range and amount of clothes in the drawer or on the shelf (e.g. socks only)
Experiment with different storage styles and layouts (e.g., vertical/horizontal) to promote search in one dimension
Hang clothes on a rail/wardrobe rather than fold them
Try hanging clothes in colour-matched sets, (e.g. red tee shirts together)
Try hanging clothes by outfit rather than item
Lay out clothes the night before
Try a spotlight or lamp in key areas in the room e.g. above drawers.
Involve your child in ironing and sorting out their belongings. (As appropriate for age.)
Store most clothing in a separate location, providing the child with a limited number of sequenced items in (say) a vertical canvas pocket system get dressed from. (With a view to building up the task.)
Use an elevated shoe rack
27. **Finds it hard to recognise an object if it is partly hidden, or viewed from an unusual angle**
Affected children adapt by spreading out their possessions to find individual items. Do not criticise
Encourage the child to be tidy and store possessions in allocated places
Where possible, ensure items are fully visible e.g., hang clothes rather than fold them.
28. **Has difficulty selecting a chosen item from a toy-box, or school tray**
Minimise the number of items to choose from
At school, ensure only a few items on the desk, in pencil the case and in school bag
Train the child in sorting, storing and being systematic
Set up together, a location in the child's room for the consistent placement of key items e.g. a compartmented box for spectacles and mobile phone, and encourage the child to return items to their places (particularly useful for older children)

Table 7.7 (continued)

Encourage your child to put things back in the same place when they have finished using them
Organise storage systems with clearly labeled drawers and boxes using pictures, photos and colours
Try using transparent containers. i.e. pencil case and school bag.
Use books/folders colour coded for each subject
29. **Finds it hard to spot objects when they are on a similar background, e.g. a white tee shirt on a white sheet or bread on a white plate**
Use contrasting colours for foreground and background
30. **Gets lost in places where there is a lot to see, e.g. in a crowded shopping centre/new places**
Have a pre-arranged meeting point to use in case of getting lost
Share a mobile communication system
Give extra practice to develop familiarity, knowledge and consistency
If the child gets lost in familiar places at home or school try using a few circle markers or brightly coloured footprints on the floor to mark specific routes, e.g. from seat to board, seat to door, or hall to bedroom
Try using bright coloured tape to highlight the child's desk in class
31. **Finds copying words or drawings time consuming and difficult**
Reduce copying demands by providing information on a printed sheet
Email or scan information to a laptop computer rather than copy it
Ensure that written material is clearly visible by meeting the acuity and contrast needs of the child
Determine the colour of ink and size of print that is most visible to the child for use on the computer and board
Reduce the visual clutter on the board providing only relevant text
Remove distracting visual information from above or beside the board
Position child facing the board directly and at the best distance to minimise visual clutter, reduce the need for head movements and give appropriate visual magnification
Permit and encourage child to use a mobile phone to photograph instructions and messages from the board rather than write them down
Make use of auditory skills and give the information verbally
Do not expect the child to write and speak, or write and listen at the same time
Provide a lap-top computer and camera system
32. **Has difficulty reading crowded text on paper, or on a computer screen, but can cope better if some of the text is covered or taken away**
Minimise the amount of visual information presented on a page or on the board: mask adjacent text
Employ voice activated software to read written material to the child
33. **Has difficulty finding letters on the keyboard but knows the alphabet**
Highlight keyboard with luminous alphabet stickers
Consider using voice activated software to reduce keyboard demands
Develop keyboard skills through programs and activities that are fun
34. **Finds it difficult to keep to task, and after being distracted finds it difficult to get back to what they were doing**
Minimise visual and auditory distractions around the work area
Encourage short periods of focused attention by breaking down the activities and presenting work tasks in short blocks,

(continued)

Table 7.7 (continued)

Vary tasks and demands e.g. sitting, standing, moving, listening, talking, looking
Give verbal reminders and encouragement e.g. "you are doing well, just one minute to go"
Give pre-arranged non-verbal reminders to assist the child to get back on task e.g. a tap on the shoulder, or a clap
Allow frequent movement breaks e.g. to hand out pencils, or deliver a message
Try a chair with arms to assist sitting balance, if required
Try a "fidget object" to help with attention when using listening skills
Encourage child to help with tasks e.g. fetch items when shopping, have a task to do at assembly
35. **May reacts angrily when other restless children cause distraction**
Design a low stimulus workspace without visual distractions for child to work in (this space should also be available to other children in the class)
Position the child near the front of the class, facing the board and teacher to reduce visual distraction and the need to look over heads, but not right at the front, as the child can be tempted to turn round more often
Arrange for the child not to sit next to the most active members of the class
36. **Bumps into things when walking and having a conversation**
Give additional verbal reminders. e.g. "there's a tree ahead of you."
Make only one demand at a time. e.g. walk, talk or listen
37. **Demonstrates difficult behaviour or distress in cluttered rooms or busy environments e.g. supermarket, shopping centres, school assembly, dining hall**
Minimise visual clutter
Pre-warn people to anticipate difficult behaviour, so appropriate measures can be taken in advance
Encourage child to help with tasks e.g. push the trolley or carry the basket
Allow regular breaks to move around
Have a quiet area with less visual clutter and visual stimulation in the home and classroom
Provide dark polaroid glasses when out and about to diminish reflections and contrast
38. **Finds it difficult to recognise close relatives**
Consistently wear identifiers e.g., top, scarf or hairstyle with easily identifiable colour, that can be seen from all directions, training the child accordingly
Practice voice recognition skills with the child
Teach children to use a mobile phone to call/text the person they are looking for
39. **May mistakenly identify strangers as people known to them**
Ensure that everyone understands that recognition of people is impaired to prevent embarrassment and inappropriate disciplining
40. **Has difficulty understanding the meaning of facial expressions**
Ensure people interacting with the child are aware of this and give supplementary verbal descriptions of their emotions (as well as not criticising the child for behaviour due to this difficulty)
Encourage the child to focus on the tone of voice and words being used
Give practice and training in recognising facial expressions
For the younger child exaggerate the voice and linked facial expressions to assist with understanding and learning

Table 7.7 (continued)

41. **Has difficulty naming common colours**
Establish if this is due to a problem with colour vision (colour blindness)
Employ conceptual linkage, by applying an appropriate descriptor before the colour name e.g. rose red, sky blue, lemon yellow, grass green, until colour concept is mastered.
42. **Has difficulty naming basic shapes, such as squares, triangles, and circles**
Practice using 3D shapes to feel and match to 2D and 3D shapes in pictures
Play at touching, feeling, exploring, imagining and naming shapes and objects
Play at constructing shapes e.g. using sand, clay, cardboard etc.
43. **Has difficulty recognising familiar objects such as the family car, classroom door**
Consider choosing a car with an unusual colour as an alternative means of identification
'Label' the car with a flag on the aerial.
'Label' the door with a tactile/visual object of reference
44. **Finds it difficult to find their way around a familiar environment**
Facilitate independent exploration (with support in the background)
Write and memorise songs and poems that describe important routes
45. **Has difficulty identifying right and left shoes**
Use salient visual or tactile markers that the child has made and has learned
46. **Finds it difficult to locate the source of a sound or voice**
Use mobile phones or similar device to communicate in busy places

Typical behaviours elucidated by history taking (Sect. 6.4.1) are listed with specific strategies to consider and evaluate (Compiled by the Vision Assessment Team at the Royal Hospital for Sick Children, Glasgow, Scotland)

7.7 Concluding Remarks

Although evidence-based intervention programmes, which also possess sufficient ecological validity, have yet to be established, there is no reason for therapeutic nihilism. On the one hand, proven principles of perceptual learning can be successfully applied to children with CVI, which can serve as useful guidelines and strategies for intervention (see also Malkowicz et al. 2006). On the other hand, it is a challenging and exciting scientific task to develop and validate new or alternative intervention programmes that not only extend treatment measures in children with CVI but also facilitate tailor-made application.

Basic research in the field of CVI needs to be complemented by research into its practical application under 'natural' conditions, aimed at developing, evaluating and implementing novel therapeutic approaches. Furthermore, CVI poses questions to basic researchers on the functional organisation of the visual brain and its cooperation with other functional brain systems, as well as on issues concerning functional plasticity of the visual brain, its essential prerequisites and the favourable and unfavourable factors that influence its development. Finally, the studies by DeGutis et al. (2011) and Incoccia et al. (2009) demonstrate that complex visual capacities as, for example, face discrimination and recognition and topographical orientation, respectively, can successfully be acquired after systematic training, despite having been congenitally impaired.

Table 7.8 summarises some relevant guidelines for intervention in children with CVI. Of course, guidelines have to be adapted to individual positive and negative performance pictures and the individual needs of the child; this applies to each of the visual impairments in question and to the sequence of implementation of the intervention components.

Family members need to be involved and integrated in the intervention process as far as it is practicable. The amount of time demanded of the child, and the type

Table 7.8 Guidelines for intervention in children with CVI, ensuring that all interventions are within the attentional, visual, physical and intellectual limitations of the child and are enjoyable and rewarding

1. Determination of cognitive requirements for intervention
Attention
(Visual) Curiosity
Learning and memory
Executive functions (self-control and self-monitoring of responses)
2. Determination of motor requirements for intervention
Eye movements (saccades, fixation, pursuit movements)
Head posture control
Hand movements (pointing, touching, grasping)
Body control and movements (sitting upright; walking)
3. Determination of visual capacities and their impairments (positive and negative picture of visual performance) as basis for the composition of tailor-made intervention programmes
Visual field
Visual acuity and contrast sensitivity
Colour and form vision
Object and face perception, including recognition
Perception, including identification of facial expression
4. Development of individual training programmes depending on (1) – (3) of guidelines
Selection of appropriate visual stimuli/visual material
Selection of appropriate tasks and response modes
Definition of successive task difficulty levels and training phases
5. Assessment of training progression (intermediate intervention goals) on the basis of regular documentation and flexible adaptation of intervention programme when required
6. Assessment of generalisation of improved visual capacities and activities to new stimulus and task conditions and contexts
7. In the context of additional functional impairments: planning of further intervention phases with special consideration of cognitive, motivation, motor, language or social difficulties
8. In the context of insufficient visual acuity: application with visual aids (including practise in how to use them) employing all the senses to best advantage
9. Ensuring that all communication is accessible and understandable in the context of the child's level of vision, using 'radio communication' for those who cannot see what is being referred to (see text)
10. Counselling of family members, kindergarten and school teachers, etc. on how they can support and include acquired visual capacities and skills into everyday life, conditions and activities, and providing them with special measures for further education

and degree of involvement, needs to be considered carefully to avoid unnecessary and excessive demands and the potential for inappropriate support for the child. Continuous supervision and feedback is needed between the child, therapist and family concerning intervention and feedback by experts in CVI measures and goals, time plan, actual stage of visual development and transfer of newly acquired skills to everyday life conditions as well as the child's mood, motivation and individual needs. The study of Schmalzl et al. (2008) is a good example of how family members can be actively and successfully involved in the intervention programme. However, it needs to be remembered that family members include, first of all, the mother, father, sister, brother, etc. of the child, and not therapists. They already have an important role in implementing any required adaptations in the child's environment, and their own behaviour, and the amount that they can cope with at any one time needs to be carefully taken into account.

A final remark concerns the parental perception of children with CVI and their possible role in intervention measures to remediate the visual disability. Jackel et al. (2010) have reported the results of a survey of 80 parents of children with CVI regarding the reception of the diagnosis and supports provided to their children, including educational supports, in the United States. The majority of responders (45 %) with children at an age of 1–7 years were content with the information about CVI and with the services provided. In contrast, the majority of parents (55 %) with children >7 years reported difficulties with obtaining appropriate services, mainly because of 'physicians' and teachers' lack of understanding, knowledge, and training with regard to CVI' (p. 620). The principal misunderstandings reported by parents were a kind of neglect of the visual impairment ('the child sees well enough'; 'the child does not have a true visual impairment because … it has a normal eye examination'; 'CVI will resolve, and your child will no longer be considered visually impaired'; p. 620); particularly in the case of concomitant disabilities, visual impairments were often disregarded. Such statements are not only unhelpful but have a high risk of preventing children's disabilities from being recognised and from their receiving the requisite appropriate individual intervention (Dutton et al. 2006). Parents and family members are essential for the successful transfer of visual improvements after systematic intervention to ADLs of children with CVI and are a unique source of information concerning the ecological validity of the intervention measures. Last, but not least, parents and families are the first and main 'significant others' for children with CVI. They are their promoters and supporters and should, therefore, be able to have professional experts as partners in intervention and (special) education. Undoubtedly, more combined special intervention and education measures are needed and warrant integration into school teaching and training programmes, but the first step to introduce and apply such measures, is knowledge of their existence, and their tailor-made application to remediate the degree and consequences of CVI and ultimately to enhance the welfare of children living with their CVI.

Profound Cerebral Visual Impairment

8

8.1 Introduction

Profound visual impairment due to CVI is relatively rare, but affected children and their families need a considerable amount of care to help bring about an optimal developmental and visual outcome. Their education is labour intensive. To train each child in skills that will afford as much autonomy as possible in later life, everyone looking after and working with affected children needs to know and be able to envision the nature and degree of the visual, motor, attentional, intellectual and communication limitations and their impact. These functions need to be assessed, and the results shared, so that all can capitalise upon the child's known abilities by always communicating and working with the child at a level within these limits, or ways to circumvent them.

8.2 Anatomy and Pathophysiology

Focal occipital damage can result from prolonged respiratory arrest, hypotension, hypoglycaemia and infarction due to occlusion of both occipital arteries, due to brain swelling kinking the posterior cerebral arteries on the tentorium cerebelli (Keane 1980). Despite profoundly impaired conscious visual functions, some children with acquired loss of vision are able to freely navigate through their environment. This presumably relates to preservation of posterior parietal and middle temporal lobe function, as it does in adults (see below) (Milner and Goodale 2006; Goodale et al. 2008).

More extensive damage can be seen as a sequel to perinatal hypoxic-ischaemic encephalopathy causing multifocal damage, or nonaccidental head injury, where the damage may be more diffuse. Additional parietal damage leads to cerebral palsy, while frontal damage impairs intellectual development, resulting in multiple disabilities accompanied by profound visual impairment (MDVI). When the thalamus is damaged, the visual prognosis is limited (Ricci et al. 2006).

J. Zihl, G.N. Dutton, *Cerebral Visual Impairment in Children: Visuoperceptive and Visuocognitive Disorders*, DOI 10.1007/978-3-7091-1815-3_8

Pathophysiology. The high metabolic activity of the occipital and posterior parietal lobes renders them particularly susceptible to bilateral injury due to hypoxia, ischaemia or hypoglycaemia (Soul and Matsuba 2010). Thus, a prolonged low oxygen level due to respiratory arrest or complications of labour, ischaemia and neonatal hypoglycaemia can all cause profound CVI. In some children, the damage is focal, primarily affecting vision, while in others generalised cerebral damage can profoundly limit not only the internal visual and mental representation of the surroundings but can also give rise to additional cerebral palsy and intellectual impairment (Bax et al. 2007; Rosenbaum et al. 2007).

8.3 Clinical Patterns

8.3.1 Isolated Occipital Injury

Isolated occipital injury in children is fortunately rare. The outcome tends to be primarily one of impaired vision. In our experience, it is more frequently acquired than congenital in origin, but can be due to focal brain injury during the first year of life. As discussed in Chap. 4, skills learned through vision that predate the brain injury may well remain unaffected, so that the later the injury, the greater the range of prior skills to seek and capitalise upon during rehabilitation.

The clinical features of focal occipital injury include reduction in visual acuity, contrast sensitivity and colour vision. Visual field impairment tends to affect the different quadrants to different degrees so that one quadrant or one half of the visual field may function better than the others. This is usually set against a background of overall visual field constriction. A common pattern is one of limited preservation of the left or right upper quadrant of the visual field. Visuomotor skills may be impaired, but in some cases are spared, resulting in the paradoxical behaviour of the affected child being fully mobile despite profound visual impairment (see letter to parents in Sect. 6.5). This type of vision is known as 'blindsight' in the adult literature (Weiskrantz 2004; Cowey 2010). Children affected in this way are usually able to compensate for, or supplement their lack of visual recognition by means of tactile skills (Boyle et al. 2005). In cases where the child has learned to understand and appreciate form and shape, and/or the alphabet, prior to brain injury, they can have the remarkable ability to move a finger over a drawing of a shape or letter (not embossed) and thereby recognise it haptically, through the nature of their movement, despite not being able to do so through vision. As reported in adults, the additional skill of imagining that they are moving their finger over the image can be developed and employed to learn to recognise shapes and even letters of the alphabet, through imagined finger following, or 'pantomiming' (Goodale and Milner 2013). This observation has the potential to be formalised as a rehabilitative strategy in cases of this nature. In cases with progressive recovery, in whom visual acuity is gradually regained, visual agnosia may continue to be a limiting factor.

8.3.2 Generalised Brain Damage

Profound visual impairment can accompany cerebral palsy. This can be due to optic atrophy, but in many cases the optic atrophy is limited, and the pupils react briskly. In these cases, cerebral visual impairment is suspected. Affected children may show no evidence of vision or may manifest intermittent and often fatiguable visual responses (Brodsky 2010). Light gazing is seen in a number of cases (Jan et al. 1990). Some children show intermittent reflex mouth opening in response to an approaching spoon from the side, but do so less often when the spoon approaches from straight ahead (Boyle et al. 2005). Parents and caregivers sometimes describe a positive response to a silent smile. This is akin to affective blindsight. (Affective blindsight is the phenomenon seen in some adults blind due to bilateral severe occipital damage, who respond to facial expressions conveying emotion, despite their low or absent vision (Andino et al. 2009)). Visual function as measured by visual evoked potentials (VEPs) may in some cases be enhanced under low luminance conditions (Good and Hou 2006), and parents may comment on their child's visual attention being greater in conditions of low lighting. In other children, no visual evoked potentials are identifiable at the normal latency of around 100 ms, yet a very small signal can be detected at 60–70 ms, suggesting that it arises from subcortical areas (Boyle et al. 2005). Additional damage to thalamic structures serving reflex attention tends to be associated with the most profound forms of CVI in which even this form of 'primitive' visual reflex may not be in evidence.

Another form of visual behaviour is for visual attention to become manifest when pattern and clutter have been completely removed. For some children, this can be achieved in a sensory room, where they become more attentive. When there is a single item to see (whether a moving light or the focally lit face of the child's mother), the child's visual attention can improve remarkably. This may also in part relate to improvement in visual behaviour in low light levels. A similar alternative strategy (that can prove effective even in some children who fail to respond in a sensory room) is to surround the affected child and carer by a monochromatic coloured and illuminated suspended curtain (Little and Dutton 2014). Following this approach, children who have sat head down and inattentive in the long term have been reported to start to look around with evident excitement and pleasure. These visual behaviours are suggestive of underlying hitherto unidentified visual disorders similar to Balint syndrome (masked by accompanying cerebral palsy and intellectual dysfunction) and also indicate that profoundly impaired visual guidance of movement (optic ataxia) may compound any associated cerebral palsy. This potentially necessitates physiotherapeutic efforts to encourage and support tactile supplementation of visually guided reach, initially while enclosed by a tent in this way. Children whose attention has been 'woken up' by being enveloped in monochromatic colour for half to one hour period during the day can continue to manifest this improvement outside the tent.

8.4 Prognosis

The prognosis for both early and late injury is unpredictable in our experience, but a feature in common is that gradual improvement in visuomotor skills can take place over a number of years, as can improvement in measured visual acuity. This means that regular assessment is needed to ensure that rehabilitational and educational provisions continue to be matched to visual functional skills, if and when they improve.

8.5 Principles of Assessment and Management

The principles of assessment and management of infants and children with multiple disabilities and visual impairment are the same whatever the age. The principal elements that need to be taken into account are vision and attention.

8.5.1 History Taking

The question inventory shown in Table 8.1 below provides information that has been shown to relate closely to estimated vision using preferential looking methods and vision evoked potentials (McCulloch et al. 2007). It can therefore be used to good advantage, particularly for children who are unable to cooperate at the times of assessment.

8.5.2 Assessment of Vision

Assessment of vision is best carried out after refraction, and prescription of appropriate spectacles as required. Many children with cerebral palsy have poor accommodation, and an appropriate near correction may be needed (McLelland et al. 2006); otherwise near vision is reduced. The provision of near correction for those with poor accommodation has been described as being followed by a rapid improvement in academic performance (Saunders KJ, 2006, personal communication). A poor pupil reaction when looking at a near target is a clear sign that impaired accommodation may be present (Saunders et al. 2008). If hyoscine skin patches are being used to diminish salivation, absence of accommodation is likely, and in children with sufficient vision, spectacles are required if the medication is to be continued (Firth and Walker 2006; Saeed et al. 2007).

For an initial formal assessment of functional vision (with both eyes open), the child is best assessed in a room free from clutter and noise. Others in the room are asked to observe in silence, unless invited to contribute. Assessment is ideally carried out when the child is calm, in a position known to be comfortable and relaxing, wearing appropriate spectacle correction and free from seizures.

Table 8.1 Inventory of questions asked for children with profound cerebral visual impairment

Visual skills inventory			
Name:			
Please help us by answering the questions relevant to your child and bring this to your next visit.			
Spectacles			
Please tick			
		Yes	No
1.	Should your child wear spectacles?		
2.	Does he/she wear them?		
Patching			
3.	Does your child wear an eye patch?		
4.	Is it difficult to patch the eye?		
5.	Do you understand why your child's eye is patched?		
Vision			
6.	Does your child follow your movements around a room when you give him/her no sound clues?		
7.	Does he/she react to you approaching him (without sound clues)?		
8.	Does he/she react to a light being switched on? (making sure there is no sound of the switch)		
9.	Does he/she screw up his eyes when taken into bright sunlight?		
10.	Does he/she return your smile when you smile without any sound?		
11.	Does your child reach for a drink bottle when you hold it in front of him/her?		
	Does he/she become excited but does not reach for the drink bottle?		
12.	Is he/she aware of a spoonful of food coming towards his/her mouth?		
	If yes do you think he/she sees it?		
	Smells it?		
	Or both?		
13:	Is he/she aware of himself in a mirror?		
	If yes at what distance: 6 feet?		
	4 feet?		
	3 feet?		
	2 feet?		
	1 foot?		
	Less?		
Please tick			
		Yes	No
14	Does your child reach for a small bright noisy object?		
	For example, rattle, slinky		
15	Does your child reach for a large bright noisy object?		
16	Does your child reach for a small bright silent object?		
17	Does your child reach for a large bright silent object?		

(continued)

Table 8.1 (continued)

18	Does he/she see a large silent bright object, e.g. ball?		
	If yes at what distance: 1 foot?		
	2 feet?		
	3 feet?		
	4 feet?		
	More?		
19	Does he/she see a small silent bright object, e.g. toy?		
	If yes at what distance: 12 inches?		
	6 inches?		
	3 inches?		
	Nearer?		
20	Does your child's vision seem better in bright light?		
	Dim light?		
21	Do you think your child knows and recognises your face?		
22	Does he/she recognise other faces of familiar people?		

Initial observation takes place as the child enters the room. The position of the eyes and their movements are observed. If the eyes move to give attention, the question is what are the features (in terms of dimensions and detail and distance away) of what is being looked at? A big silent smile is given to the child at different distances. If a reciprocal smile is evoked, the distance at which this takes place is estimated, as this may prove the only successful 'test' performed in some cases. The data in Table 8.2 provide a means of interpreting this information in terms of approximate visual acuity.

Visual field assessment entails seeking reactions in each of the visual field quadrants, using silent targets that have already been found to be visible. The aim is to find out which part of the visual field is most reproducibly receptive, so that it can subsequently be employed optimally.

Estimation of visual acuity is performed with methods chosen to match the child's visual, attentional and intellectual capacities. These include preferential looking using the acuity card procedure and assessment of visual evoked potentials designed to estimate acuity (Good 2001). Where there is hemianopia, hemi-inattention or lower visual field impairment, preferential looking methods are adapted accordingly, so that they employ the intact visual field.

Estimation of contrast sensitivity and colour vision can also be evaluated using preferential looking methods (see Chap. 6) but may not prove feasible.

8.5.2.1 Interpretation of Results

The limits at which visual attention is given reflect the optimum visual acuity under test conditions. Acuities determined by preferential looking or by visual evoked potentials can significantly overestimate functional visual acuity, and although the measures may be considered a lower limit of potential visual function under optimal

Table 8.2 Visual acuity values related to the maximum distance at which infants and young children give attention to themselves in a mirror (Bowman et al. 2010)

Age (days)	Teller acuity (cycles/degree)	Snellen acuity equivalent	Mirror distance (cm) [fixation/reflected distance (2×)]	95th percentile lower confidence limit (cm)
1.29 [31 h]	0.33	6/540	15.5 [31]	13 [26]
14.1 [2 wk]	1	6/180	38.2 [76.4]	24.5 [49]
43.7 [6 wk]	2	6/90	57.2 [115]	37 [74]
79.4 [11 wk]	3	6/60	72.5 [145]	47 [94]
126 [4.2 mo]	4	6/45	85.5 [171]	55.5 [111]
177 [5.8 mo]	5	6/36	97.5 [195]	62.5 [125]
512[a] [17 mo]	10	6/18	147 [294]	93.5 [187]
2951[a] [8 yr]	30	6/6	279 [558]	180.5 [361]

Equivalent grating, Snellen and mirror distance acuities are given for different ages. The 'fixation/reflected distance' allows one to give an approximate estimate of acuity derived from the maximum distance at which eye contact can be established

h hours, *wk* weeks, *mo* months, *yr* years

[a]Extrapolated beyond age range of study subjects

conditions, the functional acuity may be considerably lower, and this needs to be carefully taken into account.

8.5.2.2 Evaluation of Visual Attention

Volitional attention can be impaired by frontal and thalamic pathology, medication, somnolence, mood and seizures. Damage to the fronto-parietal pathways means that competition of incoming information in complex visual scenes or between the senses can lead to auditory noise and physical discomfort, swamping any hitherto evident visual responses. Eliminating clutter, the background noise and discomfort can bring about visual attention.

8.5.2.3 The Effects of Lighting

Improvement of vision and visual attention under dim lighting conditions is described in some children with profound CVI, and visual attentional responses in daylight/room lighting and diminished lighting are compared to seek evidence of this behaviour (Good and Hou 2006).

8.5.2.4 Estimation of the Temporal Limits of Perception

Children with MDVI (multiple disabilities and visual impairment) can show a variety of responses to verbal and visual information.

Parents are always asked whether the child can understand what is said. Speaking with the parents while in front of the child, while progressively slowing the voice and prolonging consonants as well as vowels, can often elicit an attentional response that is consistently lost on speeding up again (Tallal et al. 1996).

The range of speeds at which a moving target, such as a favoured toy that is known to be visible, is attended to is observed.

These functional abilities are all recorded, taught to carers and subsequently employed to best advantage.

8.6 Behaviours Associated with CVI

Rocking to and fro is commonly observed. In some children with profound visual impairment due to CVI, it appears purposeful and may compensate for akinetopsia.

Light gazing can be observed in children with profound visual impairment (Jan et al. 1990).

Distress on car journeys is sought on history taking. This can be due to a range of reasons. Some children with MDVI can be remarkably prescient in recognising when the wrong route has been taken and need to be forewarned. Others become distressed when driving through built-up or lit environments. The use of 'wrap-around' polarising ski glasses has been described by many parents as proving effective in preventing or alleviating the distress, perhaps because it diminishes the incoming flickering visual input. Headphones that either mask sound or provide favourite music are also described as proving helpful.

8.7 Management

Experiences need to be enhanced to ensure they are perceptible, attractive, meaningful and engaging. Multiply disabled visually impaired (MDVI) children show a range of visual, motor and intellectual abilities. Once these functional abilities have been elicited, they need to be employed to best advantage, particularly at school, and the following approaches, matched to the child's individual needs, can bear fruit.

Distraction is minimised by ensuring that comfort is ensured, clutter is removed and the cacophony (for them) of background sound is eliminated.

Communication with the child is clear, meaningful, referenced to the child's current and past experience, and matched to (a), the child's known vocabulary, (b), what is known the child knows and understands, and (c), the child's processing speed.

Materials used are rendered visible (where possible) by ensuring that each element of each toy or picture is matched in size to the estimated functional visual acuity. For the child with impaired movement vision (dyskinetopsia), speed of movement is maintained within the visible range, while for those who appear to see the moving image only, this too is catered for. For those with absent or very low vision, both tactile and auditory methods of affording knowledge of the surroundings are used to best advantage (Fazzi et al. 2011).

Impaired parallel processing ('simultanagnostic' visual dysfunction) is recognised. The sphere of attention reflects the distance and location at which information is perceptible with respect to acuity, visual field and attention. This dimension is determined and worked within. Tents and the sensory room environment have their place. Such approaches are applied as means of gaining, maintaining and employing attention effectively.

Eye movement disorders are taken into account. Tonic deviation of the eyes can preclude giving attention by means of central vision. Impaired pursuit, tracking and saccadic eye movements impair foveation, and this is recognised and catered for.

The speed of working with the child is matched to their speed of perceiving, attending, reacting and potentially learning. Turn taking is matched in this way so as to facilitate and optimise social interaction.

The use of language is optimised initially to ensure that it refers to the experiences of the child and thereby has meaning. Concepts primarily learned through visual experience, such as those conveyed by verbs, nouns and prepositions, are carefully communicated by affording the child direct experience of the meaning of each 'new word', for example, using the word spoon just after it has been picked up and while it is being explored.

Progression is always made through what is known that the child already knows and can do. Knowledge and understanding are gained in this way. This necessitates affording accessibility at the same time as providing meaning to the surrounding environment. The developing child with low vision is at risk of developing tactile defensiveness as a sequel to being injured. Parental training in how to help the child to initially reach out along the 'safe' adult hand as it moves to find interesting things to explore is a well-recognised technique. Parents need to be helped not to do everything for the child, but instead to encourage and bring about as much independence as possible given the individual circumstances. Advance preparation of safe environments allows the young child with very low vision to gain attention, explore and learn. As skills are learned, they are progressively capitalised upon.

Seizure activity in the visual brain is not uncommon in children with severe CVI. Loss of prior visual functional skills is a sign that seizure activity may need to be sought and treated. Moreover, grand mal seizures are commonly followed by diminished visual function for hours and sometimes days.

Training programmes founded on careful assessment, such that described by Christine Roman-Lantzy (2007), provide structure and guidance for teachers and families. By ensuring that for as much time as possible, information that the child is receiving, is being given is perceptible and manageable, the children will not miss out on their 'learning journey'. The 'jury is still out' on whether visual training programmes are effective, and future randomised trials have been advocated (Williams et al. 2014).

A Developmental Journal for babies and children with visual impairment is available for free from the British National Archive at http://webarchive.nationalarchives.gov.uk/20130401151715/https://www.education.gov.uk/publications/standard/publicationDetail/Page1/ES50#downloadableparts.

This document provides a detailed guide for professionals and parents concerning parenting and teaching approaches for children with marked visual impairment.

Conclusion

Infants with profound cerebral visual impairment need to be identified early (Dutton and Jacobson 2001; Good et al. 2001) and appropriate intervention and support provided as soon as possible. The evidence base for early intervention for these children is limited (Lueck 2006), but early intervention is known to have a positive impact on learning and development for infants and young children with other disabilities (Guralnick 1998, 2011). Parents need to train in specific parenting strategies from trained professionals who give them insight into what their child is seeing and who recognise and take into account the emotional difficulties of having had a young child with such disabilities.

Case Reports

9

In this chapter, case reports of children are presented as illustrations of the broad spectrum of cerebral visual impairments subsumed under the umbrella term CVI, which may also serve as a kind of guideline for diagnostic assessment and for intervention. Systematic and standardised procedures enable comprehensive assessment and documentation of all relevant functions, while an individualised tailor-made management strategy taking developmental stage into consideration is required for each child. This approach provides a basis for later comparison of the child's developmental stages at the time of follow-up assessment. Moreover, therapists can easily share their experiences of children with CVI, when they employ the same or at least similar standards of assessment and intervention.

As many children with CVI show additional impairments in other domains (see Chap. 5), a diagnostic and interventional approach that combines the various domains affected is apposite. Such an interdisciplinary approach often requires continuing adjustment and reconciliation of the various procedures and steps. Most children with CVI spend much of their time at home, in familiar surroundings and with familiar people; supportive practice and special education measures may therefore also be provided at home. However, the inclusion of non-professionals in the interventional program means that clear and exact information is needed as to how they can support the overall intervention in terms of enriched environments and systematic practice, as well as modify their parenting to meet both the visual and overall needs to their child. Accurate instructions and feedback on the applicability of such additional practice measures, on favourable and non-favourable stimulus and task conditions, and on outcome criteria in terms of aims of intervention are important. Regular meetings and updates from both sides can help to establish and optimise such a combined approach.

Before intervention and special education measures are planned and started, a comprehensive assessment is performed to gain a valid individual characterisation of spared and impaired functions. This diagnostic information serves as the basis for selecting appropriate intervention measures for the remediation of CVI,

J. Zihl, G.N. Dutton, *Cerebral Visual Impairment in Children: Visuoperceptive and Visuocognitive Disorders*, DOI 10.1007/978-3-7091-1815-3_9

with particular consideration of associated cognitive impairments. As longer intervention periods are usually needed, one (or more) assessments are carried out. At the end of the special intervention period, a comprehensive assessment is performed, which provides comparisons with the pre-intervention assessment, and shows the degree of improvement in the various visual functions as well as other domains. For the sake of data privacy, the childrens' names have been exchanged. We are grateful to Professor Siegfried Priglinger, former Head of the Pediatric Ophthalmology Unit in the Hospital of the Hospitaller in Linz (Austria) for reporting cases 1 and 2 and permission to report them here by JZ. Cases 3–6 are contributed by JZ, and cases 7 and 8 by GD.

9.1 Case 1: Lisa

9.1.1 Medical Diagnoses

- Hypoxic encephalopathy
- Bilateral partial optic atrophy
- Severe visual impairment
- Bilateral hypermetropic astigmatism
- Cerebral spastic tetra paresis
- Epileptic seizures
- MRI imaging showed multifocal cerebral pathology with bilateral occipital lobe infarction

Lisa had initially shown normal development, without any known visual or mental abnormalities but at the age of 4 months, she had suffered acute apnoea causing diffuse cerebral injury, and consequently multiple functional impairments, including CVI. Lisa was hospitalised for 17 months. Detailed medical examination at the age of 7.5 months revealed severe multiple disorders. At the age of 2 years she returned home to her family. At this stage, her vision was assessed in detail and regular visual intervention was started.

9.1.2 Developmental Status at the Age of 2 Years (Before Intervention)

9.1.2.1 Visual Assessment (Table 9.1)

Direct and indirect pupil responses were present. Orienting responses could be reliably elicited with a large light stimulus (a halogen lamp with a diameter of 10 cm at a distance of 80 cm). OKN was positive, when elicited with black and white stripes of at least 10 cm in width. Visual field, form, colour and object vision could not be assessed. The visual acuity was not measurable.

Table 9.1 Visual and oculomotor assessment in case 1 (Lisa) before (1st assessment) and after visual intervention (2nd assessment)

Function	1st assessment	2nd assessment
Light–dark response	+	+
Photophobia	–	–
Visual field (binocular)	(–)	(–)
Visual acuity (equivalent)	Keeler cc 2/60	Keeler sc 3/60
Colour vision	(–)	(–)
Object vision	(–)	(–)
Pupil responses	+	+
Visual lid reflex	+	+
Auditory lid reflex	+	+
Eye position	In alignment	In alignment
Convergence	(?)	(?)
Head position	Permanent rightwards	Permanent rightwards
Fixation	Central fixation (?)	Central position (?)
Nystagmus	End-gaze nystagmus	End-gaze nystagmus
Orienting responses	+	+
Oculomotor motility	No gross abnormalities	No gross abnormalities
Spontaneous exploration	–	+
Pursuit eye movements	–	(?)
Saccadic shifts	–	–
OKN	+	+

+: positive/present, (?) positive/present, but not very reliable, – negative absent, (–): not testable. For further details, see text

9.1.2.2 Further Assessment

Auditory perception: prompt and reliable responses were obtained to sounds and speech, with orienting responses towards the stimulus source, and sustained focussed attention to such stimuli. Lisa seemed to rely mainly on the audition as her principal input modality.

Tactile perception: grasp reflex was positive; she responded promptly and reliably to vibration.

Attention: there was no sign of attentional difficulties in the auditory modality.

Language: no production of utterances.

Motor functions: Quadraparesis. Head control negative, with preferred head position to the right. Sitting was possible, but only with external support of head and body control; her adopted preferred body position was supine.

Social behaviour: Lisa showed little or no social interaction.

9.1.2.3 Summary

Lisa exhibited profound developmental impairment in all modalities. Her visual capacity was limited to detection of bright light stimuli at a distance of 80 cm, indicating a severe form of CVI (corresponding to legal blindness).

The first phase of intervention comprised measures aimed at enhancing her overall mental and physical condition. Given the severity and multiplicity of functional impairments, it was clear to all experts that systematic intervention would need to take place over a considerable time before Lisa could gain any significant improvement in activities of daily life. A tailor-made intervention programme, appropriate for her developmental stage, was developed with the main aim of improving her mental and visual capacities for everyday life activities. Intervention measures were carried out for 1–2 h daily 5 days a week, where possible.

9.1.3 Intervention Plan and Outcome

9.1.3.1 First Year of Intervention

For the initial intervention, presentation of visual stimuli was accompanied by acoustic cues (noises) to indicate the location of the visual stimulus. Lisa was placed in her most comfortable head and body positions such that she was able to direct her attention and fixate straight ahead towards the screen, where large, highly saturated colour surfaces (red, green, yellow, blue, etc.) were shown to her in alternating order at a distance of 50–100 cm, until she directed her gaze towards the stimulus. By using, this procedure of stimulus presentation, Lisa could maintain her attention for at least 15 min; moving visual stimuli enhanced her attention and her attempts to fixate. In addition to this visual 'stimulation', Lisa was afforded perceptual experiences with auditory stimuli (e.g. rhythmical tunes), tactile vibrations, and gustatory and olfactory stimuli. The balanced order of presentation of stimuli in the different sensory modalities also improved Lisa's overall interest and attention span. In the next phase, Lisa was motivated to acquire her own perceptual experiences in a small room that was particularly adapted for her actual visual capacities. This room contained coloured and glittering foils and mobiles at various spatial positions and allowed diverse visual and tactile and body experiences in a spatially limited environment. Once Lisa could manage spatial orientation in this little room (and it was no longer of sufficient interest), she was given similar visual experiences in larger rooms, including her own nursery. However, for distances greater than 2 m she still relied exclusively on acoustic cues. Intervention times varied between 60 and 120 min daily (session duration: 20–30 min), depending on Lisa's daily condition.

9.1.3.2 Second Year of Intervention

Once Lisa had gained basic visual and other perceptual experiences and had shown longer periods of attention and interest, the next step in the intervention programme was systematic practice with visual fixation and visual discrimination in a room with normal daylight. For the practice with visual fixation, small light stimuli (diameter: 1 cm at a distance of 20 cm) were shown to Lisa in primary (straight ahead) position, then the position was changed to the left or right, with varying distances from the midline. Practice periods usually lasted 15 min. For practice with visual discrimination, checkerboard patterns, gratings and dot patterns on dark background were shown on slides at a distance of 20–50 cm, either singly to one side, or as a pair on either side. Intervention times varied between 60 and 120 min daily (session duration: 20–30 min), depending on Lisa's daily interest and attention level. Lisa showed slow but consistent improvements in orienting responses, fixation stability and in differential responses to stimulus patterns. In addition to the practice in the visual modality, speech therapy and physiotherapy continued to improve her language capacities and her motor functions.

After 16 months of intervention, Lisa was integrated in a kindergarten for children with special needs (by which time she was 3 years old), but the visual intervention programme was continued in addition. Lisa now preferred structured visual materials like patterns, and was very interested in differences between patterns. She could now also sit upright and control her head position, and was able to reach out and grasp for objects (ball, luminescent ring) with either hand and manipulate them with both hands together. Visual objects were always positioned in the central position in front of her to enhance integration of body and visual midline perception.

9.1.4 Developmental Status After 2 Years of Intervention

9.1.4.1 Visual Assessment (Table 9.1)

Most of the visual and oculomotor functions were unchanged, except for orienting responses that had become prompt and reliable, to weaker and smaller light stimuli (normal light with a diameter of 1 cm) at a distance of 80 cm. Fixation attempts were sometimes successful with her normal head posture. Pursuit eye movements to large (diameter: 1–2 cm) and bright light stimuli were improved, but could not always be reliably elicited. OKN could now be reliably elicited with 5 cm wide stripes.

9.1.4.2 Further Assessment

Auditory perception: prompt and reliable responses developed to noises and speech.
Tactile perception: grasp reflex positive, but reduced.
Attention: improved intensity and selectivity in the visual modality.
Language: production of utterances; comments with varying prosody were uttered to sensory stimuli.
Motor functions: quadraparesis. Head control was positive in supine position; sitting in upright position this was still impossible without external support.
Social behaviour: Lisa was now very sociable and intentionally sought social contact with other children.

9.1.5 Further Aims of Intervention and Special Education

In accord with Lisa's developmental stage and persisting quadraparesis, optic nerve atrophy and epileptic seizures, the final significant step of intervention was the maintenance of her acquired visual and mental capacities and their use in everyday life activities.

9.1.5.1 Comment

Lisa was a child with normal development until the age of 4 months when she suffered chronic brain hypoxia and consequently severe multiple functional handicaps. After systematic and regular interdisciplinary intervention for nearly 24 months Lisa showed differential improvement in several domains, but visual perceptual capacity remained low. Whether an earlier start of intervention measures would have resulted in a better outcome remains open to question. Lisa did not however possess the prerequisites that are crucial for an earlier systematic visual training, in particular concerning the control of head position and controlled gaze shifts. Furthermore, atrophy of both optic nerves may have been the principal limiting factor for the recovery of visual acuity as well as fixation accuracy. Considering these circumstances, the intervention programme can nevertheless be deemed successful, at least in part, because it facilitated Lisa to now collect visual experiences in her familiar surroundings, to manifest a degree of visual orientation in familiar rooms, to play with her favourite toys, and to interact socially with familiar people, as well as other children and adults.

9.2 Case 2: Barbara

9.2.1 Medical Diagnoses

- Severe closed head trauma, with diffuse brain injury
- Global motor impairments
- Cerebral visual impairment
- Partial atrophy of both optic nerves

Barbara was severely injured at the age of 7 months by a car while she was lying in her pushchair/pram. Her development before the accident had been normal, with no visual or mental abnormalities.

9.2.2 Status of Development at the Age of 7 Months (Before Intervention)

9.2.2.1 Visual Assessment (Table 9.2)

Visual and oculomotor functions were largely negative/absent, except for intact pupil responses and light–dark responses. Barbara's fixation was impaired by jerky horizontal nystagmus, and her head position was permanently shifted to the left side.

Table 9.2 Visual and oculomotor assessment in case 2 (Barbara) before (1st assessment) and after visual intervention (2nd assessment)

Function	1st assessment	2nd assessment
Light–dark response	(?)	+
Photophobia	–	–
Visual field (binocular)	(–)	(–)
Visual acuity (equivalent)	(–)	(?)
Colour vision	(–)	+
Object vision	(–)	(?)
Pupil responses	+ (Slowed)	+ (Prompt)
Visual lid reflex	–	+
Auditory lid reflex	+	+
Eye position	Divergent (~30°)	Divergent
Convergence	–	+
Head position	Permanent leftwards	Mostly rightwards
Fixation	–	+
Nystagmus	Jerky horizontal nystagmus	Pendular nystagmus
Orienting responses	–	+
Oculomotor motility	(–)	+
Spontaneous exploration	–	+
Pursuit eye movements	–	+
Saccadic shifts	–	+
OKN	–	–

+: positive/present, (?) positive/present, but not very reliable, – negative absent, (–): not testable. For further details, see text

9.2.2.2 Further Assessment

Auditory perception: prompt and reliable responses to sounds, with slow orienting responses towards the stimulus source.

Tactile perception: grasp reflex negative; responds promptly and reliably to vibration.

Attention: reduced attention (maintenance and concentration) in the auditory modality.

Language: production of utterances.

Motor functions: no evidence of significant motor dysfunction. Sitting was possible without external support of head and body control.

Social behaviour: Barbara showed reliable social responses, for example, smiling to friendly voices and to music.

9.2.2.3 Summary

Barbara showed profound functional impairments in all modalities. Initially her visual capacity seemed completely lost, but the apparent absence of responses even to light stimuli may also have been explained in part by her oculomotor difficulties and her severely reduced mental functions. In the context of her intact pupil responses and normal optic nerve examination her visual condition can be described as cerebral blindness. However, she subsequently showed good recovery particularly in the domains of visual curiosity, attention and motor functions.

9.2.3 Visual Intervention Programme

Visual intervention was started when Barbara was 8 months old; at this time her state of attention, her curiosity and her social interaction had improved considerably. Intervention measures were mainly carried out at home by Barbara's mother, with continuous supervision by an optometrist.

The main aim of the first phase of intervention was to enhance Barbara's visual curiosity and use of visual stimuli. Clear instructions concerning vision therapy in the familiar surroundings were given to her mother, but also to other family members. Practice with visual stimuli was carried out several times daily; duration of practice varied between 10 and 20 min.

The following visual stimulus categories (size: >20° in diameter at a distance of 30–40 cm) were initially used:

- Light spots differing in colour for eliciting and enhancing reliable orienting responses,
- Black–white patterns (gratings, checkerboard patterns) with stepwise reduction of the size of elements to match but remain well within visual discrimination as it improved,
- Coloured stimuli (red, green, blue, yellow, white, black) with high saturation for improving colour discrimination,
- High contrast pictures showing real simple objects, for improving visual interest and object vision.

Furthermore, Barbara regularly received proprioceptive, vestibular and tactile stimulation for her reliably improving somatosensory responsivity and body control. Epileptic seizures were treated with antiepileptic medication and abated by the age of 3 years.

Until her third year of life, Barbara used her near vision only to reach out and grasp for objects she could locate; after successfully grasping an object she palpated and also examined it with her mouth. From the fourth year on, Barbara began to stand upright with some support. In addition, she became able to fixate objects more often with both eyes and to focus her attention upon them; she also began to develop an increasing interest in people in general, and in faces in particular. By the age of 6 years Barbara intentionally scanned her surroundings with eye and head movements, and focused upon people and objects for increasingly longer periods. Visual orientation also developed, and Barbara became able to go for walks, albeit slowly with the help of her mother or a family member, and could discriminate between the path and lawn.

9.2.4 Developmental Status at the Age 6 Years (After Intervention)

9.2.4.1 Visual Assessment (Table 9.2)

Barbara showed improvements with respect to visual and oculomotor functions. Orienting responses to large moving and stationary visual stimuli (e.g. hand movements) could reliably be observed. A low level of visual acuity was now present; Barbara responded reliably to balls of 5 mm in diameter at a distance of 20 cm, and showed pursuit eye movements to such stimuli, provided that sufficient concentration was available. She also showed differential responses to coloured stimuli of high contrast and high saturation, and to coloured forms and objects with a diameter of 1 cm at a distance of 20 cm. Accurate fixation was present for very brief periods (1–2 s), however, this was impaired by intermittent pendular nystagmus, and by her still unstable head position, whereby the head was now mostly directed rightwards. Saccadic eye movements to moving stimuli in the periphery were consistently prompt and accurate in all directions.

9.2.4.2 Further Assessment

Audition: reliable differential responses to simple verbal instructions.

Sensorimotor functions: Eye-hand coordination was positive; Barbara could reach and grasp for food (e.g. a piece of bread or of an apple) and accurately guide her right hand with food to her mouth.

Motor functions: Very positive motor development. From her fourth year of life Barbara was able to stand upright and walk with limited support.

Language: Barbara developed several utterances and uses them as her means of communication with her family.

Social development: Her early often manifest, stereotyped behaviours disappeared, nearly completely. In the kindergarten, Barbara appeared to often become overcharged by multi-tasking conditions and showed features of auto-aggressive behaviour. Her ability to integrate with a group remained limited.

9.2.4.3 Comment

Barbara was a child with normal development until the age of 7 months when she was hit by a car and suffered severe closed head trauma with chronic hypoxia and severe multiple functional handicaps. After systematic and regular interdisciplinary intervention for nearly 6 years Barbara showed good functional recovery including in the visual domain, with improved visual orienting responses, oculomotor behaviour, visual acuity, spatial orientation and object recognition. However, language and social development were still considerably impaired. It seems that brain injury had affected, in particular, her functional system in the prefrontal and limbic structures involved in regulation and control of attention and affect. This may explain her low level of frustration tolerance and her auto-aggressive behaviour, and may also have impeded better visual and cognitive development. Furthermore, atrophy of both optic nerves may have limited further improvement in visual acuity beyond about 6/36. Nonetheless, the intervention effects can be evaluated as positive because Barbara ultimately became able to collect visual experiences of her surroundings, possessed visual orientation in familiar rooms, could play with her favourite toys, and liked social interactions with familiar people, as well as other children and adults.

9.3 Case 3: Anna

9.3.1 Medical Diagnoses

- Hypoxic encephalopathy
- Bilateral diffuse occipital injury
- Severe visual impairment (suspected cerebral blindness)
- Left-sided hemiparesis
- Severe intellectual deficit had been given as a potential prognosis

At the age of 6 years, Anna suffered blunt abdominal trauma with duodenal rupture due to a road traffic accident. During her initial medical first aid she sustained a cardiac arrest resulting in acute circulatory collapse and apnoea. Anna was hospitalised for several weeks in an intensive care unit and eventually gained full consciousness, which allowed comprehensive functional assessment. Before the accident, Anna had shown good development and had completed her first year of elementary schooling; she had been able to read and write well for her age. There was no prior history of visual or mental abnormalities.

9.3.1.1 Visual Assessment Before Intervention (Table 9.3)

Anna showed a large homonymous central scotoma, with a diameter of ~40° (see Fig. 9.1a). Visual acuity, colour vision and object vision could not be tested, although Anna reported coloured and black–white impressions when confronted with large colour or form stimuli or with large objects. Her fixation was highly unstable and inaccurate, although she tried hard to find each stimulus and keep her eyes on it. Eye alignment was slightly divergent (~10°), but no nystagmus was present. Anna tried to scan the visual environment spontaneously, but without great success.

9.3.1.2 Further Assessment

Auditory perception: positive, no abnormalities.

Tactile perception: positive, no abnormalities

Attention: intensity and selectivity were not impaired.

Memory: was not impaired. Anna could describe from memory the shape and colour of familiar objects (e.g. fruit, toys)

Language: comprehension and production of language were not impaired. Anna could describe her visual impressions in great detail.

Table 9.3 Visual and oculomotor assessment in case 3 (Anna) before (1st assessment) and after visual intervention (2nd and 3rd assessment)

Function	1st assessment	2nd assessment	3rd assessment
Light–dark response	+	+	+
Photophobia	+	+	+
Visual field (binocular)	CS (diam: ~40°)	CS (diam: ~20°)	CS (diam: ~20°)
Visual acuity	(–)	0.01 (s)	0.05 (s)
Colour vision	(–)	+	+
Object vision	(–)	(?)	(?)
Pupil responses	+ (Slowed)	+ (Prompt)	+
Visual lid reflex	+ (Slowed)	+	+
Auditory lid reflex	+	+	+
Eye position	Divergent (~10°)	Divergent (~7°)	Divergent (~6°)
Convergence	–	(?)	(?)
Head position	Left-, rightwards	Left-, rightwards	Left-, rightwards
Fixation	Highly inaccurate	+ (Eccentric)	+ (Eccentric)
Nystagmus	–	–	–
Orienting responses	+	+	+
Oculomotor motility	+	+	+
Spontaneous exploration	+	+	+
Pursuit eye movements	–	+ (Fragmented)	+ (Fragmented)
Saccadic shifts	Highly inaccurate	+ (Fragmented)	+ (Fragmented)
Visual localisation	Highly inaccurate	+ (Inaccurate)	+ (Inaccurate)
OKN	+	+	+

+: positive/present, (?) positive/present, but not very reliable, – negative absent, (–): not testable. *CS* Homonymous central scotoma, *diam* diameter. For further details, see text

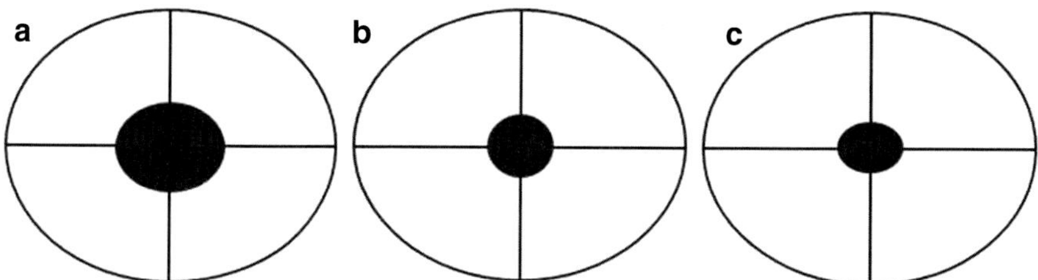

Fig. 9.1 Binocular visual field (60° plot) of Anna 6 weeks (**a**), 12 weeks (**b**) and 30 weeks (**c**) after brain injury. *Dark* areas indicate the central scotoma. Note shrinkage of the scotoma in the time period between **a** and **b**

Motor functions: left-sided hemiparesis with loss of fine motor control of the left hand; no other motor abnormalities.

Social behaviour: Anna was a friendly, curious girl, who asked questions and responded competently to questions.

9.3.1.3 Summary

Anna showed normal development until the age of 6 years. Because of her well-developed mental capacities, she had already attended elementary school and could read and write. There was no history of visual abnormalities. After her anoxic brain injury, which had mainly affected posterior brain structures, she exhibited severe visual deficits due to the loss of the central visual field, as well as left-sided hemiparesis. As her cognitive and language abilities had fully recovered 6 weeks after brain injury, systematic, regular intervention was initiated 2 weeks later. During the periods of intervention, Anna was an in-patient in a nearby hospital for children, but was transported to the Max Planck Institute of Psychiatry on a daily basis for visual training.

9.3.2 Visual Intervention Programme

Intervention measures were organised in a hierarchical order and were focused on:

- Visual localisation accuracy (fixation, pointing and grasping);
- Light–dark discrimination with increasingly demands concerning size and contrast;
- Visual orientation to improve navigation in space;
- Discrimination of forms and colours;
- Matching of visual and tactile information for object identification and recognition.

9.3.3 Visual Stimulus Materials and Task Conditions

9.3.3.1 Localisation

- Large light stimuli (diameter: 5–10 cm) at a distance of 30 cm, presented with a projector at different positions in front of Anna;
- Large objects (e.g. balls; diameter: 5 cm) with highly saturated bright colours (yellow, blue, green, red), at a distance of 30 cm on a black table.

In the first phase of practice with localisation, Anna was instructed to find a light target in front of her, fixate it and point at it but only after she could fixate it. Once she could do this more accurately, she was asked to reach for and grasp the light target. The light target was always presented at grasping distance, i.e. at 30 cm, but in different directions (midline, and in various directions to the left and right of the midline); the presentation time was about 8–10 s in the initial sessions, and 2–5 s once Anna could point at and grasp the target more accurately.

In the second phase of practice with localisation, Anna was asked to reach out for and grasp objects positioned on a desk either in front of her or at varying distances to the left or right of her midline. She was asked to look straight-ahead at first, and then to search for the object and fixate it, and eventually to grasp it. The order of presentation initially followed an order known to Anna, i.e. mid position, left, right, mid position, right, left, etc. Later, the order of positions was made unpredictable.

9.3.4 Visual Discrimination and Identification

For brightness discrimination, Anna was asked to tell the difference between pairs of light squares (presented on slides), brightness being varied by using calibrated grey filters. To practice form and colour discrimination, pairs of simple patterns (horizontal and vertical gratings of varying spatial frequency within the developing thresholds of measured visual acuity), forms (circle vs. square) and colours (circles in green vs. red, blue vs. yellow, etc.) were used. Stimuli were either paired with greys or with a stimulus of the same category, and were either identical or differed with respect to orientation and frequency (gratings), shape (form) or colour. Stimuli had a diameter of 30 cm and were always shown at a distance of 1 m in front of Anna. Anna was asked to tell whether the pair consisted of the same or different stimuli.

To make visual training more diverse and more interesting, discrimination of forms/shapes and colours was carried out alternating with practice with visual localisation. Every time that Anna felt somehow that she knew the nature of the visual stimulus, she reported it; however, she was asked to always describe the differences between stimuli first.

The following procedures of bringing about perceptual learning were used:

- Find the difference in paired stimulus presentation: (1) are the two stimuli the same or different (brightness, contours, shapes, colours), (2) which stimulus is brighter (or darker), (3) which stimulus shows a structure (e.g. grey vs. vertical or horizontal stripes, requiring an acuity of <0.02 (logMAR 1.6), (4) which stimulus is coloured, and what colour is it, (5) which stimulus is a circle or a square?
- Find similarity/identity: identify identical targets (within acuity limits) and take the odd one out. Which stimulus differs from the other two stimuli? Which stimuli are similar/identical? The position of the odd stimulus was varied systematically.
- Identify the stimulus: (1) which stimulus shows a pattern, (2) which gratings are horizontal/vertical, larger or smaller, (3) which stimulus is a circle, a square, a rectangle, a star, etc., (4) which stimulus has a definite colour (e.g. red vs. yellow), (5) which stimulus (circle or square; diameter: 5 cm) has two colours (e.g. red-yellow vs. blue), (6) which stimulus (circle or square; diameter: 5 cm) has two definite colours (e.g. red-yellow vs. green-blue).

9.3.5 Further Interventions

On account of her left-sided hemiparesis, Anna received daily physiotherapy and occupational therapy to improve motor functions and capacities including body care, dressing, eating, and mobility. When carrying out their exercises, the physiotherapist and the occupational therapist considered the actual state of Anna's visual capacities, and integrated parts of visual practice, for example, first looking at body parts and objects and fixating them briefly before moving or carrying out an action.

9.3.6 First Phase of Treatment and Outcome

The first phase of visual intervention lasted 6 weeks, with at least two treatment sessions lasting 30–45 min daily at about the same time of day (usually between 10 and 11.30 a.m.). Anna was always highly motivated to carry out the various visual and visuo-motor tasks. According to the concept of 'errorless learning', Anna was informed before each session, that she would get immediate feedback to her responses in terms of yes/no. For Anna, the best reinforcement for yes responses was operating the slide projector to show the next slide.

9.3.7 Visual Assessment (See Table 9.3)

After 6 weeks the homonymous central scotoma had become considerably smaller; the diameter was now ~20° (see Fig. 9.1b). Her near binocular visual acuity was 0.01 (single tumbling E's). Visual localisation accuracy had also improved considerably (Fig. 9.2), although saccadic and pointing/grasping responses were still inaccurate at the end of practice, indicative of early fatiguability. A similar improvement was found for her re-learning how to visually discriminate (see Figs. 9.3 and 9.4). Anna became progressively able to more accurately discriminate smaller differences in stimulus brightness, configuration (patterns), forms and colours (Table 9.4). However, discrimination performance depended crucially on stimulus size; Anna found it very difficult to fixate stimuli with a diameter <2 cm, and could not reliably discriminate or identify them.

After the first intervention period, Anna went home to familiarise herself with her earlier surroundings and get used of her, in part, regained visual and motor capacities.

9.3.8 Second Phase of Visual Intervention and Outcome

In the second phase of visual intervention, accuracy of visual localisation, visual scanning and visual search, respectively, became the main focus of systematic practice. For further improvement of visual orientation, Anna was asked to fixate visual stimuli (mainly small objects) as accurately and as quickly as possible, and then to grasp them using a single fast arm and hand movement (ballistic movement) invoking dorsal stream function. Positions of stimuli (circles and balls, diameter: 3–5 cm) were varied at random within a stimulus array of 60 (horizontal) × 40° (vertical) at a table at a distance of 30 cm. Anna was asked to obtain first a global view of the overall scene, and only then to fixate and count the stimuli she had detected. The number of stimuli was increased from 3 to 12. In a modified version

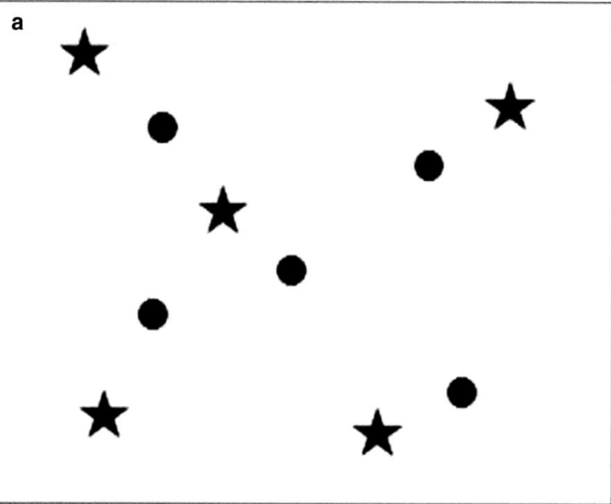

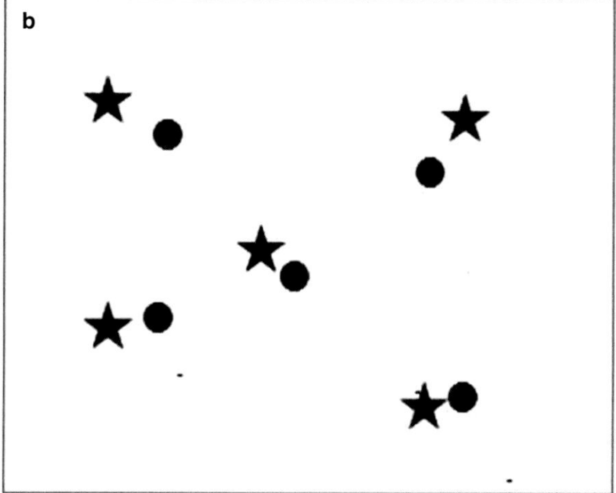

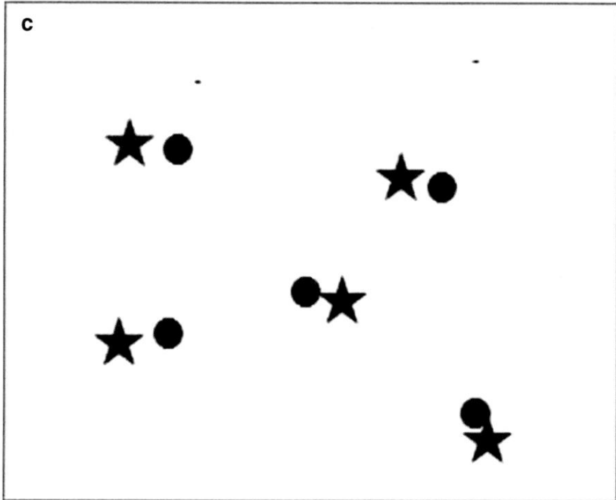

Fig. 9.2 Visual localisation (pointing responses) in Anna at three different times of assessment (**a–c**, as in Fig. 9.1). *Dots*: positions of stimuli, *Stars*: Anna's pointing responses. Stimulus diameter was 1 cm; viewing distance of 40 cm. Note improvement in localisation accuracy from **a** to **c**

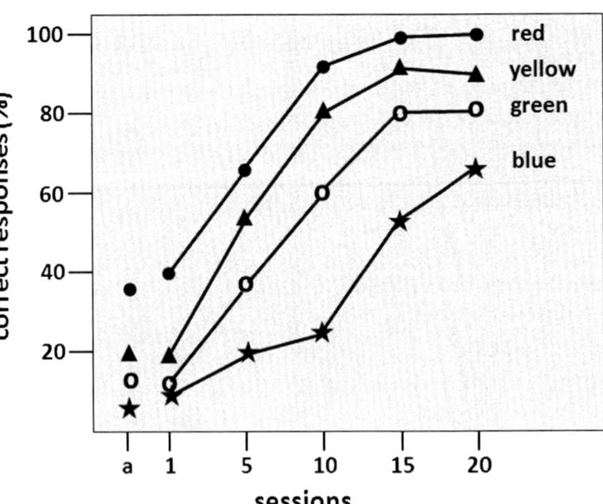

Fig. 9.3 Improvement in colour discrimination in Anna. *a*: assessment before systematic practice. In each session, Anna discriminated 60–80 pairs of colour stimuli. Note the marked overall improvement in colour discrimination, with moderate differences in the improvement between colours

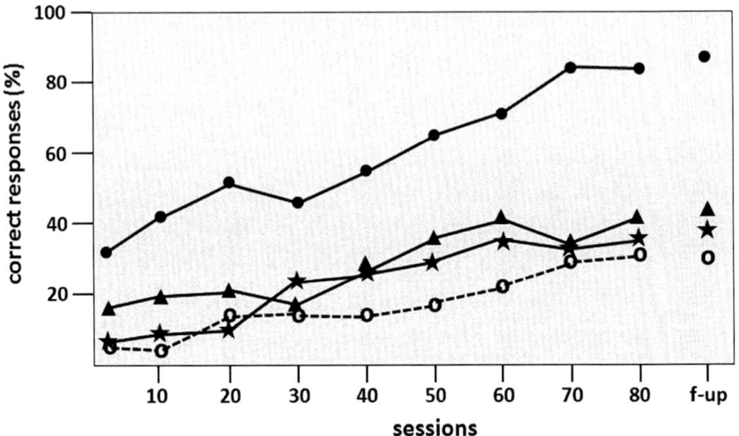

Fig. 9.4 Improvement in Anna's visual discrimination and identification performance for colours (*circles*), simple forms (*squares, triangles*), complex forms (*stars*) and letters (*open circles*). Anna showed improvement in all visual stimulus categories, but had much less difficulties to regain colour vision than form vision

of the visual scanning task, slides with dot patterns were shown at a distance of 60 cm; task and instruction were the same but Anna was asked to use a pointer to indicate the dots she had found and fixated.

In a further task version, visual search was specifically addressed by showing stimulus arrays with one target (e.g. a red circle) among several distractors (e.g. white or coloured circles, corresponding to parallel search condition). In 60 % of presentations, the target was present, for 40 %, it was absent. The set size (total number of stimuli on the screen) was systematically and progressively increased from 3 to 5, to 9, to 13 and to 15, but Anna was not informed of the total stimulus

Table 9.4 Outcome of the first visual intervention period in the case of Anna

	Before treatment	After treatment
Localisation	03	14
Brightness discrimination		
Large difference (300:10 cd/m²)	16	20
Medium difference (100:10 cd/m²)	13	19
Small difference (50:10 cd/m²)	06	15
Patterns and forms		
Gratings vs. grey	04	19
Gratings vs. gratings, frequency	01	12
Gratings vs. gratings, orientation	00	14
Circle vs. angular forms	02	18
Colours		
Colour vs. grey	11	20
Red vs. green	05	19
Blue vs. yellow	03	18
Red vs. yellow	04	19
Red vs. blue	06	20
Blue vs. green	02	17
Visual naming		
Forms (circle, square, rectangle, star)	02	16
Colours (red, green, blue, yellow)	05	18

Numbers indicate correct responses in 20 trials each. Note improvements in performance for all classes of visual stimuli after the first intervention phase. For further details, see text

Table 9.5 Improvement of visual localisation accuracy ($n=20$) and visual search performance ($n=20$) in the case of Anna

	Before practice	After practice
Localisation (hits)	09	19
Visual search		
Hits	03	07
Time (mean, in s)	46	23

Note improvement in her accuracy of visual localisation (grasping responses) and in her accuracy and speed of visual search (time for overall task) after systematic practice. For further details, see text

number. For pre–post assessments, stimulus arrays contained eight targets and seven distractors (total: 15 stimuli). Performance parameters comprised speed (search time, in seconds) and accuracy (number of hits). Table 9.5 shows the outcome of systematic practice with visual localisation and visual search. Anna improved her localisation accuracy considerably, as well as her visual search performance. These improvements allowed Anna to gain faster and more complete overview (see Fig. 9.5), which was transferable to her natural surroundings, and to navigate

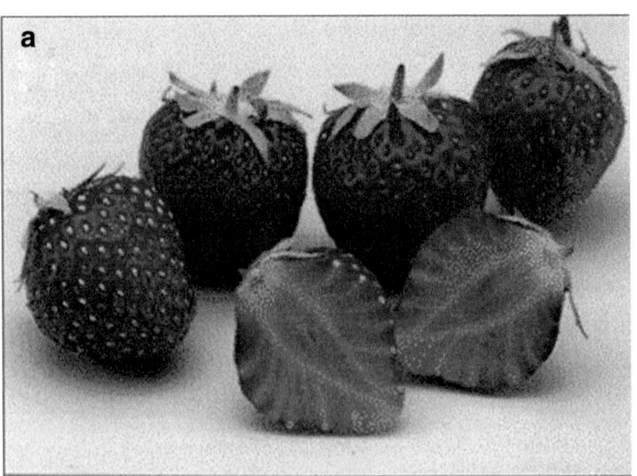

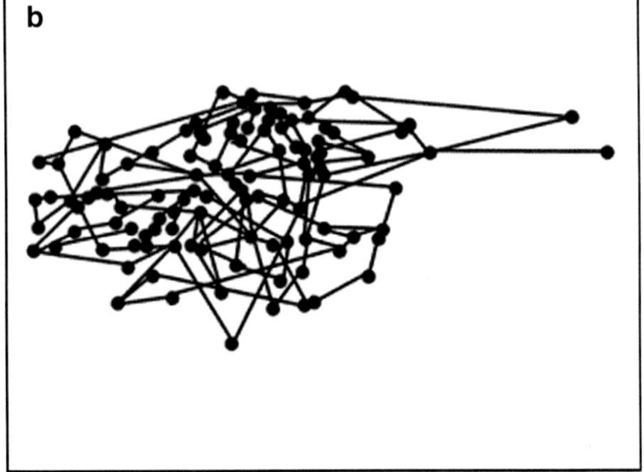

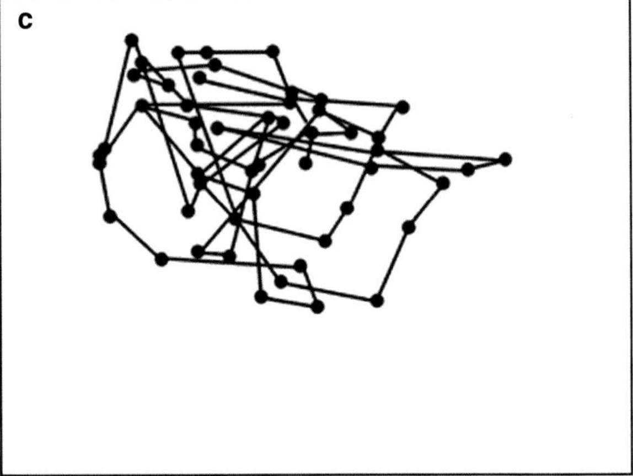

Fig. 9.5 Anna's oculomotor scanning patterns during inspection of a scene (**a**; *coloured*) containing six strawberries before (**b**) and after (**b**) the second intervention period. Anna's task was to count the objects and possibly recognise them. *Dots* in **b** and **c** indicate fixations (>0.120 s), *lines* indicate saccadic shifts. Scanning time in **b** was 59.4 s; Anna reported seeing 'three apples'. Scanning time in **c** was 28.7 s; Anna reported seeing four strawberries. Note decrease in the number of fixations and saccades, and increase in saccadic amplitudes. In addition, the scanning pattern in **c** looks better adapted to the spatial structure of the scene

Table 9.6 Outcome of systematic practice with complex forms and letters (selected items) in the case of Anna

	Before treatment	After treatment
Forms		
Open vs. filled circles	06	10
Triangle with top downwards/upwards	04	09
Cross vs. X	08	11
Open circle with black dot/cross	03	08
Square with X/x only	05	08
Letters		
O vs. I	07	10
I vs. T	06	08
L vs. D	04	06
O vs. C	05	07
L vs. T	06	09
S vs. K	05	07

Numbers indicate correct responses in 20 trials. Note that improvement in discrimination and identification performance was rather modest despite intensive systematic practice. For details, see text

better. From this time on, she preferred to find her way through the hospital corridors on her own (meanwhile she had become able to walk again, although still slowly). She also had less difficulty finding food on her plate (red with a black border), and to grasp her cup of chocolate, lemonade or water more accurately.

After systematic practice with visual localisation and visual search, training of discrimination and identification of forms and colours was carried out using smaller (size: 5 cm in diameter at a distance of 60 cm) and more complex stimuli (e.g. vertical cross vs. x; open vs. filled circle; circle with a dot (dimension within acuity level) in the centre vs. circle or dot alone, etc.). In addition, because Anna wanted also to practice with letters and digits, which she had learned prior to the accident, pairs of letters with differing degrees of similarity (e.g. O vs. I, O vs. C) were used for same-different judgments and for identification. The idea behind this was that once Anna had improved her discrimination and identification of progressively more complex forms, she would benefit from re-learning and practising letter identification.

Although some further improvement in vision was observed after 8 weeks with two sessions of 45 min each day (see Table 9.6), Anna unfortunately did not benefit in terms of reduction of the degree of her visual handicap. The diameter of the central scotoma remained more or less unchanged (Fig. 9.1c); near visual acuity was now 0.1 for simple forms (circle vs. diamond) and 0.05 for tumbling E's. Far acuity could still not be assessed because Anna could not discriminate even large targets (diameter: 10 cm) with sufficient accuracy. Furthermore, although Anna could better identify some complex forms, such as letters and digits (see Fig. 9.4) after practice, she employed guesswork rather than accurate identification, and her accuracy varied considerably between sessions. When Anna was successful, her identification time even for clearly differing letter forms such as I, O or T, took longer than 1 min, which was much too long to build a useful basis for text processing and subsequent reading. Therefore, with Anna's agreement it was decided that she would be admitted to a special education centre for visually impaired children, where she could attend school and learn Braille.

9.3.9 Summary and Comment

Anna undoubtedly has benefitted from systematic visual training, whereby it remains an open issue, whether the improvement can partly also be explained by spontaneous recovery, because intervention started soon (8 weeks) after brain injury. It can however be argued that the systematic training has at least enhanced spontaneous recovery of vision and has given Anna the chance to use her recovered visual capacities more efficiently. Although the outcome of visual intervention was limited, because Anna remained unable to correctly identify facial expressions, and could still not read words and short sentences (which she had been able to read before), her regained visual localisation and fixation, and her enlarged overview with improved visual search, enabled her to better visually grasp and understand her surroundings, and accorded her independence in everyday life activities including spatial navigation. Thus, visual intervention had at least in part a significant ecological validity.

9.4 Case 4: Florian

9.4.1 Medical Diagnoses

- Hypoxic encephalopathy, mainly affecting both occipital and frontal lobes
- Severe visual impairment (suspected cerebral blindness)
- Cerebral quadraparesis with loss of control of head and body, and ataxia
- Severe mental disability (suspected)

Florian had initially shown normal development, without any known visual or mental abnormalities, but at the age of 2 years, he suffered acute cardiac arrest causing diffuse cerebral hypoxia. He was in a comatose state for several weeks. After recovery from coma, neurological examination revealed a more or less total absence of statomotor functions and vision, but he manifested prompt responses to acoustic and somatosensory stimulation, however, without associated orienting responses. After 6 months of intensive physiotherapy, Florian had regained the ability to sit without support, and about 18 months later (i.e. at the age of about 3 years) he started walking with support. Intensive motor rehabilitation in association with concomitant global special education over the ensuing years resulted in significant improvements, including attention, language and curiosity. In contrast, vision had recovered only to the level of discrimination of light and dark.

At the age of 4 years Florian was examined concerning his visual capacities for possible specific visual intervention measures; on this occasion we also examined his cognitive capacities in more detail.

9.4.1.1 Visual Assessment at the Age of 4 Years (Table 9.7)

Florian responded promptly to visual stimuli with a diameter of >1 cm at distances of 30–50 cm. His eye alignment was slightly divergent, convergence was possible, but limited. His head position was upright with normal control. Visual fixation was possible, but inaccurate and unstable; it was more accurate for light targets than dark ones, but Florian found fixation trials (>3 s) 'very tiring'. Examination of the eyes was normal and showed normal optic nerves. Oculomotor motility was not restricted; saccadic shifts were prompt, but highly inaccurate; pursuit eye movements were absent. Confrontation testing showed concentric visual field restriction, to an extent of about 40° in both hemifields. Florian responded more slowly to stimuli presented in the central visual field (relative homonymous central scotoma?). He could correctly discriminate simple forms (circle vs. diamond) at a distance of 20 cm with assumed visual form acuity of <0.10. He could also discriminate, identify and correctly name primary colours, and could correctly discriminate between coloured and grey stimuli (diameter: 3 cm at a distance of 20 cm). In contrast, he could not discriminate between more complex forms and objects.

Table 9.7 Visual and oculomotor assessment in case 4 (Florian) at the age of 4 years (1st assessment), at 11 years (2nd assessment), and at 20 years (3rd assessment)

Function	1st assessment	2nd assessment	3rd assessment
Light–dark response	+	+	+
Photophobia	+	+	+
Visual field (binocular)	Diameter: 80°	RCS (diam: ~ 10°)	RCS (diam: ~ 3°)
Visual acuity (forms)	<0.10 (sc; 30 cm)	<0.10 (sc; 30 cm)	<0.10 (sc; 30 cm)
Colour vision	+	+	+
Object vision	(–)	+ (Large objects)	+ (Large objects)
Pupil responses	+	+	+
Visual lid reflex	+ (Slowed)	+	+
Auditory lid reflex	+	+	+
Eye position	Divergent (~3°)	Divergent (~2°)	Divergent (~2°)
Convergence	+ (Slowed)	+ (Slowed)	+ (Slowed)
Head position	Normal upright	Normal upright	Normal upright
Fixation	Inaccurate	Inaccurate	Inaccurate
Nystagmus	–	–	–
Orienting responses	+	+	+
Oculomotor motility	+	+	+
Spontaneous exploration	+ (Slowed)	+	+
Pursuit eye movements	–	+ (Fragmented)	+ (Fragmented)
Saccadic shifts	Highly inaccurate	+ (Fragmented)	+ (Fragmented)
Visual localisation	Highly inaccurate	+ (Inaccurate)	+ (Inaccurate)
OKN	+	+	+

+: positive/present, (?) positive/present, but not very reliable, – negative absent, (–): not testable. *RCS* relative central scotoma, *diam* diameter. For further details, see text

9.4.1.2 Further Assessment

Florian showed normal hearing capacities, including localisation and identification of sounds and noises. Tactile perception in particular in the hands was impaired, but motility of fingers and motor and visually guided control of finger movements was very good; Florian could manipulate toys with both hands without difficulties. Cognitive capacities and verbal comprehension and speech were normal, apart from cognitive slowing. Florian's social behaviour was also normal; there were no pronounced cognitive slowing, psychopathological symptoms.

9.4.2 Intervention Aims and Programme

The visual intervention programme was integrated in the general rehabilitation programme, and consisted of the following main components:

- Improvement of light–dark discrimination and of visual localisation (increase of accuracy of visually guided fixation, and pointing and grasping responses);
- Acquisition of visual-spatial orientation to improve navigation and mobility;
- Acquisition of basal visual discrimination ability for forms and colours;
- Matching of visual and tactile information for object identification and recognition.

The methodological approach and procedures were similar to those used for visual training with Anna. In addition to visual intervention, the other sensory modalities (audition, tactile perception, smell and taste) as well as cognitive abilities (attention, memory, language and hand motor functions) were considered and closely connected with visual impressions and activities. These intervention measures were performed daily for at least 1.5 h by a young, engaged teacher under the supervision of JZ. Physiotherapy and occupational therapy was continued.

Between 4 and 6 years of age Florian went to the regular kindergarten and was enrolled at the age of 7 years in a normal elementary school with support by a special teacher during class. Systematic visual training was continued by the same teacher as before; she reported regularly to JZ about Florian's development. Florian's visual capacities were examined again before he left elementary school at the age of 11 years, to enrol in a secondary school and eventually in a vocational school. In elementary school Florian had learned to read and write using large characters, but reading and writing was too slow and too difficult for him. Learning Braille was impossible because of the impaired tactile sensitivity and perception of his fingers. Therefore, texts were read aloud to him, and he learned to use a Dictaphone for his verbal responses. Eventually Florian was trained to use a PC system with an enlarged and specially adapted keyboard.

9.4.2.1 Visual Assessment at the Age of 11 Years (Table 9.7)

Visual field examination (Tübingen Perimeter; target diameter: 69 min of arc, target luminance: 102 cd/m^2, background luminance: 3.2 cd/m^2) revealed a relative central scotoma (diameter: ~10°); the extent of his peripheral visual field remained restricted

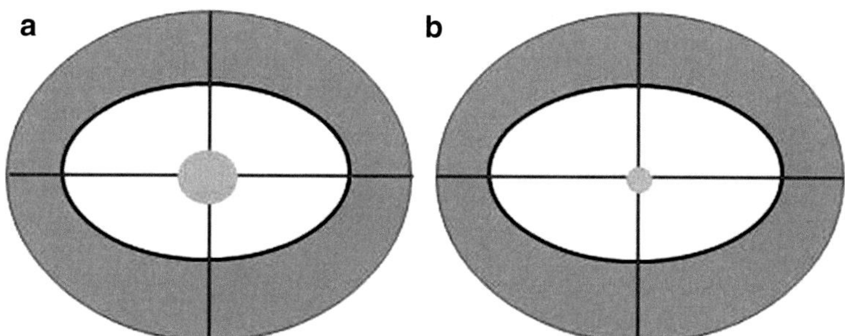

Fig. 9.6 Binocular visual field (60° plot) in the case of Florian at the age of 11 years (**a**) and at the age of 20 years (**b**) with a relative central scotoma (*grey areas*). Note the smaller size of the scotoma at the second assessment

to 40° in the left and right hemifields (see Fig. 9.6). Binocular visual form acuity for near was still <0.1; no distance visual acuity could be measured. Florian showed good colour vision (stimulus diameter: 3°); he could correctly discriminate and identify (and also name) saturated red, green, yellow, black and white hues. Florian could also accurately and promptly discriminate between grey and coloured stimuli. Form and object vision was now possible for crude shapes and large contours. Florian's eyes remained slightly divergent; convergence was positive, but limited. Florian could fixate visual stimuli (diameter: 3°) for up to 5 s, but required a long time (up to 15 s) to find the stimulus for accurate fixation (Fig. 9.7a). Spontaneous oculomotor exploration had improved in terms of speed and spatial organisation. Pursuit eye movements were possible provided the stimulus was large enough (diameter: 3°), but these were still fragmented. Saccadic eye movements had also improved, but were still inaccurate, as was visual localisation, which was also quite time-consuming (Fig. 9.7b). Florian's visually guided pointing accuracy was very low (Fig. 9.9a).

9.4.2.2 Further Visual Intervention and Follow-Up

At the age of 20 years, Florian started to work as an operator in a company with the help of a software program especially developed for his visual needs. The software transforms the keys on a touch screen into the form of symbols constructed by combinations of large forms (circle, square and triangle) and colours (e.g. red circle with black border). In a first attempt, we used fine grey contrasts for the different forms, but even after 300 trials Florian did not show any improvement in the discrimination of the virtual keys, while localisation was somehow better. Therefore we decided to use a combination of simple coloured forms (e.g. red circle, blue triangle, green square) for further practice with localisation and discrimination. The final 'touch keyboard' consisted of ten different 'keys' that enable Florian to use a software program that manages the telephone, and organisational tasks (e.g. reservations for conference rooms). The software program is supported by a voice output that gives feedback after each operation (Novak 2000).

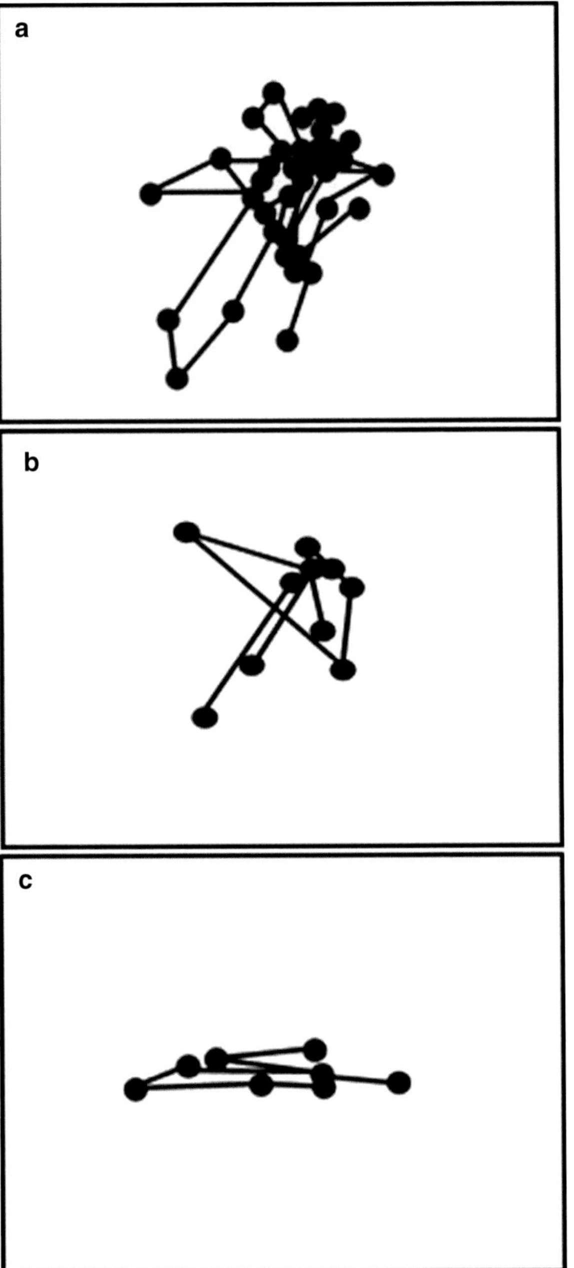

Fig. 9.7 Fixation patterns (diameter of light dot on a dark background: 2°; distance: 140 cm) in the case of Florian at the age of 11 years before (**a**) and after (**b**) systematic practice with visual localisation, and at the age of 20 years (**c**). Note effortful fixation attempts in **a** (recording period: 30 s), and improved fixation attempts in **b** (recording period: 15 s) and **c** (recording period: 9 s). *Dots* indicate fixations (fixation duration: >120 ms), *lines* represent saccadic eye shifts. Note that fixation is still inaccurate at the age of 20 years (**c**)

A crucial prerequisite for successful use of this technical aid was that the keys on the virtual keyboard required even more accurate localisation (diameter: 1 cm, distance between keys: 0.5 cm). Therefore, Florian's visual and cognitive capacities were again examined at the age of 20 years to see whether he would benefit from further visual training measures.

9.4.2.3 Visual and Cognitive Assessment at the Age of 20 Years (Table 9.7)

The relative central scotoma was unchanged. His foveal light threshold was still depressed (about 0.6 log units below normal values). Visual form acuity for near was in the same range as in the previous assessment (<0.1); far acuity could not be assessed, because Florian could only see very large stimuli (diameter: 10 cm) at a distance of 2 m. Colour discrimination was correct and fairly prompt, with occasional confusion of blue and green hues. Form and object vision were still limited to discrimination of crude black–white contours and large shapes. Florian could occasionally identify them, but usually reported only single features and could also see only one stimulus at a time (impaired parallel processing). However, he benefitted from additional information (cues) indicating that top-down processing based on previous visual experiences was possible. Fixation accuracy was improved, but still unstable and time consuming. For eventual accurate fixation he required on average 5 s (see Fig. 9.7c). Spontaneous oculomotor exploration was positive, but punctuated by saccadic dysmetria. Scenes were scanned more systematically than at the age of 11 years, but his scanning time was three- to fivefold longer than in normal age-matched subjects (see Fig. 9.8). Visual localisation had also improved, but still inaccurate and time-consuming (see Fig. 9.9c). Florian showed good visual orientation in familiar surroundings, but was helpless in unfamiliar or complex surroundings (e.g. supermarkets) with unforeseen obstacles. Independent navigation and thus mobility outside familiar surroundings were accordingly impaired. Florian's 'inner' vision of objects and scenes was now based on vivid and detailed descriptions by his parents, his older sister, his grandparents and his therapists, indicating that visual memory and this form of visual experience were spared.

9.4.2.4 Further Assessment

Prolonged maintenance of concentration was impaired; after about 20 min of demanding visual activities Florian's focused attention diminished, particularly when he was engaged in multi-tasking activities (parallel processing of several visual stimuli, storing in working memory and using this for visually guided responses). Working memory was generally impaired; Florian could retain and remember 3–4 digits (cut off: 6 digits). Logical memory (retaining a story consisting of 30 items) was also impaired; Florian could remember 12 items (cut off: 24 items). Executive functions (inductive and deductive reasoning, planning and problem solving) were normal, with high creativity and originality. Language capacities were also good. Control of fine finger movements of both hands was normal.

9.4.3 Further Intervention Programme as Special Preparation for Occupational Integration

Based on the outcome of neuropsychological assessment, emphasis in the final stage of intervention was given to the following components:

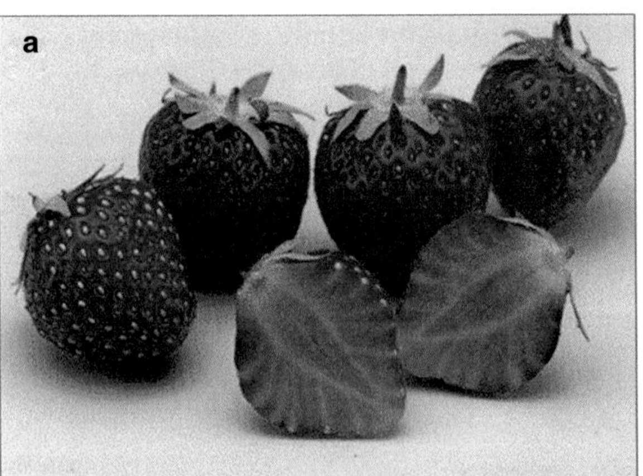

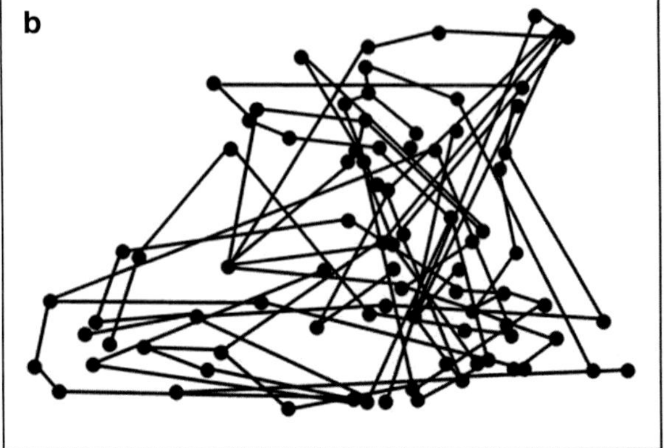

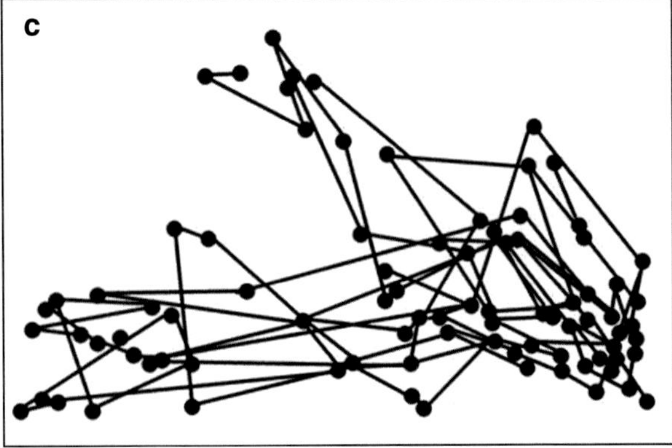

Fig. 9.8 Florian's oculomotor scanning patterns during inspection of a scene (**a**; *coloured*) containing six strawberries at the age of 11 (**b**) and of 20 years (**c**). Florian's task was to count the objects and possibly recognise them. *Dots* in **b** and **c** indicate fixations (>120 ms); *lines* indicate saccadic shifts. Scanning time in the normal subject (**b**) was 16.9 s. Florian's scanning time was 63.8 s in (**c**); he reported seeing 'two *red dots*'; his scanning time in DC was 37.3 s; he reported seeing three 'apples'. Note the decrease in the number of fixations and saccades, but incorrectly matched adaptation of the scanning pattern to the spatial structure of the scene in **b** and **c**

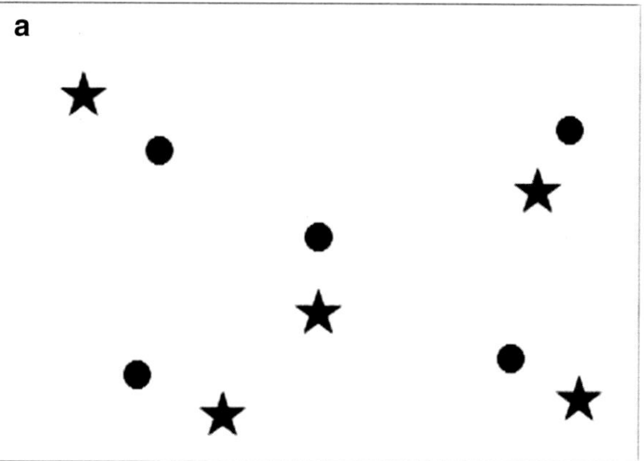

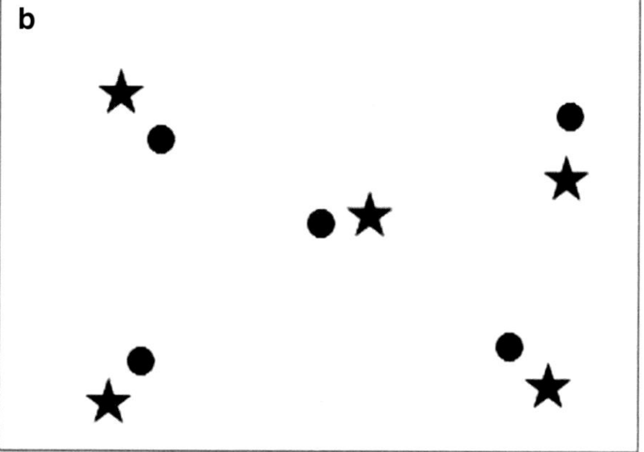

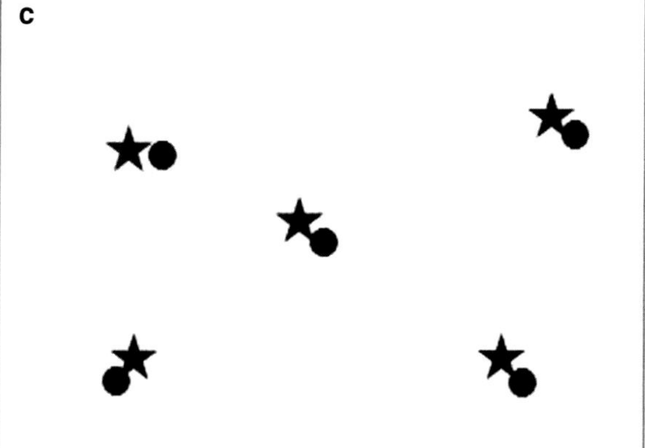

Fig. 9.9 Visual localisation (pointing responses) in Florian before (**a**) and after (**b**) systematic practice with localisation and at follow-up (9 years later; **c**). *Dots*: positions of stimuli, *stars*: Florian's pointing responses. Stimulus diameter was 1 cm; viewing distance of 40 cm. Note improvement in localisation accuracy from **a** to **c**, but still inaccurate localisation in **c**

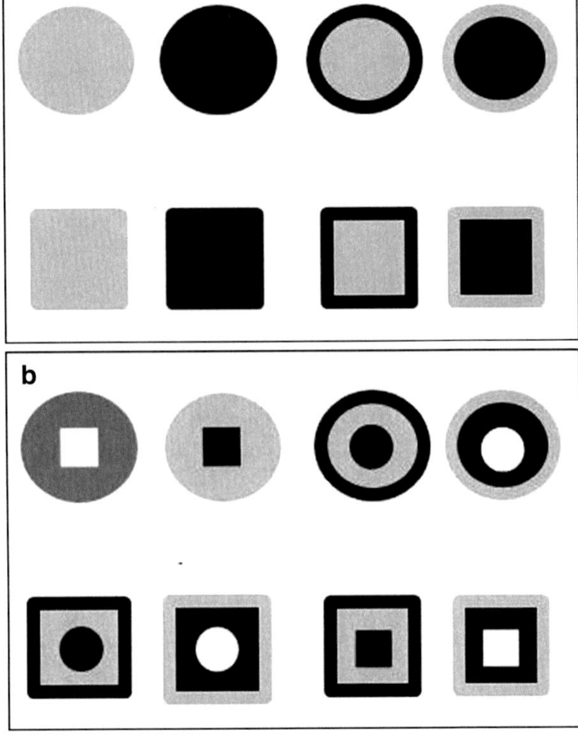

Fig. 9.10 'Buttons' varying in form and colour used for systematic practice of Florian's visual localisation and discrimination performance as the basis for using a touch screen-based keyboard. (**a**) Simple combinations of form and colour (*grey*, *white* and *black areas* indicate colours), (**b**) complex combinations of forms and colour. The virtual keyboard contained maximally 5 × 3 stimuli with a diameter of 1.5° and a spatial separation of 2.5° (Modified after Novak 2000)

- Practice with visual localisation, his intrinsic accuracy was not sufficient for using the virtual keyboard;
- Practice with discrimination of smaller coloured stimuli (single colours and combinations of colours and forms; diameter: 1 cm; see Fig. 9.10);
- Improvement of concentration with diminution of mental burden required for the planned activity;
- Practice with more independent visual orientation and navigation.

For systematic and specific practice with visual localisation and colour discrimination, a software-based training programme using a touch screen was specifically adapted (Novak 2000). Florian was given daily practice for 2–3 h, depending on his mental burden, whereby the duration of his training units was increased from 10 to 30 min, before a break of 5–10 min was introduced. In addition, attentional and verbal memory, especially in communication with others, was practiced daily for about 1 h. For improving visual navigation and mobility a special programme was performed with the help of a physiotherapist. This combined and integrated intervention programme proved successful (see Fig. 9.11). After 1 year of intensive training Florian could use the software program successfully, and navigate without difficulty within 'his' department in the company.

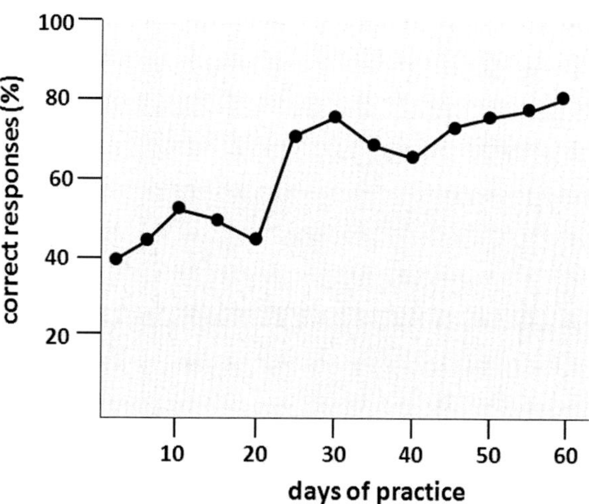

Fig. 9.11 Improvement in localisation accuracy in Florian after specific practice with the use of virtual buttons (see Fig. 9.10). Pointing responses were recorded by means of a touch screen. Note the striking increase in localisation accuracy from 40 to 80 % correct response after 60 sessions of practice (i.e. after about 4,000 trials over a period of 3 months) (Modified after Novak 2000)

9.4.3.1 Last Assessment at the Age of 30 Years

We could not find any significant changes in Florian's visual capacities, except for his improved visual localisation, fixation and visual scanning (Fig. 9.12), and colour and form discrimination (Table 9.7), but he has learned to use visual information and visual cues highly efficiently for visual orientation and navigation. He now has a guide dog, giving him greater independence.

Standardised assessment of cognition revealed normal verbal short-term (digit span forward) and working memory (digit span backward). Verbal learning (15-item word list) was below average (7 items; cut off: 10 items). Verbal long-term memory was also below cut off (5 items; cut off: 9 items) for the free recall condition, but was normal for recognition. Interestingly, logical memory (story, 30 items) was normal for immediate and delayed (after 30 min) recall.

9.4.4 Summary and Comments

At the age of 2 years, Florian had suffered severe chronic hypoxia with diffuse brain injury. The occipital and frontal structures were particularly affected. As a consequence, vision was nearly lost (only light–dark perception), while sensibility and fine motor control of both hands and cognition (attention, working memory) were particularly affected. A long-term intervention programme was developed and carried out at home and in school under regular supervision by JZ. Using modern software technology, Florian learned to use software programs with the help of a virtual key board on a touch screen, and was able to take up a job as operator and organiser of rooms for meetings.

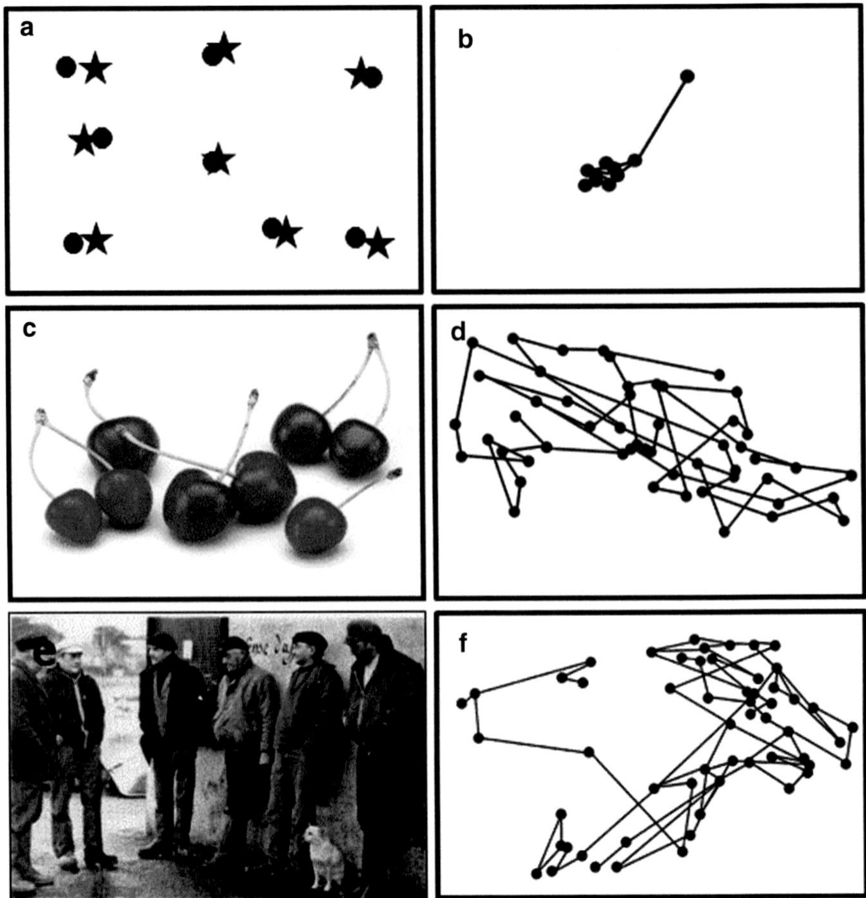

Fig. 9.12 Localisation performance (**a**; *circles*: targets; *stars*: pointing responses), fixation (**b**; 6 s), scanning of a simple scene (**c**, **d**), and scanning of a complex scene (**e**, **f**) in Florian at the age of 30 years. Note improvement of localisation and fixation accuracy in **a** and **b**. In **d**, scanning time was 27.3 s; Florian reported seeing six cherries. In **f**, scanning time was 46.2 s; Florian reported seeing four men and a dog. *Dots* indicate fixations (fixation duration: >120 ms); *lines* represent saccadic eye shifts. Note improvement of adaptation of the scanning patterns in **d** and **f** to the spatial structure of the scenes compared with scanning patterns shown in Fig. 9.8

One might argue that an intensive intervention programme over 20 years is not worth the outcome achieved. However, although vision is still severely impaired and fulfils the criteria for legal blindness, and Florian can neither read nor write, and needs support and help in many situations, he lives a relatively independent life and earns his maintenance. This does not mean that he is completely happy with his current situation. Indeed he has started to look into other professional options and opportunities, which may eventually lead to what Florian commonly refers to 'real quality of life'.

9.5 Case 5: Sarah

9.5.1 Medical Diagnoses

- Left frontal intracerebral haemorrhage
- Left-sided posterior cerebral artery occlusion and occipital lobe infarction
- Right-sided hemiparesis
- Global cognitive impairment
- Right-sided homonymous hemianopia

Nine-year-old Sarah showed normal development, and attended school with success. She suddenly fell unconscious and was immediately admitted to a Neurological Intensive Care Unit. Computerised tomography revealed intracerebral haemorrhage in the left frontal lobe, which was surgically removed. In addition, an infarction was found in the territory of the left posterior cerebral artery, possibly caused by increased intracranial pressure. Sarah showed good recovery; after 20 weeks of neurological and neuropsychological rehabilitation her mental and motor capacities had nearly returned to her premorbid level, except for maintenance of concentration (maximal 1 h) and cognitive slowing. Right-sided hemianopia persisted, and Sarah complained of difficulties with reading, but also – to a lesser extent – with overview of her visual field, particularly when playing ball with other children or cycling. Her social and affective behaviour was normal.

9.5.2 Visual Assessment at 20 Months After Surgical Intervention (Age: 11 Years)

Visual field: Quantitative testing with the Tübingen perimeter revealed right-sided homonymous hemianopia, with sparing of 2° along the horizontal axis. Field of gaze showed an extent of 32° in the right and 48° into the left hemifield (Fig. 9.13).

Visual search/visual scanning: Sarah's visual search performance (parallel condition) was normal with respect to accuracy (hits), but was below age-appropriate values with respect to speed (Fig. 9.14). Her oculomotor scanning pattern was accurate, but characterised by small saccades and many re-fixations, and associated higher time demand (Fig. 9.15a).

Reading: Reading performance (reading aloud) was 132 words per minute (wpm), which was below the expected performance for the same age and education level (cut off: 150 wpm). Impaired reading was caused by the parafoveal visual field loss, as evidenced by the typically altered associated eye movement pattern (Fig. 9.16a).

Other visual and oculomotor functions: Visual acuity, contrast sensitivity, space and object perception were normal, as were oculomotor functions including fixation and pursuit eye movements.

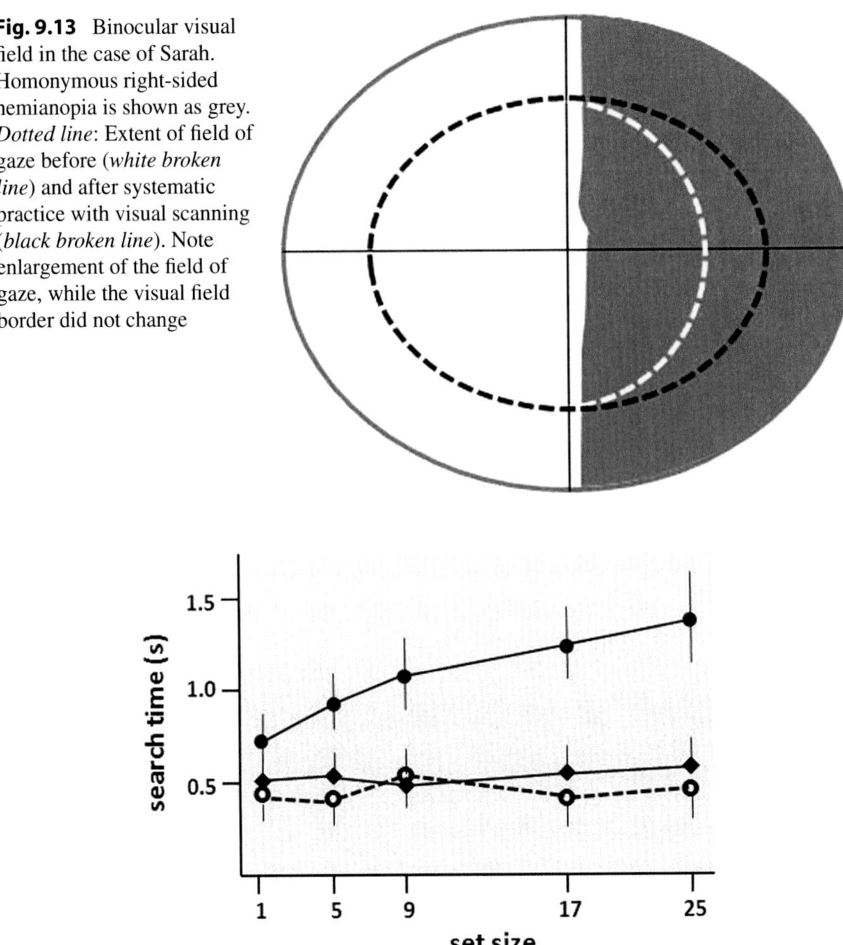

Fig. 9.13 Binocular visual field in the case of Sarah. Homonymous right-sided hemianopia is shown as grey. *Dotted line*: Extent of field of gaze before (*white broken line*) and after systematic practice with visual scanning (*black broken line*). Note enlargement of the field of gaze, while the visual field border did not change

Fig. 9.14 Visual search performance in the parallel condition in Sarah before (*closed circles*) and after systematic practice (*diamonds*) for different set sizes. *Open circles*: data from a healthy girl of the same age. Note that Sarah's serial search changed into parallel after practice, and was comparable with performance of the normal subject. In addition, standard variation (indicated by *vertical lines*) decreased after practice, indicating higher consistency and stability of search performance. Search accuracy was between 90 and 100 % in both subjects for all conditions

9.5.3 Intervention and Outcome

The main aim of intervention was improvement of text processing speed and visual scanning to gain a quicker and more complete overview of even complex scenes. Treatment procedures were identical to those for adults with right-sided hemianopia with difficulties with overview and reading (hemianopic dyslexia) (see Zihl 2011). For practice with scanning, visual search tasks were used to improve parallel and serial scanning of scenes, consisting of arrays of letters and forms. Sarah's task was

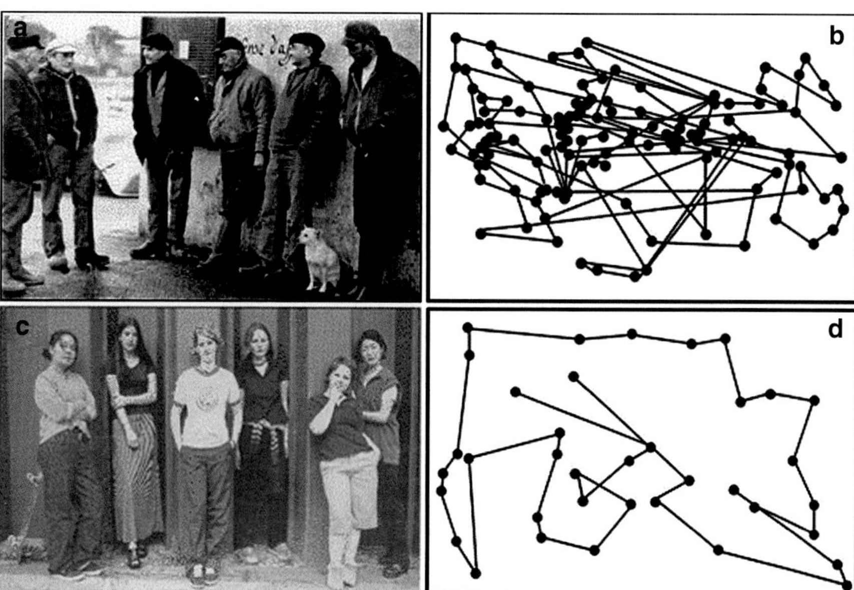

Fig. 9.15 Oculomotor scanning patterns of Sarah during the inspection of different scenes with similar spatial configuration before (**a**) and after (**b**) systematic practice with scanning. On both occasions, Sarah reported all relevant details of the scene, but required less time after (**b**, 18.3 s) than before practice (**a**, 49.5 s). Note the decrease in the number of fixations (*dots*; fixation duration: >120 ms) and saccades as well as the better adaptation of the oculomotor scanning pattern to the spatial structure of the scene after practice

to find a predefined target among an increasing number of distractors, as quickly as possible, whereby the level of difficulty was adjusted according to the actual level of performance. To improve text-processing speed, words of increasing length were presented for a defined time, which was successively decreased. Sarah was instructed to fixate the beginning of the word presented and then to shift her gaze to the end of the word. She was asked not to use a letter-by-letter or syllable-by-syllable reading strategy, but to 'grasp' the word as a whole (Gestalt), and then to read it with understanding. The first training sessions were carried out in Munich with JZ, and then Sarah was provided with the software programs and she performed and practiced at home with her older sister with overview from JZ. Training sessions (duration: 45 min) were performed at least three times a week for both visual search and reading.

After 2 months of regular visual training, search and reading performance were examined again. While the visual field did not show any change (field sparing: 2°), the field of view had enlarged and extended now to 46° (intact left hemifield: 48°; see Fig. 9.13). Visual search performance had improved, indicating that global visual processing was established again (Fig. 9.14), which apparently allowed Sarah to also compensate better for the hemianopia (Fig. 9.15b). Reading performance had reached 166 wpm and thus was in the normal range; improvement was paralleled by the reading eye movement pattern (Fig. 9.16b).

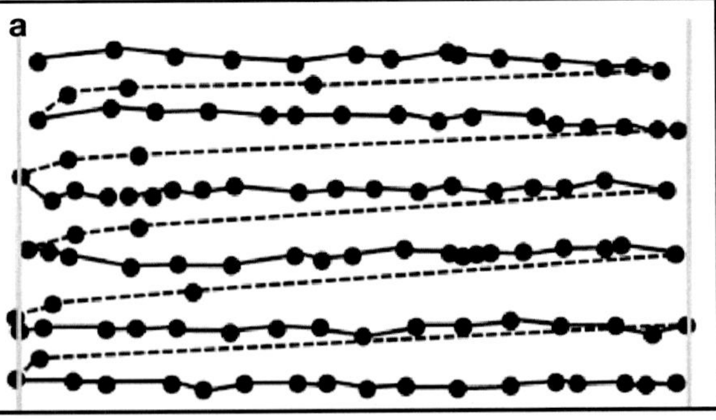

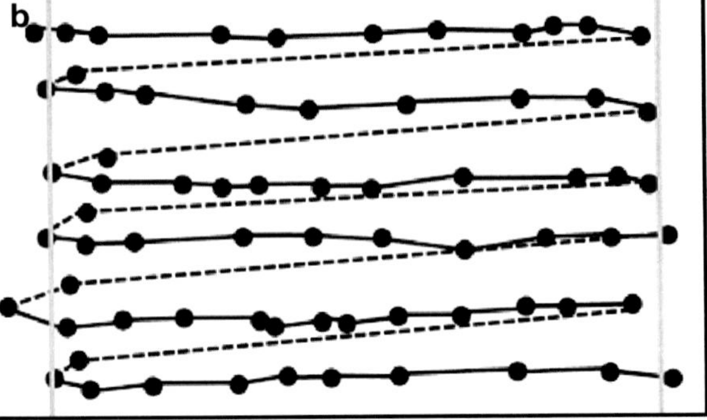

Fig. 9.16 Eye reading patterns of Sarah before (**a**) and after systematic practice (**b**) with text processing to reduce the severity of hemianopic dyslexia. *Dots* indicate fixation positions (fixation durations >0.2 s), *lines* saccadic shifts. Grey vertical lines indicate left and right margins of lines of text (not visible during recording). Reading performance before practice (**a**): 92 words per minute, after practice: 154 words per minute. *Dots* indicate fixations (fixation duration: >120 ms), *lines* denote saccadic eye shifts. Note the decrease in the number of fixations and increase in the length of saccadic movements in the reading direction (from left to right)

Sarah reported far fewer visual difficulties after training, but still complained that she often needed too much time for satisfactory visual performance compared with others, for example in sports.

9.5.4 Comment

The persistent complete homonymous hemianopia was associated with visual difficulties comparable to that in adult hemianopes: in 'grasping' fast scenes, and particularly longer words. Unfortunately, no data were available on Sarah's scanning and reading performance at the time of rehabilitation, but it appears very likely that Sarah had already improved her scanning and reading capacities before the specific training using our software programs. However, the observation that Sarah still had significant visual difficulties 12 months after the end of general rehabilitation, i.e. 17 months after her brain injury that had ostensibly resolved after 2 months of specific visual training, provides evidence for the efficacy of this type of intervention.

Meanwhile, Sarah lives the normal life of a 17-year-old teenager, with high engagement in school, in sports and social activities.

9.6 Case 6: Paul

9.6.1 Medical Diagnoses

- Suspected CVI (preterm)
- Global visual difficulties
- Developmental visual dyslexia

Paul was a 9-year-old boy with normal development and school performance, apart from reading and sports. Although he liked football very much, he was not accepted as a team player because he was 'too slow' and quite often could not find the ball or the team mate who was in a better position to score a goal. Neurological and psychological examinations were negative, except for a mild clumsiness of his right hand, slowed reading performance and difficulties with complex visuo-constructive tasks (e.g. copying complex figures).

9.6.1.1 Visual Assessment

Visual field: Quantitative testing with the Tübingen perimeter revealed a normal, age-appropriate visual field extent for light, colour and form.

Visual search/visual scanning: The visual field of view (extent of search field with eye shifts allowed) was 46° in both hemifields. Paul was unable to search for targets in parallel, although his performance was normal with respect to accuracy (hits) (Fig. 9.17). His oculomotor scanning pattern was accurate, but characterised by small saccades and an increased number of fixations, resulting in reduced speed (Fig. 9.18c).

Reading: Reading performance was 61 words per minute (wpm), which was far below the expected performance for the same age and education level (cut off: 140 wpm).

Other visual and oculomotor functions: Visual acuity, contrast sensitivity, space and object perception were normal, as were oculomotor functions including fixation and pursuit eye movements.

9.6.2 Intervention and Outcome

The main aim of intervention was to improve Paul's visual scanning/visual search and text processing speed. Treatment procedures were identical to those used for Sarah (case 5) and for adults with text processing difficulties because of hemianopia (Zihl 2011). The reason for using the same type of text processing practice was the

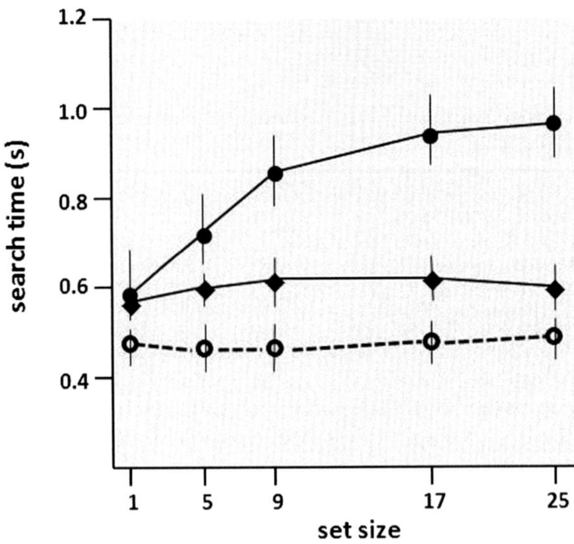

Fig. 9.17 Visual search performance in the parallel condition in Paul before (*closed circles*) and after systematic practice (*diamonds*) for different set sizes. *Open circles*: data from a healthy boy of the same age. Note that Paul's serial search changed into parallel after practice, and was comparable with the performance of the normal subject. In addition, standard deviation (indicated by *vertical lines*) decreased after practice, indicating improved consistency and stability of search performance. Search accuracy was between 90 and 100 % in both subjects in all conditions

consideration, that an impaired integration of letter and word stimuli is the main underlying cause for the reading problem. Training sessions usually lasted 45 min (breaks included) and were performed daily for a period of 4 weeks. Because Paul wanted to read better and faster – he liked reading books very much – we started with practice of his text processing. After Paul had gained a much better performance in reading, we switched to practicing visual search.

After intervention, his reading performance became 105 wpm (before: 61 wpm), i.e. reading speed had increased by 75 %, but was still far from an age-appropriate performance (140 wpm). His visual search performance had improved and parallel search was possible, indicating that his global processing mode was now in the age-appropriate range of performance (Fig. 9.17). His improvement in visual search performance was paralleled by his improved oculomotor scanning (Fig. 9.18d).

9.6.3 Comment

Paul showed a combination of impaired visual search and text processing. Although he could somehow manage the demands of school despite his severe reading impairment, he was quite unhappy because of his marginal marks in German language. After intervention, he started to read books with enthusiasm, and although one could certainly argue, that his reading speed was still very low, it was a big step for Paul

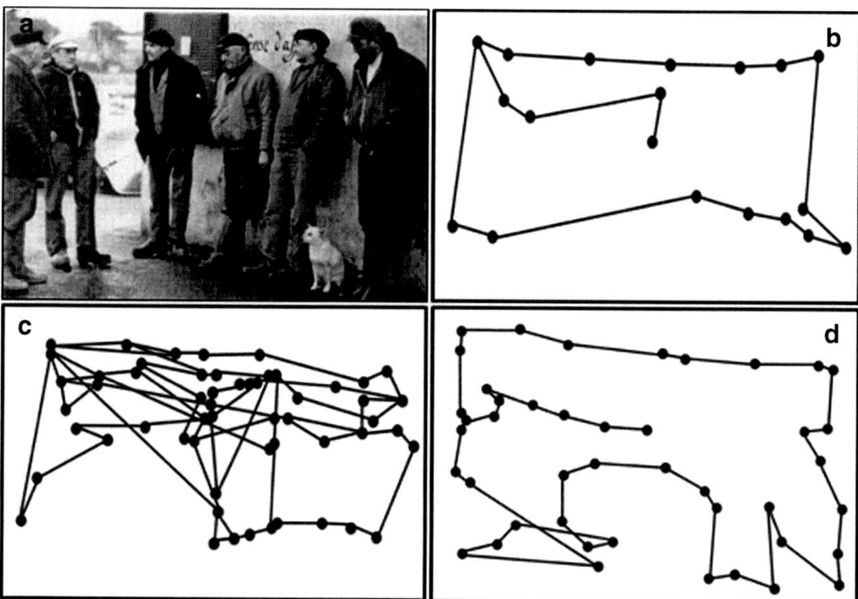

Fig. 9.18 Oculomotor scanning patterns during the inspection of a scene (**a**) by a healthy boy (**b**; scanning time: 9.9 s) and by Paul before (**c**; scanning time: 29.6 s) and after (**d**) systematic practice with scanning (scanning time: 17.8). On both occasions, Paul reported all relevant details of the scene before and after practice. *Dots* indicate fixations (fixation duration: >120 ms), *lines* denote saccadic eye shifts. Note the decrease in the number of fixations (*dots*) and saccades as well as the better adaptation of the oculomotor scanning pattern to the spatial structure of the scene after practice. However, even after practice Paul still required about double the time compared to the normal subject

who had, for the first time in his life, the feeling that now he could read really fast! We examined Paul again 2 years later and found a further significant gain – his reading performance was now 146 wpm, which was close to the cut-off value of 150 wpm. Thus, Paul has undoubtedly benefitted from specific and systematic intervention measures, which had not required much time. Meanwhile he is enrolled in a grammar school – and is attaining good marks not only in languages, but also in sport.

9.7 Case 7: Ben

9.7.1 Medical Diagnoses

- Hypoxic ischaemic encephalopathy complicating delivery
- Bilateral posterior parietal infarction
- Right visual inattention
- Possibility of a Balint syndrome picture emerging

9.7.2 Introduction

It has been argued that the 'earlier the better' when it comes to managing CVI, but the paradox is that the earlier the presentation and intervention, the more difficult it is to make a diagnosis, and to objectively construct, administer and audit the outcome of any specific therapeutic strategies. Ben's is a case in point.

Ben was 10 months old when first seen by the author as a friend of the family (such an early presentation, would not otherwise have come to the author's attention). At the time of birth, he had sustained a traumatic delivery, and had required resuscitation. Subsequent MRI brain imaging was reported as showing evidence of extensive multifocal hypoxic ischaemic encephalopathy, primarily affecting the posterior parietal region on both sides, more extensively so on the left than the right side. Despite his adverse prognosis, Ben's visits to the eye department had shown him to have normal eye movements and alignment, and normal development of visual acuities. No gross motor deficits were evident at that stage, and his language development was not delayed.

9.7.3 History from Ben's Mother (9 March 2012)

'Although Ben easily met basic milestones (such as bringing his hands together and to his mouth and being able to bat at toys on his play gym, early babbling and smiling), his development appeared to have stalled, primarily because he was showing no interest in reaching out for, or exploring objects (other than inconsistently batting at one of the toys on his play gym). This meant that at 10 months of age, he did not use his arms because he has no real interest in exploring his surroundings. The physiotherapist had been unable to find anything wrong with physical development or muscle tone. He moved his arms and legs purposefully – he just would not do much with them! He chewed his hands all the time and, if an object was put into his hands, he would take it and bring it to his mouth, but he never reached out for an object himself. He babbled very well and responds well socially to us (clapping, waving, responding to his name), and met his milestones in this regard. It was his lack of coordinated movements and interest in exploring his surroundings which concerned us most of all.'

9.7.3.1 Visual Assessment

Visual field: Ben turned to look at large single targets revealed to him from behind an occluder in each of the four quadrants of his visual fields.

Eye movements: Ben's eyes were aligned normally. Pursuit and saccadic eye movements were intact to both horizontal and vertical optokinetic nystagmus. He had no optical errors requiring spectacles. However, he could not be encouraged to reach out for any moving targets.

Visual search/visual scanning: When identical targets were introduced in mirror image positions on both sides, Ben consistently failed to look at the target on his right side. He returned smiles from two metres, but could not transfer his gaze to a second person to his right, despite consistently being able to do so to his left side.

9.7.4 Intervention and Outcome

Report written for Ben's mother as a sequel to the above informal assessment:

- Use the left side of his vision for his teaching and education at this stage
- Help Ben to enhance his awareness of his right side during dedicated sessions say two or three times a day, in which he is in an environment with nothing to attract attention to his left, while toys/real items are provided for him on his right.
- Most children with Ben's condition are 'one thing at a time people', because they can only process a limited number of entities at once. Exceed their threshold and they can become distressed and unable to perceive well.
- Remove pattern and clutter from his environment. Single items of meaning can then be presented, perhaps initially on his left to gain knowledge and awareness of what items are, then for longer on his right to help him find and explore them.
- He also shows evidence of lack of auditory attention to his right. This may account for why he was thought to have poor hearing in his right ear on recent behavioural assessment.
- He tends to reach only with his left hand. (You noticed that when his left hand was immobilised with a drip while he was in hospital however, that this reversed within 4 days, but subsequently reverted.)
- Ben is likely to have difficulty in seeing and listening in crowded and noisy environments, so it is worthwhile decluttering and depatterning his environments at present. This is likely to enable him to perceive specific single items, rather than his being surrounded by what for him is likely to be a 'visual cacophany'.
- Ben appears to be processing information more slowly than one would expect. Match your communication with him to his response/acknowledgement rate, so that what you convey becomes perceptible to him.
- His attention is intermittent and of relatively short duration. Try to look out 'through his eyes'. Give clear simple words to match what he looks at and what he touches or reaches for, in order to enhance his moments of lucidity, and thereby consistently build up his understanding and knowledge.
- It is important to sing songs and it is worth using a sing song voice. This is because the processing of language through song takes place in different locations in the brain to the processing of language through speaking. Song is therefore likely to enhance his language acquisition.
- I explained that these ideas are founded on the concept of neuroplasticity of the brain. Thus by creating environments that are clutter and pattern free for the present, in the direction in which he is attending, he is likely to feel most comfortable and learn the most from the series of single things that are presented to him (perhaps having pre-prepared them in a basket the previous evening). It also helps to limit extraneous sounds.
- Videos like Spot the Dog in which single large moving images on a plain background are presented are likely to have the greatest educational benefit. It is also appropriate to place him, perhaps on a reclining baby seat very close to the TV programmes that his brother is watching, with the TV to his left. (Children with his difficulty typically get very close to the TV to watch it, probably so that they see single elements, without crowding.)

9.7.5 Progress Report: 19 March 2012 (Written by Ben's Mother)

We had already created a sensory area (or Little Room) for Ben some weeks previously, which we called 'The Ben Den'. It comprised a travel cot with a colourful play gym with six or seven brightly coloured toys dangling from it, as well as a bright red rope light, about five other bright toys and lights dotted around, a foil blanket and a book playing music (which we put behind Ben). There were a lot of different colours, lights and sounds in The Ben Den. It also had mesh sides which enabled Ben to see out in to the living room, which had a lot of his brother's toys lying around. Ben enjoyed being in The Ben Den, but made no real progress in terms of his movement or reaching out. He only ever reached for one object and it was the parrot which dangled directly above his head and was within very easy reach. His range of movement was very poor.

Following your visit, we transformed The Ben Den by removing everything and putting it all into a box by the side of The Ben Den. We covered up the mesh sides with a plain white sheet, so that Ben could not see out in to the living room. We took one toy at a time from the box and put it in to The Ben Den.

Ben was even more pleased with his new Den and it was not long before he was taking the single object we had left in the Den and reaching for it (even though we left it so that he had to reach some distance to get it) and playing with it with both hands. This is something he had never done before.

We would leave Ben on his own in the Den to work out how to get the toy, without distractions. I think, previously, we had been hovering over him too much and had not afforded him all the time he needed to be able to work out what to do.

Once Ben started reaching out for objects, he began doing it more and more over the following days. However, it became clear that he could only reach while lying down. He was not able to reach while in the sitting position. The physiotherapist examined him and, again, said that there was no reason why he should not be able to reach for objects while sitting and that she considered the problem to be habitual. Ben does not sit confidently without support, so we could not put him in the sitting position in The Ben Den, as he would quickly throw himself back in to the lying position.

As well as decluttering The Ben Den, we decluttered the entire living room and moved most of David's toys up in to David's bedroom (with the strict instruction that he is to only bring down toys to play with one at a time). We sat Ben up in his highchair in the decluttered living room and put the tray on to the highchair and placed one object on the tray in front of him. We turned the highchair away from the window, because staring out of windows at the daylight is one of Ben's favourite distractions. The first object was a toy which I had borrowed from the special needs toy library for children with visual and sensory impairments. It is a large simple toy with silver beads which plays a tune. Again, giving Ben just one toy and plenty of time to work out what he needed to do meant that he was soon reaching out and playing with the toy with both hands while in the sitting position. Since starting off with the large toy for children with special needs, we have moved on to using smaller toys such as a colourful monkey, which he now holds on to with both hands while eating his dinner. As his confidence in reaching out for objects has grown, he has become more able to 'multi-task' and cope with more than one thing at a time and he needs less time to focus on reaching, because it is becoming second nature.

We plan to use this approach to move him on to other stages of exploring objects:

- Creating a plain environment;
- Without distractions;
- Using one simple object;
- Leaving plenty of time for Ben to work out what to do;
- First to his good side (the left) and then to his bad side (the right) once he is more confident.

As well as encouraging him to reach for objects, we have been spending some time reading, speaking and singing to him. We do this in his bedroom which we have cleared and kept as plain as possible to allow him to concentrate. We have taken down all the posters and put all the toys in to the cupboard so that the room has no visual distractions. We try to set aside time for one of us to go to Ben's room alone with Ben away from the noise of his brother. We have chosen five books for him, which are all very similar "That's Not My… Monkey/Dinosaur/Tiger…" He is showing a real interest in these books – looking intently at the pages and helping to turn the pages with his hands. We had not previously been able to get him to show any interest in books, but we had always read to him downstairs in the living room amongst all the toys and clutter and normally when David was there and the TV was on.

I read to him from his 'good side' (the left) to capture his interest in the books, but I have found that it has also been possible to read from the right, provided that there is nothing to distract him. The main problem at the moment is that we have a black out blind in Ben's bedroom and I draw the blind, but he seems to focus on the chinks of light which shine through the sides of the blind. I plan to try either moving to another part of the room for his story time or putting up material around the edges of the blind.

We are also showing him objects from a box of objects and saying the names of the objects (ball, teddy, book). This is going quite well, but one thing I have noticed is that his attention span is very short and this is not his favourite activity. I think I will have to think of a way to make it a bit more interesting, or maybe we just need to shorten the 'learning sessions' for Ben.

We have also been trying to speak to Ben in simple, sing song language and encouraging him to make eye contact with us. We are also babbling back to him. We are doing this all the time with Ben now and hope that it is going to become second nature to us. We talk to him about everyday activities using a couple of simple words in a sing song voice (e.g. Ben's Bath, Ben's Spoon). I do think he is starting to babble more and more and it is almost starting to sound sentence like. He has no real words yet though.

9.7.6 Follow-Up

During the ensuing 2 years, Ben has made good progress. He went through a stage of reaching for patterns on plates as if they were three-dimensional, but this has abated. He now shows no signs of lack of attention to his right. He has developed good hand eye coordination and now reaches out accurately. He copes well in a crowded nursery. He is now walking despite slight diplegia which later became evident. He is being reviewed for the possible emergence of additional perceptual deficits.

9.7.7 Conclusion

Ben's reported brain pathology was in the distribution seen in children who manifest features of Balint syndrome. Ben's lack of visual and auditory attention to his right provided clinical evidence of left posterior parietal pathology, while his failure to reach out was hypothesised as being due to a combination of possible 'simultanagnostic' visual dysfunction and optic ataxia. The clear verbatim reports written by Ben's mother provide compelling evidence that the changes recommended to Ben's parenting was followed by a rapid change for the better in Ben's development. No harm could come from limiting and pacing the amount of stimulation given to Ben, and this appears to have led to considerable benefits. The younger the child, the greater the need, and the greater the potential efficacy of appropriate parental intervention, but the more difficult it is to validate its efficacy.

9.8 Case 8: Nicola

9.8.1 Medical Diagnoses

- Spontaneous rupture of a vascular malformation in the left occipito-parietal region at 16 years of age
- Right homonymous hemianopia
- Additional hitherto unrecognised 'simultanagnostic' visual dysfunction, with late diagnosis

9.8.2 Introduction

Nicola's presentation and 'assessment' were unusual. She is a teacher of visually impaired children, and presented to the author immediately after a lecture concerning CVI in children that he had given, explaining that she too had the same visual symptoms that had just been described. Her case is presented as an autobiographical account.

9.8.3 Patient Autobiography

My journey started in June 1996 when I suffered a brain haemorrhage caused by an arteriovenous malformation. I was sixteen at the time. After surviving through the initial few days and then the surgery 8 days after the haemorrhage, I walked out of hospital 3 weeks later with my only known side effect being a right-sided homonymous hemianopia. Aside from the hemianopia, I was completely unaware of how much damage had actually been caused by this haemorrhage. I also did not fully comprehend how much my life would change as a result. The doctors informed us that it would take me 10 years to fully recover. I don't think they actually knew that and they were wrong. My recovery will not be complete until I fully understand what effects this 'incident' had on other parts of my brain, not just the left occipital lobe where the malformation was located.

The neurosurgeons explained the basics of what had happened. Then with the help of the local doctor who had been the first doctor on the scene and had undoubtedly saved my life, we were able to understand it better at an emotional level. However no one could tell us why it had happened, other than that it was a blood vessel malformation that could have burst at any time. A suggestion was made that because I had been a competitive swimmer and had put myself under so much pressure it occurred when I was that young. But it could have happened at any time; it was a ticking time bomb that we knew nothing about. Once I was well enough to leave the hospital, my parents and I were sent out into the world unequipped for the aftermath of this haemorrhage.

What followed was years of unexplained battles and difficulties with many aspects of my life, which apparently was to be expected after a serious brain injury. During this time I saw countless specialists, all of whom attempted to 'fix' me, but none who actually explained to me the bigger picture to help me to understand what was going on. This started to change when I began a career in educating children who are blind and visually impaired. I was then lucky enough to hear a keynote speech at a conference about cerebral visual impairment. The speaker started talking about things that children with this condition would tend to do and they were things that I did. Things like having difficulty finding specific items in a cluttered environment or having difficulty with processing visual and auditory information at the same time. Unbeknown to me at the time, this was the moment that my recovery would truly begin.

I introduced myself to the speaker after the lecture and in a sense spent the next hour learning about myself. He was able to explain to me why I struggle to find my child in a crowd and why spending time in a congested shopping mall is exhausting for me. For the first time in 17 years I realised that what I did and who I am is normal considering the insult my brain had received. I was not crazy, I was not weird and most importantly I am not less of a human being because of the things I can't do. Gaining this knowledge and understanding of my condition was enlightening. I now embrace my disability and feel able to let people know when I am having difficulty with certain situations, such as not coping in a busy supermarket. This has also helped me to realise that I am not the only one with this condition; other people experience the same difficulties that I do. I now feel that I can use this newfound knowledge to help others, especially children and their families who are only at the start of their journey into cerebral visual impairment.

So with the help of the lecturer I have embarked on a journey of self-discovery to find strategies and techniques to make my life easier. My first lesson was an introduction to 'blindsight', a phenomenon that I had already experienced but did not understand. For me blindsight is the ability to unconsciously detect visual stimuli in my right field of vision. My task was to therefore make this unconscious function become a more conscious function. So after a year of focusing my attention on detecting and interpreting any movement on my right hand side, I have already become more conscious of visual activity occurring around me, which had been something I had previously been unable to do. This has recently been validated, by using both simple and diagnostic visual field tests, which have demonstrated that I am in fact seeing more into the right field than ever before.

Another suggestion was that I train myself to read books vertically downwards and not horizontally. The reason for this seemed so obvious but had never occurred to me. This way, instead of only the first word of each sentence being visible without scanning, I could view the whole line. This means that only what I have already read moves into my right visual field. To achieve this, I firstly read each morning for 3 weeks for about 30 min at a time. By using a Kindle I was able to increase not only the font size but also the line spacing, which reduced the visual clutter for me. Once I felt comfortable with reading this way in the morning, I then tried reading this way at a more relaxed time of day, such as bedtime. It took about 6 weeks for me to be able to read this way and I now find it just as relaxing as reading the normal way. I am now able to read for longer periods of time and do not feel the visual fatigue that I had grown accustomed to. For a book lover, this in itself is exciting.

I have also put together a photo essay of different environments, highlighting scenes that I find complex and difficult, through to scenes that I find simple and relaxing. By doing this, it has helped me to understand and demonstrate to others how different environments affect my visual abilities. These photos are now being used by educators of the visually impaired to demonstrate what it is like having this condition. Another simple suggestion that I have tried is turning my body about fifteen degrees to the right when reading, sitting at a table or viewing into the distance. Professor Dutton felt that this might actually increase my field of view to the left. I experimented with this and even though it feels unnatural he is in fact correct.

So from this personal experience the question has to be, would the last 18 years of my life have been any different if I had had this knowledge and understanding earlier? The simple answer is yes. Knowledge is power and when you are feeling powerless and isolated, being able to understand yourself and your capabilities better is life changing. For 18 years I have been searching for answers and fighting to be 'fully recovered'. At times it has felt like this haemorrhage has haunted me, constantly following me around and causing unrelenting difficulties in my life. I suddenly went from a happy carefree teenager to that girl that had a brain haemorrhage. Not a day goes by without me being reminded of what happened; however I have now learned to embrace my differences and uniqueness because I understand who I am again.

9.8.4 Comment

Nicola's case highlights the importance of neuropsychological assessment and proper management at the time of visual brain injury. It also demonstrates the need for patients to be afforded an in-depth understanding of their visual symptoms, so that they can be empowered to recognise their own visual disorders and themselves take action to ameliorate any adverse impact that these disorders may have.

Erratum to: Visual Disorders

Erratum to:
Chapter 4 in: J. Zihl, G.N. Dutton, *Cerebral Visual Impairment in Children: Visuoperceptive and Visuocognitive Disorders*, DOI 10.1007/978-3-7091-1815-3_4

Figure 4.3c on page 75 was published incorrectly. Please find the correct version of Figure 4.3:

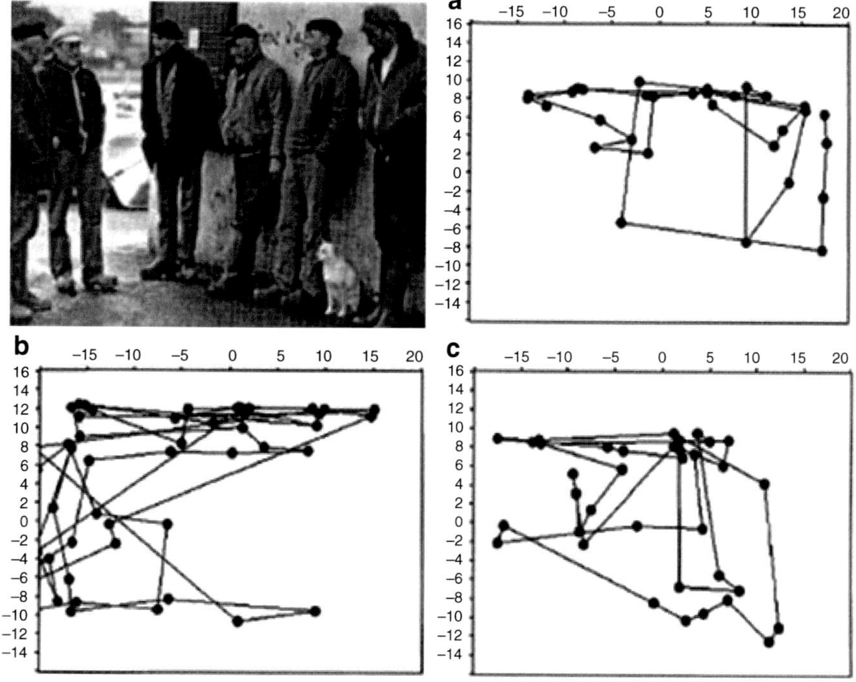

The online version of the original chapter can be found under
DOI 10.1007/978-3-7091-1815-3

Josef Zihl
LMU Munich
Department of Psychology
München
Germany

Gordon N. Dutton
Department of Visual Science
Glasgow Caledonian University
Glasgow
UK

J. Zihl, G.N. Dutton, *Cerebral Visual Impairment in Children: Visuoperceptive and Visuocognitive Disorders*, DOI 10.1007/978-3-7091-1815-3_10

Glossary

Ability Denotes the capability to perform defined tasks.

Accommodation The facility of the eye to focus upon near targets.

Accommodative esotropia Convergent strabismus due to long-sightedness (hypermetropia). The eyes accommodate to compensate for the hypermetropia. Inability to suppress the associated convergence of the eyes results in esotropia.

Achromatopsia Inability to perceive and differentiate colours.

Activity Entails the application of abilities to attain a specific goal in the context of the social model of disability.

ADD (attention deficit disorder) A cognitive disorder characterised by difficulty maintaining attention on a stimulus or activity and to regulate attention according to task demands.

Agnosia A visual-cognitive disorder characterised by inability to recognise and identify familiar visual stimuli (objects, faces, letters, places, etc.) by vision only, despite sufficiently available visual and cognitive capacities. (This term does not apply to difficulties with assigning labels/names to visual stimuli (Visual anomia)).

Aicardi syndrome A genetic disorder characterised by the combination of absence of or diminution in the size of the corpus callosum with infantile spasms due to seizures and a characteristic pattern of multifocal discrete atrophic patches in the retina and underlying choroid. Aicardi syndrome is associated with other structural-developmental brain disorders such as microcephaly, enlarged ventricles or focal lack of brain tissue (porencephalic cysts).

Akinetopsia Inability to perceive visual stimuli in motion, despite normal visual field, visual acuity, spatial contrast sensitivity, temporal resolution (accurate perception of the order of succession of stimuli) and normal field of attention.

Alertness Is the state of active attention, i.e. being watchful and prompt to detect, analyse and respond to stimuli, which is characterised by high sensory awareness.

Anisometropia Refractive optical error which differs between the two eyes.

Anosognosia Lack of awareness of and insight into an obvious functional impairment because the subject is unable to detect the mismatch between assumed/expected function and the real functional status. Anosognosia typically occurs in about 30 % of subjects with hemiplegia and (visual) neglect (mainly after

J. Zihl, G.N. Dutton, *Cerebral Visual Impairment in Children: Visuoperceptive and Visuocognitive Disorders*, DOI 10.1007/978-3-7091-1815-3

right-hemisphere injury) or homonymous hemianopia (irrespective of the side of brain injury).

Apraxia Difficulty performing learned purposeful actions despite the requisite physical capacity. This can affect simple movements (e.g. gestures) on command after verbal instruction or by imitation (ideomotor apraxia) or complex movements (e.g. preparing a cup of tea, dressing) (ideational apraxia). The latter form is explained as loss of the action plan (impairment of Procedural memory).

Apraxia of gaze See Gaze apraxia.

Associate learning Is the process by which an association between two stimuli or between a response and a stimulus is learned.

Astereopsis Severe impairment or lack of Stereopsis.

Astigmatism Refractive error of the eye in which the optical error in one meridian is different from the optical error in the meridian at 90° to it. The commonest cause is the cornea being more curved in one meridian than the other.

Attention A state of Alertness, which allows the person to stay in a state of readiness to respond (Internal attention) and to focus on stimuli in the environment (External attention). Attention can vary with respect to quantity/Intensity and quality/Selectivity. Attention also denotes the allocation of mental processing and general cognitive resources.

Attention span Denotes the length of time a person can be attentive to one subject and/or the amount of material that can be processed during a restricted period of time.

Autistic spectrum disorder A pervasive disorder with the onset before the age of 3 years, which is characterised by impaired development in social perception, social interaction and communication, with limited activities and interests, often associated with repetitive, stereotyped and inflexible use of routines and rituals.

Balint syndrome Results from bilateral posterior parietal injury and associated disconnection of fronto-parietal fibre tracts. A neuropsychological condition characterised by marked limitation in the number of entities that can be seen at the same time leading to restriction of the Field of attention, Oculomotor (ocular) apraxia and Optic ataxia. The syndrome can vary in severity from mild to severe; the resulting impairments are omission of parts of the surroundings, difficulties with intentionally shifting gaze to locations of interest or to external stimuli and impaired visual guidance of grasping movements and movement of other parts of the body. In addition, those affected exhibit Spatial disorientation and have difficulties with reading, writing, copying, dressing, etc.

Bilateral homonymous hemianopia Homonymous loss of vision in both visual hemifields with sparing of the central visual field; also called 'tunnel vision'.

Binocular vision Three-dimensional perception of the surroundings brought about by the combined slightly differing visual input from each of the two eyes.

Biological motion perception Visual perception of the kinds of motion performed by humans and animals (e.g. hand, head and body movements; movements of the tail of cats and dogs; galloping or cantering of horses).

Blindsight The capacity to detect and locate visual stimuli presented in a perimetrically blind visual field region (e.g. in the anopic hemifield) in conditions of forced guessing without awareness or associated visual experience. Blindsight is assumed to be mediated by extra-geniculo-striate visual pathways, e.g. the Visual midbrain, or is due to residual vision in spared striate cortex or to processing in extrastriate visual cortical areas.

Blurred vision See Visual blurring.

Bottom-up processing The processing of stimulus input from the retina to higher cortical levels of processing.

Brain plasticity The capacity of the brain to adapt its functions to altered environmental (or task) conditions by experience (Environment-dependent plasticity) and Learning (Practice-dependent plasticity) and to compensate for functional alterations of the brain, e.g. after injury or in pathophysiological states (Functional compensation).

Brodmann area Is a region of the Cerebral cortex, which is defined by its structure and organisation of cells (so-called cytoarchitecture). Brodmann areas were originally defined and numbered by the German neuroanatomist Korbinian Brodmann who in 1909 described 47 different cortical areas.

Brodmann's area An area of the Cerebral cortex that is characterised by differences in the form and arrangement of nerve cells (neurons) from neighbouring areas. The original map of Brodmann contains 47 different cortical areas.

Capacity The amount of available mental processing function required to perform a task or Activity.

Categorisation The process of grouping stimuli, events, people or experiences into classes based on characteristics shared by members of the same class (category) and on the basis of features that distinguish the members of one class from another; also called classification.

Central nervous system (CNS) The brain and spinal cord.

Central scotoma Focal lack of central visual function, classified as relative scotoma, i.e. reduced central visual function, and absolute scotoma, i.e. absence of central visual function.

Central visual field A loose term referring approximately to the central 20° of the visual field.

Cerebral achromatopsia Acquired severe impairment or loss of colour perception, which typically results from injury to ventromedial occipital cortex; also labelled acquired colour blindness. Colours can no longer be discriminated and coloured stimuli appear as being pale and washed out or as shades of grey.

Cerebral amblyopia Lack of colour and form vision associated with depression of light vision in Homonymous central or peripheral visual field regions (Homonymous hemiamblyopia).

Cerebral blindness Profound complete or incomplete lack of vision due to visual brain dysfunction. (Also commonly referred to as cortical blindness.)

Cerebral cortex The layer of grey matter that covers the outside of the brain and consists of six layers of neurons. Regional differences in the cytoarchitectonic characteristics led Brodmann to the categorisation of the cerebral cortex into distinct areas (Brodmann's areas).

Cerebral dyschromatopsia Acquired mild to moderate impairment of colour perception resulting in difficulties with fine colour hue discrimination.

Cerebral hypoxia Lack of oxygen supply to the brain, which can be brought about by impaired blood flow or impaired oxygenation due to severe respiratory disorders.

Cerebral palsy Loss or impairment of motor function caused by damage or abnormal development of the brain before, during or immediately after birth.

Cerebral visual disorder Cerebral visual dysfunction; Cerebral visual impairment.

Cerebral visual dysfunction Lack of perceptual visual functions as a sequel to damage or abnormal development of the brain.

Cerebral visual impairment Deficient visual function as a sequel to damage or malfunction of the retrogeniculate visual pathways (optic radiations, occipital cortex, and visual associative areas) commonly also affecting oculomotor control.

Cerebrovascular disease A range of disorders interfering with the blood supply to the brain leading to brain damage. This may be generalised or focal, profound or mild.

Chorioretinitis (retinochoroiditis) Focal damage to the retina and underlying choroid due to inflammation. The term is applied to both active disease and subsequent scarring. Causes include toxoplasmosis, cytomegalovirus and herpes simplex infection, which can cause damage to the brain.

Classical conditioning A type of learning in which a neutral stimulus (conditioned stimulus, CS) is paired with a stimulus which elicits a response (unconditioned stimulus, UCS) when the CS is presented; also called Pavlovian conditioning.

Classification See Categorisation.

Closed head trauma Blunt injury to the head. Bruising (contusion) of the brain of varying severity can result.

Cognition Umbrella term for all forms of higher-order mental processes that enable processing, selection, storing and evaluation of information but also guiding and monitoring activities, i.e. Perception, Attention, Learning and Memory, Executive function and Praxis.

Cognitive visual impairment The impairment of cognitive capacities that are involved in and depend on visual perception, e.g. Visual spatial attention, Visual perceptual learning and Visual memory, and Visual recognition.

Colour vision The ability to distinguish visual stimuli on the basis of their wavelengths (colour (a fully saturated hue), hues).

Colour contrast vision The ability to distinguish tints (colours to which white has been added (e.g. light blue)) and shades (colours to which black has been added (e.g. navy blue)).

Compensation See Functional compensation

Concept formation The process by which we abstract a common percept or idea from single, particular experiences through learning characteristic or defining features of a particular category or class of stimuli or ideas; see also Categorisation.

Congenital Present at the time of birth (whether acquired, developmental or inherited in origin).

Congenital colour vision deficiency Usually refers to inherited disorders of colour vision discrimination due to specific abnormal development of retinal cones. Impaired red and green discrimination are most common, affecting up to 8 % of men on account of sex-linked inheritance. However, cerebral visual impairment from birth can also impair the ability to discriminate colours.

Congenital oculomotor apraxia (Cogan syndrome) Impairment in the ability to make horizontal fast eye movements associated with disordered structure of the cerebellar vermis. Intermittent rapid horizontal head movements or head thrusting is commonly observed. The condition tends to abate spontaneously into teenage years.

Constancy See Perceptual constancy.

Contrast sensitivity A measure of spatial resolution of the visual system to detect subtle differences between regular light and dark elements (e.g. gratings or vertical stripes) of a given size. Contrast sensitivity is best for gratings with spatial frequencies of 4–8 cycles per degree (one cycle is a pair of light and dark stripes) and is lower for both lower and higher frequencies. Reduction of contrast sensitivity may cause Visual blurring and 'foggy vision'.

Convergence The ability to turn both eyes in towards the nose. Reflex convergence occurs when looking at a near target in order to maintain the target upon the fovea of the retina of each eye.

Convergence insufficiency Impaired ability to bring about reflex convergence of the eyes to view near targets.

Curiosity The spontaneous impulse or desire to investigate the physical and social surroundings for information, particularly for novel or interesting stimuli. Young children with high visual curiosity explore their environments using gaze shifts and, for near, also engage in manipulatory hand activities to explore and inspect stimuli of interest.

Dark adaptation The capacity of the retina to increase its sensitivity to light under darkened conditions. The retinal cones adapt for levels of lighting in which colour can be perceived; the retinal rods adapt further under dark conditions where colour cannot be seen. Full dark adaptation is slow and takes half an hour. (That is why one cannot see when walking into a cinema, but can see to walk out).

Declarative memory Refers to the memory of episodes (episodic memory) and knowledge (semantic memory) that can be consciously recalled when requested to remember; also called explicit memory.

Deficit Nonspecific term referring to lack of a function (e.g. a visual field deficit refers to an area of deficient visual field).

Developmental dyslexia Is an umbrella term for various types of difficulties with the acquisition of reading. Typically reading development lags behind other cognitive development, and reading is limited and characterised by slow reading.

Developmental plasticity The enhanced capacity of the brain to adapt to the environment by specific experience ('experience-expectant plasticity'). Periods of high developmental plasticity ('sensitive periods') are characterised by increased sensitivity to sensory experiences, resulting in fast and highly effective learning, and at the same time by increased vulnerability, because development may be impaired. For example, if the visual cortex is deprived from visual input, because of clouding of the lens of the eye or retinal disease, neurons in the visual cortex cannot develop their normal sensitivity; connections in the visual cortex will not develop (properly), and thus visual function cannot develop normally.

Developmental prosopagnosia The specific inability to learn to recognise frequently seen faces (e.g. of parents, grandparents, friends) as familiar, despite normal visual functions and cognitive capacities, which typically occurs after abnormal brain development of or injury to occipito-temporal structures in the right hemisphere or in both hemispheres. Also called congenital prosopagnosia.

Developmental visual agnosia A specific type of visual agnosia characterised by the inability to learn to recognise frequently seen visual stimuli (objects, faces, places, letters) despite normal visual functions and cognitive capacities, which typically occurs after abnormal brain development of or injury to Visual association areas in the posterior brain. Also called congenital visual agnosia.

Developmental visual dyslexia A specific type of visual agnosia which is characterised by the inability to learn the significance of letters and/or the integration of letters into words. Also called congenital dyslexia.

Dioptre A measure of the power of a lens, which is the reciprocal of the focal length of a lens (e.g. a one dioptre lens will bring a parallel beam of light to a focus at one metre, while a two dioptre lens will focus the light at half of a metre.) Positive values refer to convex lenses, while negative values refer to concave lenses.

Diplegia Term commonly used to describe the pattern of cerebral palsy in which there is weakness of the lower limbs.

Disability Impairment of Ability.

Disorder Lack of order or organisation.

Divergence The act of change in the position of the eyes from being convergent to look at a near target to becoming aligned to look at a distant target.

Dorsal pathway Denotes the visual pathway from the Striate cortex to the Posterior parietal cortex (occipito-parietal route), also known as the 'WHERE' pathway, because this pathway is specialised for the analysis of visual spatial information, which is used for the visual guidance of actions.

Dorsal route See Dorsal pathway.

Down syndrome Or trisomy 21 is a genetic disorder caused by the presence of all or part of an additional third copy of chromosome 21.

Dyschromatopsia Defective colour vision.

Dysfunction Visual dysfunction can be used to describe the outcome of developmental perceptual disorders.

Dyslexia Specific disorder of reading, either congenital or acquired; see Developmental dyslexia; Hemianopic dyslexia.

Dysmetric saccadic movements Fast eye movements that do not reach the target and require compensatory saccades to do so. These can be observed clinically.

Early developmental disorder Impairment of child development observed during early life.

Ecological validity Denotes the degree to which observed behaviour/performance reflects the behaviour/performance of a subject in the 'real world', i.e. the degree to which diagnostic findings can be generalised (or extended) to natural, everyday life settings.

Encephalomalacia Literally means softening of the brain, but the term is used to refer to outcome of degenerative disorders affecting the structure of the brain.

Emmetropia Having no optical error and, therefore, normal sighted.

Emotion Simple or complex discrete and consistent responses to internal or external events which have a particular significance for the individual. Emotions are brief in duration and consist of a coordinated set of nonverbal (e.g. mimics, gestures) and verbal responses and of physiological reactions (e.g. increase in blood pressure). Basic emotions are surprise, happiness, anger, disgust, fear and sadness; also called affect. See also Mood.

Encephalopathy Any extensive brain disorder.

Environment-dependent plasticity Denotes the influence of environmental stimuli on Brain plasticity; without adequate environmental stimulation, learning processes in the domains of perception and action cannot take place properly.

Epilepsy A group of conditions in which disturbance of the electrical activity of the brain results in impairment and disorder in a range of brain functions, including consciousness, movement, sensation and vision.

Episodic memory The memory for events and episodes with respect to time, place and other details; personal memories are stored in the autobiographical memory.

Esotropia A condition in which the eyes are turned in. Also known as convergent strabismus or convergent squint.

Executive function Umbrella term comprising processes/functions of organising, adapting and monitoring/controlling of mental processes and actions.

Exotropia A condition in which the eyes are turned out. Also known as divergent strabismus or divergent squint.

Experience-dependent plasticity Denotes the influence of experience (learning) on Brain plasticity; without systematic and specific experience with environmental stimuli, learning processes in the domains of perception and action cannot take place properly.

External attention Attention guided by the selection and modulation of spatial and temporal properties and modality of sensory input.

Extrageniculate visual pathways Retinal afferents projecting to the visual midbrain (superior colliculus, posterior thalamus) and hence to Extrastriate visual areas and to the parietal, temporal and frontal cortex.

Extrastriate cortex See Extrastriate visual areas.

Extrastriate visual areas Visual cortical areas outside the Striate (primary) visual cortex; also called prestriate cortex or visual association areas.

Face perception Sensory and cognitive processes involved in the processing of (unfamiliar and familiar) faces and of Facial expressions.

Face recognition The identification of an individual's face on the basis of specific and characteristic facial features, enabled by repeated identification of the same face.

Facial expression The sum of nonverbal social signals produced by the movement of facial muscles that reflects the individual's emotional state.

Foetal alcohol spectrum disorders A term describing the permanent birth defects caused by maternal consumption of alcohol during pregnancy.

Field of attention The distribution of attention in the field of vision, which enables the individual to detect stimuli in the corresponding sector of the surroundings and allows Global perception of a scene, with coarse spatial resolution.

Field of gaze The extent of visual processing when moving the eyes and head.

Figure-ground discrimination The ability to discriminate an object from its surroundings; also called figure-ground perception.

Fixation The ability to maintain the direction of the eyes to look at a target.

Fixation inaccuracy Inaccuracy of the ability of the eyes to look at a target.

Fixation nystagmus To and fro movement of the eyes which is evident when a target is being looked at.

Flash-evoked visual potential Electrical signals recorded from electrodes placed on the back of the head and extracted from background brain activity in response to flashes of light directed at the eyes; mainly generated in subcortical visual structures.

Foggy vision See Visual blurring

Form perception The ability to judge the shape, size, texture, etc. of an object by vision or touch; also called form discrimination.

Fovea The central depression in the retina populated by cone photoreceptors, responsible for the high resolution colour perception at the centre of the visual field.

Foveal sparing A term referring to retinal disease that is paracentral, causing a Paracentral scotoma.

Fragile X syndrome A specific disorder of the X chromosome that most commonly affects males (females usually being spared by having a second normal X chromosome). The mutation impairs normal neural development. It is the most widespread single gene cause of autism.

Functional compensation The substitution of impaired or lost capacities by other functions, e.g. vision by touch.

Functional specialisation Sensory cortical areas are specialised in processing and coding for specific pieces of sensory information.

Functional vision The way vision with both eyes open is employed in everyday life. Assessment of functional vision determines impact of the limits of visual function on everyday life and is employed as a means of ensuring that these limits are dealt with by strategies that minimise their impact.

Fusional vergence The act of converging or diverging the eyes to ensure that the two incoming images are integrated.

Ganglion cells The cell bodies on the surface of the retina whose neurons synapse with the bipolar cells in the retina and the cells in the lateral geniculate bodies whose neurons comprise the optic radiations.

Gaze apraxia Is the impairment in using eye movements in a purposeful action, despite the intact capacity to carry out the eye movements.

Geographical orientation Is the ability to recognise the spatial arrangements of places, paths and rooms/buildings by using familiar Landmarks.

Gestalt The integration of elements into an entire perceptual configuration.

Gestalt principles Principles of perception, which describe and explain the tendency to perceive/interpret certain configurations at the level of the whole, rather than details of a given object, e.g. symmetry, similarity, grouping, continuity, closure.

Global perception Overall perception of a scene or an object, without focusing on details (Local processing).

Global processing See Global perception.

Grating A stimulus that consists of regular parallel light and dark elements.

Habilitation A strategy of facilitating the use of all intact capabilities in a child who has impaired functions from around the time of birth, to bring about optimal development.

Handicap Disability causing difficulty in bringing about actions.

Hemianopic dyslexia Refers to impairment of reading at the level of text processing because of a restricted reading span due to parafoveal visual field loss.

Hemiplegia Disability moving one side of the body.

Hemispherectomy Therapeutic surgical removal of one hemisphere of the brain.

Heterotopia Location of brain tissue in an abnormal focal position.

Heterotropia An alternative term for strabismus or squint.

History taking A structured approach of questioning, listening and interpreting the responses of patients or those who are close to them, to gain as much information as possible to guide diagnosis, therapy and rehabilitation.

Holoprosencephaly Failure of the forebrain to completely divide into two halves.

Homonymous central loss of vision See Homonymous loss of vision.

Homonymous loss of vision Denotes loss of vision due to injury to the visual pathways behind the Optic chiasm, in which the distribution is very similar in both Visual fields. As a rule, the more similar (or congruous) the pattern of visual field loss, the closer the injury to the Striate cortex.

Homonymous hemiachromatopsia The loss of colour vision in both corresponding (e.g. left-sided) halves of the visual field, while light and form vision are spared.

Homonymous hemiamblyopia The loss of colour and form vision in corresponding (e.g. left-sided) halves of the visual field for each eye, while light vision is depressed.

Homonymous hemianopia The loss of vision in the same half of the visual field of each eye, e.g. in both left halves of the visual field.

Homonymous quadranopia The loss of vision in the same quadrant of the visual field of each eye, e.g. in both upper or lower left quadrants of the visual field; also called quadrantanopia.

Horizontal pursuit Movement of the eyes as they follow a moving target.

Hydrocephalus Impaired drainage of cerebrospinal fluid leading to its retention. In children, expansion of the lateral ventricles with damage to the lining white matter is a common outcome.

Hypermetropia or long-sightedness A condition in which incoming light is not brought to a focus sufficiently to be in focus on the retina. Convex spectacle lenses are used to compensate.

Hyperopia An alternative term for Hypermetropia.

Hypometric saccades (hypometria) Fast eye movements that are short of the target.

Impairment The outcome of disorder or lack of function.

Infarction Death of tissue resulting from absence of blood supply.

Intensity Of attention refers to the quantitative components of attention, i.e. level of attention and duration of a given attentional level.

Intermittent saccadic failure The transient absence of externally triggered saccades.

Internal attention The selection, modulation and maintenance of internally generated 'information' and of actions.

Intervention The action and technique, respectively, to deal with the issues and problems of a patient or a client.

Joint attention Attention directed by two or more people on the same object, action, event or person at the same time; also called shared attention.

Kinaesthetic information Information that is conveyed to the brain in response to the movement of one's body, comprising the nature, direction, speed and the initial and final locations of the movement.

Kinetic perimetry Instrumental assessment of the extent of the visual fields using a bowl perimeter and a moving visual target. The lines drawn join points of equal retinal sensitivity and are known as isopters.

Landmark Is a recognisable natural or man-made feature used for navigation.

Learning Is the process of acquisition of new knowledge or modifying and reinforcing existing knowledge, behaviours or skills, with progress over time, due to regular and systematic repetition; changes produced by learning are relatively persistent.

Learning by insight Is a form of cognitive learning, whereby inductions and deductions as well as problem solving combined with previous experiences and learned behaviour play important roles.

Letter agnosia Is a selective type of visual agnosia, which is characterised by the loss of recognition of the significance of letters and/or the integration of letters into words.

Light adaptation Is the capacity of the retina to adapt to increased levels of illumination.

Lissencephaly Literally meaning 'smooth brain', is caused by defective neuronal migration between the 12th and 24th weeks of gestation resulting in lack of brain folds (or gyri).

Local processing Detailed analysis of a scene or an object (Global processing).

logMAR The logarithm of the minimum angle of resolution is a measure of visual acuity and comprises an angular measure of the smallest maximum contrast (black vs. white) target that can be discriminated.

Long-term memory Is the final stage of memory, in which information can be stored for long periods of time.

Loss of vision Acquired absence or lack of ability to see.

Low vision A term usually applied to those who have impaired visual acuities.

Macropsia Is a form of dysmetropsia, in which visual stimuli (e.g. objects) appear larger than normal.

Macular sparing Is a term applied to those whose bilateral occipital lobe damage (usually due to occlusion of the posterior cerebral arteries) has spared central visual function within a diameter of ~9° visual angle. (In a sense, it is not the maculae that are spared, but the input from the maculae that is.)

Maladaptation Adaptive strategies resulting from pathology that exacerbate rather than compensate for the resulting disabilities.

Memory Includes all processes which allow us to encode information, create a permanent record, and retrieve stored information.

Mental functions Is an umbrella term for processes of the mind, i.e. cognition, emotion, motivation.

Mesopic vision Partially dark-adapted vision at the level at which cone adaptation is maximal.

Micropsia Is a form of dysmetropsia, in which stimuli appear smaller than normal.

Milestone Is a developmental stage, which a child is expected to have reached at a given age.

Minimum separable or discriminable Refers to visual acuity and denotes the measure of separation at which elements of high-contrast images can be seen or discriminated.

Model learning Observational learning.

Mood Denotes more diffuse, longer-lasting emotional states.

Motion perception Is a genuine visual capacity that allows the direct analysis of the direction and speed of moving visual stimuli.

Motivation Is the impulse or desire ('drive') which gives purpose or direction to actions. External factors for motivation ('extrinsic motivation') are rewards or disincentives, for example punishment and its avoidance, respectively; internal factors ('intrinsic motivation') are individual interests, pleasure and positive self-reinforcement (satisfaction).

Movement vision See Motion perception.

Multitasking Is the performance of handling more than one task at a time.

Myopia or short-sightedness A condition in which incoming light is brought to a focus in front of the retina. Near targets can be seen, but distant targets are blurred. Concave spectacle lenses are used to compensate.

Neonatal Shortly after birth or newborn.

Neurofibromatosis (type 1) A genetically inherited autosomal dominant disorder in which the nerve tissue grows tumours.

Neuroplasticity Refers to adaptation of neural pathways and structures which are due to changes in behaviour, environment and neural processes as well as changes resulting from injury due to learning processes; see also Brain plasticity.

Non-declarative memory Denotes unconscious memories such as skills (e.g. learning to ride a bicycle); also called procedural memory.

Non-organic visual dysfunction Is impairment or loss of vision without evidence for an organic dysfunction of the peripheral and/or central components of the visual system; also called 'psychogenic' or 'functional' visual disorder.

Nystagmus Is a congenital or acquired involuntary, persistent, rapid and oscillatory to and fro movement of the eyes.

Observational learning Is learning of new responses or behaviours, without reinforcement, by observing the response/behaviour of another person that serves as a model.

Occipital cortex Is the most posterior lobe of the brain, which contains the structures for processing and coding of visual information; see also Visual brain.

Occipital encephalocele Congenital sac-like protrusion of the brain through an opening at the back of the skull.

Oculomotor scanning Use of eye movements (Saccades, Fixations) to scan the visual surrounding or a visual stimulus array (scene, object); see also Scanning pattern.

Oculomotor system The neural system that brings about eye movements.

OKN See Optokinetic nystagmus.

Operant conditioning Is the use of consequences (e.g. positive reinforcement) to modify the occurrence and form of a given behaviour.

Optic ataxia Impaired visual guidance of movement of the limbs and body related to bilateral damage in the posterior parietal territory of the brain.

Optic atrophy Pallor of the optic nerves seen by ophthalmoscopy.

Optic chiasm Is the part of the afferent visual system where the optic nerves partially cross.

Optic nerve hypoplasia Congenital small size of the optic nerves.

Optic radiation Is the part of the visual pathways from the Optic chiasm to the Striate cortex.

Optokinetic nystagmus (OKN) Reflex to and fro movement of the eyes in response to moving targets. OKN can be tested horizontally and vertically in response to moving black and white stripes or other repeating targets in the appropriate directions in front of the eyes.

Optotypes Letters, shapes or images used for testing visual acuity.

Orienting response Is an immediate response (e.g. gaze shift) to a novel or significant stimulus or stimulus change in the environment that is typically preceded by a shift in covert attention.

Orthophoria The eyes are straight and do not deviate even when one is covered.

Pachygyria A congenital malformation of the cerebral hemispheres with wide brain folds or gyri.

Paracentral scotoma An area of lack of vision close to the centre of the visual field.

Parallel processing Is the ability to simultaneously process several stimuli.

Paroxysmal ocular deviations Rapid pathological eye movements, which are commonly upwards and to one side that are most often seen in children with quadriplegic cerebral palsy.

Pattern perception Is the discrimination and identification, respectively, of a set of stimuli arranged in a certain regular form, e.g. contours, figures, objects, faces, words, melodies.

Pattern-evoked visual potential Electrical signals recorded from electrodes placed on the back of the head and extracted from background brain activity in response to equiluminant patterns such as alternating chequerboards, while viewed by the eyes; mainly generated in cortical structures of the visual system.

Perception Is the conscious outcome of processing stimulus information that includes observing, discriminating and identifying.

Perceptual constancy Tendency to see familiar stimuli (e.g. objects, faces, letters) as having the same (or at least a very similar) shape, size, colour or location regardless of changes in the angle of perspective, lighting or distance. Perceptual constancy is responsible for the ability to identify objects under various conditions; it is reduced by limited experience with the stimulus and by reducing environmental cues that aid in stimulus identification.

Perceptual learning Denotes improvement of skills in perception by learning, comprising detection, localisation, discrimination, identification/recognition and categorisation.

Perimetry See Kinetic perimetry.

Perinatal The time period between 22 weeks' gestation to 7 days after birth.

Peripheral visual field Refers to the full extent of the capacity to perceive targets in the periphery of the visual fields. When tested by moving large peripheral targets, it can extend to 100° temporally, is bounded by the profile of the nose nasally, and inferiorly allows detection of the movement of one's own feet. (This extent of the visual field is not detected by formal periphery, yet is of considerable functional importance.)

Periventricular leucomalacia (PVL) A form of white matter brain injury due to ischaemic damage adjacent to the lateral ventricles. This is considered a neuropathological term, and for this reason the term periventricular white matter pathology may be applied to describe the appearance seen by means of MRI scanning.

Periventricular white matter pathology See Periventricular leucomalacia.

Peroxisomal disorders A class of medical conditions caused by defects of peroxisome function including the progressive brain disorder of adrenoleucodsytrophy.

Photopic vision The state of visual adaptation in conditions of good lighting.

PL See Preferential looking.

Planning Is the process of thinking about and developing and organising the activities required to achieve a desired goal of action; also called forethought.

Polymicrogyria A descriptive term applied to the condition in which there are multiple small convolutions on the brain instead of the normal pattern of gyri. The functions affected depend on the distribution of the disorder.

Porencephaly Cysts or cavities within the cerebral hemisphere resulting from resorption of the damaged brain after prior pathology such as ischaemia, haemorrhage or abnormal development.

Posterior parietal cortex Is part of parietal cortex which contains a multimodal representation of space, which serves as the basis for the visual guidance of movements of eyes, head, arms and hands in space and facilitates visual search.

Postural control Is the ability to control the position of one's body, including head lifting and holding, sitting up and walking.

Practice-dependent plasticity Is the capacity of the brain to develop and adapt actions to cope with environmental challenges or task demands by learning due to systematic practice; without systematic learning, processes in the domains of perception and action cannot take place properly; see also Brain plasticity; Environmental-dependent plasticity.

Praxis Denotes skilled actions or acts.

Preferential looking (PL) Is an experimental method in developmental psychology. An infant is habituated to a particular stimulus; then a second, new stimulus is shown, which differs from the habituated stimulus with respect to a specific feature (e.g. size, colour, form). If the infant now looks for longer at the new stimulus, it is suggestive that the infant can discriminate between the two stimuli. See also Visual preference paradigm. Preferential looking is now used routinely to estimate visual acuities in young children and those who are otherwise unable to cooperate with the use of other methods.

Prematurity Birth before 37 weeks' gestation.

Problem solving Is the use of rules in a (more or less) systematic manner to find a solution to a problem and thereby to reach a definite goal, because cognitive or action procedures from past experience are not successful to cope with, e.g. a task.

Procedural memory Is the memory for action plans and action routines; also called implicit memory.

Prosopagnosia Is a specific type of Visual agnosia, which is characterised by the acquired loss of the ability to recognise visually familiar faces and learn new faces; it occurs typically after bilateral or (less frequently) unilateral occipito-temporal injury.

Pure alexia Is a specific type of Visual agnosia, which is characterised by the acquired loss of the significance of letters and/or the integration of letters into words.

Pursuit eye movements Coordinated tracking by the eyes of a slowly moving visual target ($\leq$30 deg/s).

Quadriplegia/tetraplegia Impaired ability to move all four limbs.

Reading Is the cognitive process of decoding symbols (letters, numbers and digits) to derive meaning from the text at the semantic level after processing the text at the visuo-sensory, pre-semantic level.

Reading span Is the spatial and temporal width of text processing at the pre-semantic level and at the semantic level, where text material is semantically processed for comprehension.

Receptive field Is the region of space that elicits a response from a neuron.

Refractive error An abnormality of optics of the eye such as Myopia, Hypermetropia and Astigmatism.

Refraction anomaly Unspecified Refractive error.

Reliability Is a psychometric measure that denotes the consistency of a measure; high reliability means that the measure produces similar results under consistent conditions.

Retina The inner receptive lining of the eye.

Retinopathy (of prematurity) Abnormal vascular growth of the retina seen in very premature infants that is screened for and treated prophylactically by laser treatment. Progression of the disorder leads to retinal detachment (previously known as retrolental fibroplasia) and loss of vision.

Saccades See saccadic eye movements.

Saccadic eye movements Fast eye movements.

Scanning pattern Is the pattern of oculomotor activity that is used to process and perceive a scene or an object; it is characterised by an organised scan path, i.e. a sequence of Saccades and Fixations; see also Oculomotor scanning.

Schizencephaly A grey matter-lined cleft in the brain occurring as a rare developmental abnormality of brain tissue.

Scotoma A focal area of lack of vision in the visual field.

Scotopic vision Dark adapted vision; see Dark adaptation.

Selective attention Is the cognitive process of selectively concentrating on one stimulus or aspect of a stimulus, or part of the environment, while ignoring other stimuli.

Selectivity Of attention refers to the qualitative aspect of attention, i.e. focussing of attention (concentration), dividing of attention (divided attention), and flexibility of attention.

Semantic memory Is the memory for knowledge and facts and is part of the Declarative memory.

Sensitive periods Denote periods in child development that are characterised by increased sensitivity to external stimuli, such as in emotional and social environments (e.g. social interactions). Deprivation of appropriate stimuli or an appropriate environment may have deleterious effects on the further development of a function.

Sensitivity Is the ability/readiness to respond to external stimuli.

Short-term memory Is the capacity for holding a limited number (7 ± 2) of stimuli (or items) for a short period of time, without further processing (e.g. repeating a number of digits).

Simultanagnosia Is the inability of an individual to perceive more than a single stimulus or object at a time. Because the 'agnostic' nature of this disorder is unclear, the term 'impaired parallel processing' may be preferred to denote this visual-attentional disorder.

Smooth pursuit eye movements See Pursuit eye movement.

Social perception Is the perception of social signals, e.g. facial expressions, gestures, body position and movements, and voice, that help to understand the 'state of mind' of another individual.

Social signals See Social perception.

Space blindness Is the loss of the ability to process correctly visual information about the position of stimuli in space and of spatial relationships of objects in space, which can occur after bilateral posterior brain injury.

Spastic diplegia Impairment of movement of the legs in which increased muscle tone results in stiffness and tightness.

Spastic movements The nature of movement of the limbs in which there is increased muscle tone.

Spatial attention Is the distribution of attention in space; it can be globally distributed (Global processing) or locally focused (Local processing).

Spatial contrast sensitivity See Contrast sensitivity.

Spatial contrast vision See Contrast sensitivity.

Spatial disorientation Is the inability to correctly determine one's own location in space and adjustment this location with reference to Landmarks in the same space.

Spatial frequency Is the number of repeating elements in a pattern per unit distance, e.g. black and white vertical bars per degree of visual angle, usually expressed as cycles per degree (c/deg).

Spatial orientation Is the perception of one's own location in space and its adjustment with reference to objects (Landmark) in the same space.

Spatial vision Perception of spatial properties of visual stimuli, e.g. position, orientation of contours, spatial configuration of figures, objects and scenes.

Spontaneous adaptation Is the ability of an individual to adapt the behaviour to changes in the environment or in the own behavioural repertoire, i.e. in the case of functional impairment due to a disordered state of the brain (e.g. in brain developmental disorders or after brain injury) without systematic and specific practice.

Spontaneous recovery Is the recovery of function without intervention.

Squint An alternative term to Strabismus.

Stereoacuity See Stereoscopic acuity.

Stereopsis The perception of depth brought about when a scene is perceived by the two eyes.

Stereoscopic acuity A measure of the least angular disparity in depth between images seen by the two eyes that leads to perception of depth.

Stimulus salience Effectiveness of a stimulus to elicit a response.

Strabismus Misalignment of the eyes.

Striate cortex First cortical area which receives retinal input from the thalamus (geniculo-striate pathway); also called primary visual cortex, Brodmann's area 17, visual area 1, V1.

Striate (primary) visual cortex Is the discrete region in the posterior occipital lobes of the brain that receives input directly from the eyes via the Optic radiations, which serves primary visual functions, e.g. light detection; also labelled Brodmann area 17 or V1 (visual area 1). (When this part of the brain is sectioned, a light brown line, or stria, is observed, from which the term striate is derived).

Substitution of function Replacement of a severely impaired or lost function by another function, e.g. visual field loss by gaze shifts.

Take-the-odd-one-out paradigm Experimental method to assess stimulus discrimination and simple categorisation. Typically three stimuli (e.g. colours) are presented, two identical (standard stimuli) and one different (odd) stimulus. The subject's task is to find the odd stimulus, which does not match with the two other stimuli; also called oddity learning.

Tetraplegia See Quadriplegia.

Text processing Is the act of processing text material (letters, numbers); essential prerequisites are an intact central visual field, a sufficiently high visual acuity and contrast sensitivity, accurate form discrimination, ability to integrate letters/numbers to larger elements and regular shifting of fixation in the direction of processing. Text processing is the main basis for understanding of text material; see also Reading.

Top-down processing Is the processing of information guided by intention or expectation (what a stimulus might be).

Topographagnosia Specific loss of spatial and geographical orientation, because familiar landmarks, places, paths and rooms can no longer be recognised; occurs typically after right-sided posterior-parietal but also hippocampal injury. Also called topographical disorientation or topographical agnosia.

Trial-and-error learning Is a type of learning in which an individual successively tries various (random) responses until one response is successful in achieving the goal.

Turner syndrome A chromosomal disorder affecting females in which one of the two X chromosomes is missing.

Useful field of view (UFOV) Is the space a subject is spontaneously observing and searching for visual stimuli with eye movements; also called Field of gaze.

Validity Is a psychometric measure that indicates the degree to which a test or measurement accurately assesses or reflects what it purports to assess.

Ventral pathway Denotes the visual pathway from the Striate cortex to the temporal cortex (occipito-temporal route), which analyses and codes information about features (e.g. form, figural details, colour) of visual stimuli (objects, faces); also called the WHAT pathway.

Ventral route See Ventral pathway.

Vergence Horizontal movement of the eyes in opposite directions; see Convergence and Divergence.

Ventral route See Ventral pathway.

Vestibular ocular reflex (VOR) The balance system served by the inner ear accords subconscious knowledge of the vertical and horizontal; these data inform the vestibular system in the midbrain, which automatically aligns the eyes to the horizon in total darkness. Rotation of the head in an unconscious person brings about such righting (doll's eye) movements if brainstem function is intact.

Viral encephalitis Infection of the brain by virus (e.g. herpes simplex virus or cytomegalovirus).

Visual acuity A measure of the resolution of central vision at maximum contrast (black/white).

Visual adaptation The capacity of the retina to change its sensitivity to light; see Dark adaptation; Light adaptation.

Visual agnosia Is the specific loss of the ability to recognise stimuli in the visual modality, despite spared visual and cognitive functions.

Visual anomia Is the difficulty to associate visual stimuli (e.g. colours) with their proper names.

Visual association areas See Extrastriate visual areas.

Visual association cortex See Extrastriate visual areas.

Visual blurring Is observed when discrete boundaries between image components are not seen as distinct, but instead merge into one another. This can be caused by refractive error and disorder of the eyes or visual pathways.

Visual brain Is an umbrella term for all visual cortical areas and their fibre connections.

Visual contrast sensitivity See spatial contrast sensitivity.

Visual crowding A level of complexity of the visual scene that leads to impaired visual search and a sense of discomfort.

Visual curiosity Curiosity in the visual modality, characterised by active and spontaneous Visual exploration of the surroundings and attending at visual stimuli.

Visual deprivation Lack of visual experience during early life that leads to impaired visual function due to amblyopia.

Visual discomfort A subjective sense of discomfort brought about by visual conditions that are at the limit of the individual's capacity to process the information.

Visual exploration Is the intentional activity of the eyes and the head to explore the visual environment or a stimulus display.

Visual function Is the ability to process visual stimuli of a particular dimension, e.g. form, colour or motion.

Visual hallucination A visual perception in the absence of any visual stimulus.

Visual illusion A misperception of visual stimuli.

Visual impairment See Cerebral visual impairment.

Visual localisation Is the ability to locate the position of a visual target.

Visual memory Is the capacity to remember visual experiences.

Visual midbrain Denotes the upper posterior midbrain area including the superior colliculi that serves reflex visual function (e.g. reflexive saccadic orienting responses to visual stimuli).

Visual neglect Is a type of sensory neglect in the visual modality which is characterised by (a) the absence of visual activities including exploration of the contralateral space, typically left from the line of sight; (b) the shift of the subjective midline (and thus the line of sight) to the ipsilateral side; and (c) incomplete mental spatial representation of scenes and objects, which is associated with omissions of left-sided objects or details of objects when asked to draw from memory.

Visual object agnosia Specific loss of recognition of familiar objects in the visual modality, despite sufficient visual and cognitive functions; recognition of the same object in other (e.g. auditory or tactile) modalities is intact; very rare type of Visual agnosia.

Visual perceptual learning Learning in the visual modality; Perceptual learning.

Visual preference paradigm An experimental technique for the study of visual discrimination in infants in which the time spent on a particular stimulus is used as an indicator for preference.

Visual recognition Is the ability to recognise familiar stimuli (e.g. objects) by visual perception.

Visual search Is the process of detecting a target stimulus among distractor stimuli. If the target differs qualitatively from distractors, it pops out, and search time is independent of the number of stimuli in the display (set size); this search type is called a parallel search mode. If the target and distractors are similar, then the subject has to search for the target in a serial fashion (serial search mode).

Visual space perception Is the sum of abilities to process and comprehend spatial properties of the environment and of objects, i.e. position, distance, direction, spatial relationships between stimuli; see also Spatial vision.

Visual spatial attention Is attention in space in the visual modality; see Attention.

Visual spatial orientation Is Spatial orientation by means of vision.

Visual working memory Is the working memory for visual information; Working memory.

Visuo-construction Is the ability to construct two- or three-dimensional visual configurations, e.g. a square or a cube, by drawing or assembling parts into a complete structure; also called visuo-constructive ability.

VOR See Vestibular ocular reflex.

West syndrome An early onset triad of infantile spasms, a typical electroencephalographic pattern of hypsarrythmia and arrest of psychomotor development, which may first present in early infancy as the child not showing visual behaviour.

WHAT pathway Occipito-temporal route that is specialised for the processing of visual object properties; also called the Ventral route.

WHERE pathway Occipito-parietal route that is specialised for the processing of visuospatial information; also called the Dorsal route.

Williams syndrome An autosomal dominant genetic condition affecting chromosome 7q, with distinctive facies, supravalvular aortic stenosis, neonatal hypocalcaemia and a loquacious personality. The common visual dysfunction is that of impaired dorsal stream functions.

Working memory Is the ability to actively process information in temporary storage, with a phonological loop for the manipulation of verbal content and a visuospatial scratch pad for retaining of visual information; the central executive coordinates these two 'slave systems' and deploys attentional resources between them.

References

Abrahamsson M, Fabian G, Andersson AK, Sjöstrand J (1990) A longitudinal study of a population based sample of astigmatic children. I. Refraction and amblyopia. Acta Ophthalmol 68:428–434

Abramov I, Gordon J (2006) Development of color vision. In: Duckman RH (ed) Visual development, diagnosis, and treatment of the pediatric patient. Lippincott Williams & Wilkins, Philadelphia, pp 143–170

Ackerley R, Barnes GR (2011) The interaction of visual, vestibular and extra-retinal mechanisms in the control of head gaze during head-free pursuit. J Physiol 589:1627–1642

Adams RJ, Courage ML (1995) Development of chromatic discrimination in early infancy. Behav Brain Res 67:99–101

Adams RJ, Courage ML (2002) Using a single test to measure human contrast sensitivity from early childhood to maturity. Vision Res 42:1205–1210

Adams RJ, Hall HL, Courage ML (2005) Long-term visual pathology in children with significant perinatal complications. Dev Med Child Neurol 47:598–602

Ahmed M, Dutton GN (1996) Cognitive visual dysfunction in a child with cerebral damage. Dev Med Child Neurol 38:736–739

Aicardi J (2009) Malformations of the central nervous system. In: Aicardi J (ed) Diseases of the nervous system in childhood, 3rd edn. Mac Keith Press, London, pp 41–102

Allen D, Banks MS, Norcia AM (1993) Does chromatic sensitivity develop more slowly than luminance sensitivity? Vision Res 33:2553–2562

Amso D, Johnson SP (2006) Learning by selection: visual search and object perception in young infants. Dev Psychol 42:1236–1245

Anderson P (2002) Assessment and development of executive function (EF) during childhood. Child Neuropsychol 8:71–82

Anderson SL (2003) Trajectories of brain development: point of vulnerability or window of opportunity? Neurosci Biobehav Rev 27:3–18

Anderson P, Anderson V, Garth J (2001a) Assessment and development of organizational ability: the Rey Complex Figure Organizational Strategy Score (RCF-OSS). Clin Neuropsychol 15:81–94

Anderson V, Northam E, Hendy J, Wrennall J (2001b) Developmental neuropsychology. Psychology Press, Hove

Anderson V, Spencer-Smith M, Wood A (2011) Do children really recover better? Neurobehavioural plasticity after early brain insult. Brain 134:2197–2221

Andersson S, Persson EK, Aring E, Lindquist B, Dutton GN, Hellstrom A (2006) Vision in children with hydrocephalus. Dev Med Child Neurol 48:836–841

Andino SLG, de Peralta Menendez GR, Khateb A, Landis T, Pegna A (2009) Electrophysiological correlates of affective blindsight. Neuroimage 44:581–589

Ardila A (2008) On the evolutionary origins of executive functions. Brain Cogn 68:92–99

Ariel R, Sadeh M (1996) Congenital visual agnosia and prosopagnosia in a child: a case report. Cortex 32:221–240

Aring E, Gronlund MA, Hellstrom A, Ygge J (2007) Visual fixation development in children. Graefes Arch Clin Exp Ophthalmol 245:1659–1665

Arnott SR, Thaler L, Milne JL, Kish D, Goodale MA (2013) Shape-specific activation of occipital cortex in an early blind echolocation expert. Neuropsychologia 51:938–949

Arnsten AF, Rubia K (2012) Neurobiological circuits regulating attention, cognitive control, motivation, and emotion: disruptions in neurodevelopmental psychiatric disorders. J Am Acad Child Adolesc Psychiatry 51:356–367

Arroyo S, Lesser PR, Poon WT, Webber WR, Gordon B (1997) Neuronal generators of visual evoked potentials in humans: visual processing in the human cortex. Epilepsia 38:600–610

Arteberry ME, Craton LG, Yonas A (1993) Infants' sensitivity to motion-carried information for depth and object properties. In: Granrud CE (ed) Visual perception and cognition in infancy. Erlbaum Assoc, Hillsdale, pp 215–234

Ashby J, Rayner K (2006) Literacy development: insights from research on skilled reading. In: Dickinson DK, Neuman SB (eds) Handbook of early literacy research, vol 2. Guilford, New York, pp 52–63

Aslin RN, Smith LB (1988) Perceptual development. Annu Rev Psychol 39:435–473

Astle AT, Webb BS, McGraw PV (2011) Can perceptual learning be used to treat amblyopia beyond the critical period of visual development? Ophthal Physiol Opt 31:564–573

Atkinson J (2000) The developing visual brain. Oxford University Press, Oxford

Atkinson J, Braddick O (1979) New techniques for assessing vision in infants and young children. Child Care Health Dev 5:389–398

Atkinson J, Braddick O (2007) Visual and visuocognitive development in children born prematurely. Prog Brain Res 164:123–149

Atkinson J, Nardini M (2008) Visuospatial and visuomotor development. In: Reed J, Warner-Rogers J (eds) Child neuropsychology. Blackwell, Oxford, pp 183–217

Atkinson J, Anker S, Braddick O, Nokes L, Mason A, Braddick F (2001) Visual and visuospatial development in young children with Williams syndrome. Dev Med Child Neurol 43:330–337

Atkinson J, Anker S, Rae S, Weeks F, Braddick O, Rennie J (2002a) Cortical visual evoked potentials in very low birthweight premature infants. Arch Dis Child Fetal Neonatal Ed 86:F28–F31

Atkinson J, Anker S, Rae S, Hughes C, Braddick O (2002b) A test battery of child development for examining functional vision (ABCDEFV). Strabismus 10:245–269

Avery RA, Ferner RE, Listernick R, Fisher MJ, Gutmann DH, Liu GT (2012) Visual acuity in children with low grade gliomas of the visual pathway: implications for patient care and clinical research. J Neurooncol 110:1–7

Avidan G, Tanzer M, Behrman M (2011) Impaired holistic processing in congenital prosopagnosia. Neuropsychologia 49:2541–2552

Ayton LN, Abel LA, Fricke TR, McBrien NA (2009) Developmental eye movement test: what it is really measuring? Optom Vis Sci 86:722–730

Bahrick LE, Hernandez-Reif M, Flom R (2005) The development of infant learning about specific face-voice relations. Dev Psychol 41:541–552

Bailey JE, Neitz M, Tait DM, Neitz J (2004) Evaluation of an updated HRR color vision test. Vis Neurosci 21:431–436

Bajandas FJ, McBeath JB, Smith JL (1975) Congenital homonymous hemianopia. Am J Ophthalmol 82:498–500

Balcer LJ, Liu GT, Bilaniuk L, Volpe NJ, Galetta SL, Molloy PT et al (2001) Visual loss in children with neurofibromatosis type 1 and optic pathway gliomas: relation of tumor location by magnetic resonance imaging. Am J Ophthalmol 131:442–445

Ball G, Boardman JP, Rueckert D, Aljabar P, Arichi T, Merchant N et al (2012) The effect of preterm birth on thalamic and cortical development. Cereb Cortex 22:1016–1024

Baltes PB (1997) On the incomplete architecture of human ontogeny – selection, optimization, and compensation as foundation of developmental theory. Am Psychol 52:366–380

Bane MC, Birch EE (1992) VEP acuity, FPL acuity, and visual behavior of visually impaired children. J Pediatr Ophthalmol Strabismus 29:202–209

Banks MS, Shannon E (1993) Spatial and chromatic visual efficiency in human neonates. In: Granrud CE (ed) Visual perception and cognition in infancy. Erlbaum Assoc, Hillsdale, pp 1–46

Banton T, Bertenthal BI (1996) Infants' sensitivity to uniform motion. Vision Res 36: 1633–1640

Barca L, Cappelli FR, Di Giulio P, Staccioli S, Castelli E (2010) Outpatient assessment of neurovisual functions in children with cerebral palsy. Res Dev Disabil 31:488–495

Barlow KM, Thomson E, Johnson D, Minns RA (2005) Late neurologic and cognitive sequelae of inflicted traumatic brain injury in infancy. Pediatrics 116:e174–e185

Barnard NA (1989) Visual conversion reaction in children. Ophthalmic Physiol Opt 9:372–378

Barnet AB, Manson JI, Wilner E (1970) Acute cerebral blindness in childhood. Neurology 20:1147–1156

Barnikol UB, Amunts K, Dammers J, Mohlberg H, Fieseler T, Malikovic A et al (2006) Pattern reversal visual evoked responses of V1/V2 and V5/MT as revealed by MEG combined with probabilistic cytoarchitectonic maps. Neuroimage 31:86–108

Baroncelli L, Braschi C, Spolidoro M, Begenisic T, Sale A, Maffei L (2010) Nurturing brain plasticity: impact of environmental enrichment. Cell Death Differ 17:1092–1103

Barrett LF, Bar M (2009) See it with feeling: affective predictions during object perception. Philos Trans R Soc Lond B Biol Sci 364:1325–1334

Barrett J, Fleming AS (2011) All mothers are not created equal: neural and psychobiological perspectives on mothering and the importance of individual differences. J Child Psychol Psychiatry Allied Disciplines 52:368–397

Barrouillet P, Gavens N, Vergauwe E, Gaillard V, Camos V (2009) Working memory span development: a time-based resource-sharing model account. Dev Psychol 45:477–490

Barton JJS (2008) Prosopagnosia associated with a left occipitotemporal lesion. Neuropsychologia 46:2214–2224

Barton JJ (2011) Disorders of higher visual function. Curr Opin Neurol 24:1–5

Barton JJS, Cherkasova MV, Press DZ, Intriligator JM, O'Connor M (2003) Developmental prosopagnosia: a study of three patients. Brain Cogn 51:12–30

Barton JJ, Hefter RL, Cherkasova MV, Manoach DS (2007) Investigations of face expertise in the social developmental disorder. Neurology 69:860–867

Bassi L, Ricci D, Volzone A, Allsop JM, Srinivasan L, Pai A et al (2008) Probabilistic diffusion tractography of the optic radiations and visual function in preterm infants at term equivalent age. Brain 131:573–582

Bax MC, Flodmark O, Tydeman C (2007) Definition and classification of cerebral palsy. From syndrome toward disease. Dev Med Child Neurol Suppl 109:39–41

Bedell HE (2000) Perception of a clear and stable visual world with congenital nystagmus. Optom Vis Sci 77:573–581

Bedny M, Saxe R (2012) Insights into origins of knowledge from the cognitive neuroscience of blindness. Cogn Neuropsychol 29:56–84

Behrmann M, Aidan G, Marotta JJ, Kimchi R (2005) Detailed exploration of face-related processing in congenital prosopagnosia: 1. Behavioral findings. J Cogn Neurosci 17: 1130–1149

Ben-Artsy A, Glicksohn J, Soroker N, Margalit M, Myslobodsky M (1996) An assessment of hemineglect in children with attention-deficit hyperactivity disorder. Dev Neuropsychol 12:271–281

Bennet DM, Gordon G, Dutton GN (2009) The useful field of view test, normative data in children of school age. Optom Vis Sci 86:717–721

Ben-Schachar M, Dougherty RF, Deutsch GK, Wandell BA (2011) The development of cortical sensitivity to visual word forms. J Cogn Neurosci 23:2387–2399

Benson NC, Butt OH, Datta R, Radoeva PD, Brainard DH, Aguirre GK (2012) The retinotopic organization of striate cortex is well predicted by surface topology. Curr Biol 22:2081–2085

Berardi N, Pizzorusso T, Maffei L (2000) Critical periods during sensory development. Curr Opin Neurobiol 10:138–145

Berenbaum SA, Moffat S, Wisniewski A, Resnick S (2003) Neuroendocrinology: cognitive effects of sex hormones. In: De Haan M, Johnson MH (eds) The cognitive neuroscience of development. Psychology Press, Hove/New York, pp 207–235

Berlucchi G (2011) Brain plasticity and cognitive rehabilitation. Neuropsychol Rehabil 21:560–578

Berman R, Colby C (2009) Attention and active vision. Vision Res 49:1233–1248

Berridge KC, Kringelbach ML (2013) Neuroscience of affect: brain mechanisms of pleasure and displeasure. Curr Opin Neurobiol 23:294–303

Best JR, Miller PH (2010) A developmental perspective on executive function. Child Dev 81:1641–1660

Bi H, Zhang B, Tao X, Harwerth RS, Smith EL, Chino YM (2011) Neuronal responses in visual area V2 (V2) of macaque monkeys with strabismic amblyopia. Cereb Cortex 21:2033–2045

Billingsley RL, Lang FF, Slopis JM, Schrimsher GW, Ater JL, Bartlett DM (2002) Visual-spatial neglect in a child following sub-cortical tumor resection. Dev Med Child Neurol 44:191–200

Birch EE, Bane MC (1991) Forced choice preferential looking acuity of children with cortical visual impairment. Dev Med Child Neurol 33:722–729

Birch EE, Salomao S (1998) Infant random dot stereoacuity cards. J Paediatr Ophthalmol Strabismus 35:86–90

Bistricky SL, Ingram RE, Atchley RA (2011) Facial affect processing and depression susceptibility: cognitive biases and cognitive neuroscience. Psychol Bull 137:998–1028

Black JE (1998) How a child builds its brain – some lessons from animal studies of neural plasticity. Prev Med 27:168–171

Bloch H, Carchon I (1992) On the onset of eye-head coordination in infants. Behav Brain Res 49:85–90

Blythe HI, Liversedge SP, Joseph HS, White SJ, Rayner K (2009) Visual information capture during fixations in reading for children and adults. Vision Res 49:1583–1591

Boden C, Giaschi D (2007) M-stream deficits and reading-related visual processes in developmental dyslexia. Psychol Bull 133:346–366

Bodis-Wollner I, Diamond SP (1976) The measurement of spatial contrast sensitivity in cases of blurred vision associated with cerebral lesions. Brain 99:695–710

Boelens H (1992) Effect of identity versus oddity training on novel matching-to-sample responding after naming. Psychol Rep 71:307–320

Bonnier C, Marique P, Van Hout A, Potelle D (2007) Neurodevelopmental outcome after severe traumatic brain injury in very young children: role for subcortical lesions. J Child Neurol 22:519–529

Boot FH, Pel JJM, van den Steen J, Evenhuis HM (2010) Cerebral visual impairment: which predictive visual dysfunctions can be expected in children with brain damage? A systematic review. Res Dev Disabil 31:1149–1159

Borchert MS, Sadun AA, Sommers JD, Wright KW (1987) Congenital ocular motor apraxia in twins. J Clin Neuroophthalmol 7:104–107

Bosse ML, Tainturier MJ, Valdois S (2007) Developmental dyslexia: the visual attention span deficit hypothesis. Cognition 104:198–230

Bova SM, Fazzi E, Giovenzana A, Montomoli C, Signorini SG, Zoppello M, Lanzi G (2007) The development of visual object recognition in school-age children. Dev Neuropsychol 31:79–102

Bova SM, Giovenzana A, Signorini SG, La Piana R, Uggeti C, Bianchi BE, Fazzi E (2008) Recovery of functions after early acquired occipital damage. Dev Med Child Neurol 50:311–315

Bowman R, McCulloch DL, Law E, Mostyn K, Dutton GN (2010) The 'mirror test' for estimating visual acuity in infants. Br J Ophthalmol 94:882–885

Boyle NJ, Jones DH, Hamilton R, Spowart KM, Dutton GN (2005) Blindsight in children: does it exist and can it be used to help the child? Observations on a case series. Dev Med Child Neurol 47:699–702

Braddick O, Atkinson J (2011) Development of human visual function. Vision Res 51:1588–1609

Braet W, Wagemans J, Op de Beeck HP (2012) The visual word form area is organized according to orthography. Neuroimage 59:2751–2759

Brambati SM, Termine C, Ruffno M, Danna M, Lanzi G, Stella G, Cappa SF, Perani D (2006) Neuropsychological deficits and neural dysfunction in familial dyslexia. Brain Res 1113:174–185

Bravarone FV, Fea A, Chiado Piat L, Porro G, Ponzetto M, Cortassa F (1993) Preferential looking techniques yield important information in strabismus amblyopia follow up. Doc Ophthalmol 83:307–312

Breznitz Z, Shaul S, Horowitz-Kraus T, Sela I, Nevat M, Karni A (2013) Enhanced reading by training with imposed time constraint in typical and dyslexic adults. Nat Commun 4:1486

Broadbent H, Westall C (1990) An evaluation of techniques for measuring stereopsis in infants and young children. Ophthal Physiol Opt 10:3–7

Brodsky MC (2010) Pediatric neuro-ophthalmology, 2nd edn. Springer, New York

Brodsky MC, Fray KJ, Glasier CM (2002) Perinatal cortical and subcortical visual loss: mechanisms of injury and associated ophthalmologic signs. Ophthalmology 109:85–94

Brown AM (1990) Development of visual sensitivity to light and color vision in human infants: a critical review. Vision Res 30:1159–1188

Brown JK, Minns RA (1993) Non-accidental head injury, with particular reference to whiplash shaking injury and medico-legal aspects. Dev Med Child Neurol 35:849–869

Brunsdon R, Coltheart M, Nickels L, Joy P (2006) Developmental prosopagnosia: a case analysis and treatment study. Cogn Neuropsychol 23:822–840

Brunsdon R, Nickels L, Coltheart M, Joy P (2007) Assessment and treatment of childhood topographical orientation: a case study. Neuropsychol Rehabil 17:53–94

Bucci MP, Nassibi N, Gerard CL, Bui-Quoc E (2012) Immaturity of the oculomotor saccade and vergence interaction in dyslexic children: evidence from a reading and a visual search task. PLoS One 7:e33458

Bulens C, Meerwaldt JD, van der Wildt GJ, Keemink J (1989) Spatial contrast sensitivity in unilateral cerebral ischaemic lesions involving the posterior visual pathway. Brain 112:507–520

Bunt AH, Minckler DS, Johanson GW (1977) Demonstration of bilateral projection of the central retina of the monkey with horseradish peroxidase neuronography. J Comp Neurol 171: 619–630

Burgess PW, Gonen-Yaacovi G, Volle E (2011) Functional neuroimaging studies of prospective memory: what have we learnt so far? Neuropsychologia 49:2246–2257

Burrage MS, Ponitz CC, McCready EA, Shah P, Sims BC, Jewkes AM et al (2008) Age and schooling-related effects on executive functions in young children: a natural experiment. Child Neuropsychol 14:510–524

Bushnell IWR (2011) Mother's face recognition in newborn infants: learning and memory. Infant Child Dev 10:67–74

Caldarelli M, Massimi L, Tamburrini G, Cappa M, Di Rocco C (2005) Long-term results of the surgical treatment of craniopharyngioma: the experience at the Policlinico Gemelli, Catholic University, Rome. Childs Nerv Syst 21:747–757

Callens M, Whitney C, Tops W, Brysbaert M (2013) No deficiency in left-to-right processing of words in dyslexia but evidence for enhanced visual crowding. Q J Exp Psychol 66:1803–1817

Candy TR (2006) Development of the visual system. In: Duckman RH (ed) Visual development, diagnosis, and treatment of the pediatric patient. Lippincott Williams & Wilkins, Philadelphia, pp 7–33

Candy TR, Bharadwaj SR (2007) The stability of steady state accommodation in human infants. J Vis 7:1–16

Cannon MW (1983) Evoked potential contrast sensitivity in the parafoveal: spatial organization. Vision Res 23:1441–1449

Catherwood D, Skoien P, Holt C (1996) Colour pop-out in infant response to visual arrays. Br J Dev Psychol 14:315–326

Cattaneo Z, Renzi C, Casali S, Silvanto J, Vecchi T, Papagno C et al (2014) Cerebellar vermis plays a causal role in visual motion perception. Cortex 58:272–280

Cavezian C, Vilyaphonh M, Vasseur V, Caputo G, Laloum L, Chokron S (2013) Ophthalmic disorder may affect visuo-attentional performance in childhood. Child Neuropsychol 19:292–312

Celesia GG, Polcyn RD, Holden JE, Nickles RJ, Gytley JS, Koeppe RA (1982) Visual evoked potentials and positron emission tomography of regional cerebral blood flow and cerebral metabolism: can the neuronal potential generators be visualized? Electroencephalogr Clin Neurophysiol 54:243–256

Cetinkaya A, Oto S, Akman A, Akoya YA (2008) Relationship between optokinetic nystagmus response and recognition visual acuity. Eye (Lond) 22:77–81

Chandna A, Karki C, Davis J, Doran RM (1989) Preferential looking in the mentally handicapped. Eye (Lond) 3:833–839

Charman WN (2004) Aniso-accommodation as a possible factor in myopia development. Ophthalmic Physiol Opt 24:471–479

Charman WN, Voisin L (1993) Astigmatism, accommodation, the oblique effect and meridional amblyopia. Ophthalmic Physiol Opt 13:73–81

Cheung SH, Fang F, He S, Legge GE (2009) Retinotopically specific reorganization of visual cortex for tactile pattern recognition. Curr Biol 19:596–601

Chi JG, Dooling EC, Gilles FH (1977) Gyral development of the human brain. Ann Neurol 1:86–93

Chiricozzi F, Chieffo D, Battaglia D, Iuvone L, Acquafondata C, Cesarini L et al (2005) Developmental plasticity after right hemispherectomy in an epileptic adolescent with early brain injury. Childs Nerv Syst 21:960–969

Choi SY, Kim Y, Oh SW, Jeong SH, Kim JS (2012) Pursuit-paretic and epileptic nystagmus in MELAS. J Neuroophthalmol 32:135–138

Chugani HT (1998) A critical period of brain development: studies of cerebral glucose utilization with PET. Prev Med 27:184–188

Chugani HT, Muller RA, Chugani DC (1996) Functional brain reorganization in children. Brain Dev 8:347–356

Chun MM, Golomb JD, Turk-Browne NB (2011) A taxonomy of external and internal attention. Annu Rev Psychol 62:73–101

Cioni G, Bertuccelli B, Boldrini A, Canapicchi R, Fazzi B, Guzzetta A et al (2000) Correlation between visual function, neurodevelopmental outcome, and magnetic resonance imaging findings in infants with periventricular leucomalacia. Arch Dis Child Fetal Neonatal Ed 82:F134–F140

Cioni G, Bertuccelli B, Boldrini A, Canapicchi R, Fazzi B, Guzzetta A et al (2006) Contrast sensitivity function. In: Duckman RH (ed) Visual development, diagnosis, and treatment of the pediatric patient. Lippincott Williams & Wilkins, Philadelphia, pp 52–68

Cioni G, D'Acunto G, Guzzetta A (2011) Perinatal brain damage in children: neuroplasticity, early intervention, and molecular mechanisms of recovery. Prog Brain Res 189:139–154

Clavadetscher JE, Brown AM, Ancrum C, Teller DY (1988) Spectral sensitivity and chromatic discriminations in 3- and 7-weeks old human infants. J Opt Soc Am A 5:2093–2105

Clearfield MW, Osborne CN, Mullen M (2008) Learning by looking: infants' social looking behavior across the transition from crawling to walking. J Exp Child Psychol 100:297–307

Coldren JT, Colombo J (1994) The nature and process of preverbal learning: implications from nine-month-old infants' discrimination problem solving. Monogr Soc Res Child Dev 59:1–75

Cole M, Cole SR (2001) The development of children, 4th edn. Worth Publ, New York

Colenbrander A (2009) The functional classification of brain-damage-related vision loss. J Vis Impair Blind 103:118–123

Colenbrander A (2010) What's in a name? Appropriate terminology of CVI. J Vis Impair Blind 104:583–585

Colombo J (2001) The development of visual attention in infancy. Annu Rev Psychol 52:337–367

Connolly DM, Barbur JL, Hosking SL, Moorhead IR (2008) Mild hypoxia impairs chromatic sensitivity in the mesopic range. Invest Ophthalmol Vis Sci 49:820–827

Cooke RW, Foulder-Hughes L, Newsham D, Clarke D (2004) Ophthalmic impairment at 7 years of age in children born very preterm. Arch Dis Child Fetal Neonatal Ed 89:F249–253

Corbetta M, Miezin FM, Dobmeyer S, Shulman GL, Petersen SE (1991) Selective and divided attention during visual discrimination of shape, color, and speed: functional neuroanatomy by positron emission tomography. J Neurosci 11:2383–2402

Corbetta M, Miezin FM, Shulman GL, Petersen SE (1993) A PET study of visuospatial attention. J Neurosci 13:1202–1226

Corkum V, Moore C (1998) Origins of joint visual attention in infants. Dev Psychol 34:28–38

Costa MF, Ventura DF (2012) Visual impairment in children with spastic cerebral palsy measured by psychophysical and electrophysiological grating acuity tests. Dev Neurorehabil 15:414–424

Courage ML, Howe ML (2004) Advances in early memory development research: insights about the dark side of the moon. Dev Rev 24:6–32

Cowey A (1994) Cortical visual areas and the neurobiology of higher visual processes. In: Farah MJ, Ratcliff G (eds) The neuropsychology of high-level vision. Erlbaum, Hillsdale, pp 3–31

Cowey A (2010) The blindsight saga. Exp Brain Res 200:3–24

Craft S, White DA, Park TS, Figiel G (1994) Visual attention in children with perinatal brain injury: asymmetric effects of bilateral lesions. J Cogn Neurosci 6:165–173

Creavin AL, Brown RD (2009) Ophthalmic abnormalities in children with Down syndrome. J Pediatr Ophthalmol Strabismus 46:76–82

Cregg M, Woodhouse JM, Pakeman VH, Saunders KJ, Gunter HL, Parker M et al (2001) Accommodation and refractive error in children with Down syndrome: cross-sectional and longitudinal studies. Invest Ophthalmol Vis Sci 42:55–63

Cummings MF, van Hof-van Duin J, Mayer DL, Hansen RM, Fulton AB (1988) Visual fields in young children. Behav Brain Res 29:7–16

Cuomo J, Flaster M, Biller J (2012) Right brain: a descriptive account of two patients' experience with and adaptations to Balint syndrome. Neurology 79:e95

Currie DC, Manny RE (1997) The development of accommodation. Vision Res 37:1525–1533

Dain SJ, Ling BY (2009) Cognitive abilities of children on a gray seriation test. Optom Vis Sci 86:E701–E707

Dalla Via P, Opocher E, Pinello ML, Calderone M, Viscardi E, Clementi M et al (2007) Visual outcome of a cohort of children with neurofibromatosis type 1 and optic pathway glioma followed by a pediatric neuro-oncology program. Neuro Oncol 9:430–437

Dalrymple KA, Corrow S, Yonas A, Duchaine B (2012) Developmental prosopagnosia in childhood. Cogn Neuropsychol 29:393–418

Damaraju E, Huang Y-M, Feldmann Barett E, Pessoa L (2009) Affective learning enhances activity an functional connectivity in early visual cortex. Neuropsychologia 47:2480–2487
Damato BE (1985) Oculokinetic perimetry: a simple visual field test for use in the community. Br J Ophthalmol 69:927–931
Daniel PM, Whitteridge D (1961) The representation of the visual field on the cerebral cortex in monkeys. J Physiol 159:203–221
Danker JF, Anderson JR (2010) The ghosts of brain states past: remembering reactivates the brain regions engaged during encoding. Psychol Bull 136:87–102
Dannemiller JL, Friedland RL (1989) The detection of slow stimulus movement in 2- to 5-month-olds. J Exp Child Psychol 47:337–355
Das M, Bennett DM, Dutton GN (2007) Visual attention as an important visual function: an outline on manifestations, diagnosis and management of impaired visual attention. Br J Ophthalmol 91:1556–1560
Das M, Spowart K, Crossley S, Dutton GN (2010) Evidence that children with special needs all require visual assessment. Arch Dis Child Fetal Neonatal Ed 95:888–892
Davidson S, Quinn GE (2011) The impact of pediatric vision disorders in adulthood. Pediatrics 127:334–339
Daw NW (2006) Visual development, 2nd edn. New York, Springer
De Haan M (2008) Neurocognitive mechanisms for the development of face processing. In: Nelson CA, Luciana M (eds) The handbook of developmental cognitive neuroscience, 2nd edn. MIT Press, Cambridge, MA, pp 509–520
De Haan EH, Campbell R (1991) A fifteen year follow-up of a case of developmental prosopagnosia. Cortex 27:489–509
De Haan EHF, Cowey A (2011) On the usefulness of 'what' and 'where' pathways in vision. Trends Cogn Sci 15:460–466
De Haan M, Johnson MH (eds) (2013) The cognitive neuroscience of development. Psychology Press, Hove/New York
De Haan M, Nelson CA (1998) Discrimination and categorisation of facial expressions of emotion during infancy. In: Slater A (ed) Perceptual development. Visual, auditory, and speech perception in infancy. Psychology Press, Hove, pp 287–309
De Luca M, Burani C, Paizi D, Spinelli D, Zoccolotti P (2010) Letter and letter-string processing in developmental dyslexia. Cortex 46:1272–1283
De Schoenen S, Mancini J, Camps R, Maes E, Laurent A (2005) Early brain lesions and face-processing development. Dev Psychobiol 46:184–208
Deco G, Rolls ET (2005) Attention, short-term memory, and action selection. Prog Neurobiol 76:235–256
Defoort-Dhellemmes S, Moritz F, Bouacha I, Vinchon M (2006) Craniopharyngioma: ophthalmogic aspects at diagnosis. J Pediatr Endocrinol 19(Suppl 1):321–324
DeGutis J, DeNicola C, Zink T, McGlinchey R, Milberg W (2011) Training with own-race faces can improve processing of other-race-faces: evidence from developmental prosopagnosia. Neuropsychologia 49:2505–2513
Dehaene S, Cohen L (2011) The unique role of the visual word form are in reading. Trends Cogn Sci 15:254–262
Del Guidice E, Grossi D, Angelini R, Crisanti AF, Latte F, Fragassi NA et al (2000) Spatial cognition in children. I. Development of drawing-related (visuo-spatial and constructional) abilities in preschool and early school years. Brain Dev 22:362–367
Delaney SM, Dobson V, Mohan KM (2005) Measured visual extent varieties with peripheral stimulus flicker rate in very young children. Optom Vis Sci 82:800–806
Deng W, Pleasure J, Pleasure D (2008) Progress in periventricular leucomalacia. Arch Neurol 65:1291–1295
Dennis M (2000) Developmental plasticity in children: the role of biological risk development, time, and reserve. J Commun Disord 33:321–332
Desimone R, Ungerleider LG (1989) Neural mechanisms of visual processing in monkeys. In: Boller F, Grafman F (eds) Handbook of neuropsychology, vol 2. Elsevier, Amsterdam, pp 267–299

Di Filippo G, Zoccolotti P (2012) Separating global and specific factors in developmental dyslexia. Child Neuropsychol 18:356–391
Distler C, Bachevalier J, Kennedy C, Mishkin M, Ungerleider LG (1996) Functional development of the cortico-cortical pathway for motion analysis in the macaque monkey. A C-2 deoxyglucose study. Cereb Cortex 6:184–195
Dobkins KR (2009) Does visual modularity increase over the course of development? Optom Vis Sci 86:E583–E588
Dobler VB, Manly T, Verity C, Woolrych J, Robertson IH (2003) Modulation of spatial attention in a child with developmental unilateral neglect. Dev Med Child Neurol 45:282–288
Dobson V, Brown AM, Harvey EM, Narter DB (1998) Visual field extent in children 3.5–30 months of age tested with a double- arc LED perimeter. Vision Res 38:2743–2760
Dogru M, Shirabe H, Nakamura M, Taoka K, Naomura K, Yamamoto M (2001) Effect of retinopathy of prematurity on resolution acuity development in 1–3 year old children. J Pediatr Ophthalmol Strabismus 38:144–148
Donahue SP, Haun AK (2007) Exotropia and face turn in children with homonymous hemianopia. J Neuroophthalmol 27:304–307
Donnelly N, Cave K, Greenway R, Hadwin JA, Stevenson J, Sonuga-Barke E (2007) Visual search in children and adults: top-down and bottom-up mechanisms. Q J Exp Psychol 60:120–136
Dormal G, Leopore F, Collignon O (2012) Plasticity of the dorsal "spatial" stream in visually deprived individuals. Neural Plast. Article ID 687659, 12 pages
Dowdeswell HJ, Slater AM, Broomhall J, Tripp J (1995) Visual deficits in children born at less than 32 weeks gestation with and without major ocular pathology and cerebral damage. Br J Ophthalmol 79:447–452
Drummond SR, Dutton GN (2007) Simultanagnosia following perinatal hypoxia – a possible pediatric variant of Balint syndrome. J AAPOS 11:497–498
Dubowitz LMS, Mushin J, De Vries L, Arden GB (1986) Visual function in the newborn infant: is it cortically mediated? Lancet 327:1139–1141
Duchaine BC, Nakayama K (2005) Dissociations of face and object recognition in developmental prosopagnosia. J Cogn Neurosci 17:249–261
Duchaine BC, Nakayama K (2006) Developmental prosopagnosia: a window to content-specific face processing. Curr Opin Neurobiol 16:166–173
Duchowny MS, Weiss IP, Majlessi H, Barnet AB (1974) Visual responses in childhood cortical blindness after head trauma and meningitis: a longitudinal stuffy of six cases. Neurology 24:933–940
Duckman RH (2006) Visual acuity in the young child. In: Duckman RH (ed) Visual development, diagnosis, and treatment of the pediatric patient. Lippincott Williams & Wilkins, Philadelphia, pp 34–51
Duckman RH, Du JW (2006) Development of binocular vision. In: Duckman RH (ed) Visual development, diagnosis, and treatment of the pediatric patient. Lippincott Williams & Wilkins, Philadelphia, pp 124–142
Dumas TC (2005) Developmental regulation of cognitive abilities: modified composition of a molecular switch turns on associative learning. Prog Neurobiol 76:189–211
Dumoulin SO, Wandell BA (2008) Population receptive field estimates in human visual cortex. Neuroimage 39:647–660
Duncan J, Humphreys GW (1989) Visual search and similarity. Psychol Rev 96:433–458
Dutton GN (2002) Visual problems in children with damage to the brain. Vis Impair Res 4:113–121
Dutton GN (2003) Cognitive vision, its disorders and differential diagnosis in adults and children: knowing where and what things are. Eye (Lond) 17:289–304
Dutton GN (2009) "Dorsal stream dysfunction" and "dorsal stream dysfunction plus": a potential classification for perceptual visual impairment in the context of cerebral visual impairment? Dev Med Child Neurol 51:168–172
Dutton GN (2013) The spectrum of cerebral visual impairment as a sequel to premature birth: an overview. Doc Ophthalmol 127:69–78
Dutton GN, Bax M (eds) (2010) Visual impairment in children due to damage to the brain. MacKeith Press, London

Dutton GN, Jacobson LK (2001) Cerebral visual impairment in children. Semin Neonatol 6:477–485
Dutton G, Ballantyne J, Boyd G, Bradnam M, Day R, McCulloch D et al (1996) Cortical visual dysfunction in children: a clinical study. Eye (Lond) 10:302–309
Dutton GN, Saaed A, Fahad B, Fraser R, McDaid G, McDade J et al (2004) Association of binocular lower visual field impairment, impaired simultaneous perception, disordered visually guided motion and inaccurate saccades in children with visual dysfunction – a retrospective observational study. Eye (Lond) 18:27–34
Dutton GN, MacKillop ECA, Saidkasimova S (2006) Visual problems as a result of brain damage in children. Br J Ophthalmol 90:932–933
Dutton GN, Calvert J, Ibrahim H, Macdonald E, McCulloch DL, Macintyre-Beon C, Spowart K (2010) Structured clinical history taking for cognitive and perceptual visual dysfunction and for profound visual disabilities due to damage to the brain in children. In: Dutton GN, Bax M (eds) Visual impairment in children due to damage to the brain. MacKeith Press, London, pp 117–128
Dutton GN, Bowman R, Fazzi E (2014) Visual, oculomotor and refractive disorder in children with cerebral palsy: diagnosis characterisation and management. In: Dan B, Mayston M, Paneth N, Rosenbloom L (eds) Cerebral palsy: science and clinical practice. Mac Keith Press, London
Eacott MJ, Crawley RA (1999) Childhood amnesia: on answering questions about very early life events. Memory 7:279–292
Eckert MJ, Abraham WC (2013) Effects of environmental enrichment exposures on synaptic transmission and plasticity in the hippocampus. Curr Top Behav Neurosci 15:165–187
Eckstein MP (2011) Visual search: a retrospective. J Vis 11:14, 1–36
Eden GF, Stein JF, Wood HM, Wood FB (1994) Differences in eye movements and reading problems in dyslexic and normal children. Vision Res 34:1345–1358
Ekici B, Caliskan M, Tatli B, Aydinli N, Ozmen M (2011) Rapidly progressive subacute sclerosing panencephalitis presenting with acute loss of vision. Acta Neurol Belg 111:325–327
Ekstrom AB, Tulinius M, Sjostrom A, Aring E (2010) Visual function in congenital and childhood myotonic dystrophy type 1. Ophthalmology 117:976–982
Elam KK, Carlson JM, DiLalla EF, Reinke KS (2010) Emotional faces capture spatial attention in 5-year-old children. Evol Psychol 8:754–767
Ellemberg D, Lewis TL, Liu CH, Maurer D (1999) Development of spatial and temporal vision during childhood. Vision Res 39:2325–2333
Ellsworth CP, Muir DW, Hains SM (1993) Social competence and person-object differentiation: an analysis of the still-face effect. Dev Psychol 29:63–73
Endo A, Fuchigami T, Hasegawa M, Hashimoto K, Fujita Y, Inamo Y, Mugishima H (2012) Posterior reversible encephalopathy syndrome in childhood: report of four cases and review of the literature. Pediatr Emerg Care 28:153–157
Eriksson K, Kylliäinen A, Hirvonen K, Nieminen P, Koivikko M (2003) Visual agnosia in a child with non-lesional occipito-temporal CSWS. Brain Dev 25:262–267
Evans GW (2006) Child development and the physical environment. Annu Rev Psychol 57:423–451
Evenson KA, Lindquist S, Indredavik MS, Skranes J, Brubakk AM, Vik T (2009) Do visual impairments affect risk of motor problems in preterm and low birth weight adolescents? Eur J Paediatr Neurol 13:47–56
Facoetti A, Lorusso ML, Paganoni P, Umilta C, Mascetti GG (2003) The role of visuospatial attention in developmental dyslexia: evidence from a rehabilitation study. Cogn Brain Res 15:154–164
Fantz RL (1964) Visual experience in infants: decreased attention to familiar patterns relative to novel ones. Science 146:668–670
Fantz RL, Fagan JF (1975) Visual attention to size and number of pattern details by term and preterm infants during the first six months. Child Dev 46:3–18
Fantz RL, Oddy JM (1959) A visual acuity test for infants under six months of age. Psychol Rec 9:159–164
Farah M (2000) The cognitive neuroscience of vision. Blackwell Publishers Ltd., Oxford

Farnsworth D (1943) The Farnsworth-Munsell 100-hue and dichotomous tests for colour vision. J Opt Soc Am 33:568–578

Farran EK, Jarrold CH (2003) Visuospatial cognition in Williams syndrome: reviewing and accounting for the strengths and weaknesses in performance. Dev Neuropsychol 23:173–200

Fazzi E, Signorini SG, Bova SM, La Piana R, Ondei P, Bertone C et al (2007) Spectrum of visual disorders in children with cerebral visual impairment. J Child Neurol 22:294–301

Fazzi E, Bova S, Giovenzana A, Signorini S, Uggetti C, Bianchi P (2009) Cognitive visual dysfunctions in preterm children with periventricular leukomalacia. Dev Med Child Neurol 51:974–981

Fazzi E, Signorini SG, Bomba M, Luparia A, Lanners J, Balottin U (2011) Reach on sound: a key to object permanence in visually impaired children. Early Hum Dev 87:289–296

Fazzi E, Signorini SG, La Piana R, Bertone C, Misefari W, Galli J, Balottin U, Bianchi PE (2012) Neuro-ophthalmological disorders in cerebral palsy: ophthalmological, oculomotor, and visual aspects. Dev Med Child Neurol 54:730–736

Fedrizzi E, Inverno M, Bruzzone MG et al (1996) MRI features of cerebral lesions and cognitive functions in preterm spastic diplegic children. Pediatr Neurol 15:207–212

Fedrizzi E, Anderloni A, Bono R, Bova S, Farinotti M, Inverno M, Savoiardo S (1998) Eye-movement disorders and visual-perceptual impairment in diplegic children born preterm: a clinical evaluation. Dev Med Child Neurol 40:682–688

Fedrizzi E, Facchin P, Marzaroli M, Pagliano E, Botteon G, Percivalle L, Fazzi E (2000) Predictors of independent walking in children with spastic diplegia. J Child Neurol 15:228–234

Fei-Ying Ng F, Kenney-Benson GA, Pomerantz EM (2004) Children's achievement moderates the effects of mothers' use of control and autonomy support. Child Dev 75:764–780

Fellenius K, Ek U, Jacobson L (2001) Reading strategies in children with cerebral visual impairment caused by periventricular leukomalacia. Int J Disabil Dev Educ 48:283–302

Ferretti G, Mazzotti S, Brizzolara D (2008) Visual scanning and reading ability in normal and dyslexic children. Behav Neurol 19:87–92

Ferro JM, Martins IP, Távora L (1984) Neglect in children. Ann Neurol 15:281–284

Ferziger NB, Nemet P, Brezner A, Feldman R, Galili G, Zivotofsy AZ (2011) Visual assessment in children with cerebral palsy. Visual assessment in children with cerebral palsy: implementation of a functional questionnaire. Dev Med Child Neurol 53:422–428

Fielder AR, Russell-Eggitt IR, Dodd KL, Mellor DH (1985) Delayed visual maturation. Trans Ophthalmol Soc U K 104:653–661

Fielder AR, Gresty MA, Dodd KL, Mellor DH, Levene MI (1986) Congenital ocular motor apraxia. Trans Ophthalmol Soc U K 105:589–598

Findlay JM, Gilchrist ID (2003) Active vision: the psychology of looking and seeing. Oxford University Press, Oxford

Fiorentini A, Berardi N (1997) Visual perceptual learning: a sign of neural plasticity at early stages of visual processing. Arch Ital Biol 135:157–167

Firth AY, Walker K (2006) Visual side-effects from transdermal scopolamine (hyoscine). Dev Med Child Neurol 48:137–138

Fischer ML, Cole RG (2000) Functional evaluation of the adult: optometric and ophthalmologic evaluations. In: Silverstone B, Lang MA, Rosenthal BP, Faye EE (eds) The Lighthouse handbook on vision impairment and vision rehabilitation. Oxford University Press, Oxford, pp 833–853

Flodmark O, Jan JE, Wong PKH (1990) Computed tomography of the brains of children with cortical visual impairment. Dev Med Child Neurol 32:611–620

Fox R, McDaniel C (1982) The perception of biological motion by human infants. Science 218:486–487

Frank V, Torres F (1979) Visual evoked potentials in the evaluation of 'cortical blindness' in children. Ann Neurol 6:126–129

Franklin A, Davies IR (2004) New evidence for infant colour categories. Br J Dev Psychol 22:344–377

Frebel H (2006) CVI?! How to define and what terminology to use: cerebral, cortical or cognitive visual impairment. Br J Vis Impair 24:117–120

Freeman RD (2010) Psychiatric considerations in cortical visual impairment. In: Dutton GN, Bax M (eds) Visual impairment in children due to damage to the brain. MacKeith Press, London, pp 174–180

Frigerio E, Burt DM, Gagliardi C, Cioffi G, Martelli S, Perrett DI, Borgatti R (2006) Is everybody always my friend? Perception of approachability in Williams syndrome. Neuropsychologia 44:254–259

Fukushima J, Hatta T, Fukushima K (2000) Development of voluntary control of saccadic eye movements. I. Age-related changes in normal children. Brain Dev 22:173–180

Fulton AB, Hansen RM (1987) The relationship of retinal sensitivity and rhodopsin in human infants. Vision Res 27:697–704

Gabrieli JD (1998) Cognitive neuroscience of human memory. Annu Rev Psychol 49:87–115

Gale CR, O'Callaghan FJ, Godfrey KM, Law CM, Martyn CN (2004) Critical periods of brain growth and cognitive function. Brain 127:321–329

Garon N, Bryson SE, Smith IM (2008) Executive function in preschoolers: a review using an integrative framework. Psychol Bull 134:31–60

Garrett AS, Menon V, MacKenzie K, Reiss AL (2004) Here's looking at you, kid: neural systems underlying face and gaze processing in fragile X syndrome. Arch Gen Psychiatry 61:281–288

Gava L, Valenza E, Turati C (2009) Newborns' perception of left–right spatial relations. Child Dev 80:1797–1810

Gelbart SS, Hoyt CS, Jastrebski G, Marg E (1982) Long-term visual results in bilateral congenital cataracts. Am J Ophthalmol 93:615–621

Geldof CJ, Oosterlaan J, Vuijk PJ, Vries MJ, Kok JH, Wassenaer-Leemhuis AG (2014) Visual sensory and perceptive functioning in 5-year-old very preterm/very-low-birthweight children. Dev Med Child Neurol 56:862–868

Germano E, Gagliano A, Curatolo P (2010) Comorbidity of ADHD and dyslexia. Dev Neuropsychol 35:475–493

Germine L, Cashdollar N, Düzel E, Duchaine B (2011) A new selective developmental deficit: impaired object recognition with normal face recognition. Cortex 47:598–607

Ghasia F, Brunstrom J, Gordon M, Tychsen L (2008) Frequency and severity of visual sensory and motor deficits in children with cerebral palsy: gross motor classification scale. Invest Ophthalmol Vis Sci 49:572–580

Giaschi D, Jan JE, Bjornson B, Young SA, Tata M, Lyons CJ et al (2003) Conscious visual abilities in a patient with early bilateral occipital damage. Dev Med Child Neurol 45:772–781

Gibson JJ (1979) The ecological approach to visual perception. Houghton Mifflin, Boston

Gilbert CD, Li W (2013) Top-down influences on visual processing. Nat Rev Neurosci 14:350–363

Gilbert CD, Li W, Piech V (2009) Perceptual learning and adult cortical plasticity. J Physiol 587:2743–2751

Gillen JA, Dutton GN (2003) Balint's syndrome in a 10-year-old male. Dev Med Child Neurol 45:349–352

Giza CC, Prins ML (2006) Is being plastic fantastic? Mechanisms of altered plasticity after developmental traumatic brain injury. Dev Neurosci 28:364–379

Gizewski ER, Gasser T, de Greiff A, Boehm A, Forsting M (2003) Cross-modal plasticity for sensory and motor activation patterns in blind subjects. Neuroimage 19:968–975

Glezer LS, Jiang X, Riesenhuber M (2009) Evidence for highly selective neuronal tuning to whole words in the "visual word form area". Neuron 62:199–204

Goldberg MC, Maurer D, Lewis TL (2001) Developmental changes in attention: the effects of endogenous cuing and of distractors. Dev Sci 4:209–219

Goldstein EB (2010) Sensation and perception, 8th edn. Thomson Wadsworth, Belmont

Goldstone RL (1998) Perceptual learning. Annu Rev Psychol 49:585–612

Goncalves Carrasquinho S, Teixeira S, Cadete A, Bernardo M, Pego P, Prieto I (2008) Congenital ocular motor apraxia. Eur J Ophthalmol 18:282–284

Good WV (2001) Development of a quantitative method to measure vision in children with chronic cortical visual impairment. Trans Am Ophthalmol Soc 99:253–269

Good WV, Hou C (2006) Sweep visual evoked potential grating acuity thresholds paradoxically improve in low-luminance conditions in children with cortical visual impairment. Invest Ophthalmol Vis Sci 47:3220–3224

Good WV, Jan JE, Burden SK, Skoczenski A, Candy R (2001) Recent advances in cortical visual impairment. Dev Med Child Neurol 43:56–60

Good WV, Hou C, Norcia AM (2012) Spatial contrast sensitivity vision loss in children with cortical visual impairment. Invest Ophthalmol Vis Sci 53:7730–7734

Goodale MA (2011) Transforming vision into action. Vision Res 51:1567–1587

Goodale MA, Milner AD (2010) Two visual streams: interconnections do not imply duplication of function. Cogn Neurosci 1:65–68

Goodale M, Milner D (2013) Sight unseen: an exploration of conscious and unconscious vision, 2nd edn. Oxford University Press, Oxford

Goodale MA, Westwood DA (2004) An evolving view of duplex vision: separate but interacting cortical pathways for perception and action. Curr Opin Neurobiol 14:203–211

Goodale MA, Wolf ME, Whitwell RL, Brown LE, Cant JS, Chapman CS, Witt JK, Arnott SR, Khan SA, Chouinard PA, Culham JC, Dutton GN (2008) Perception and action: how dissociated are they? Preserved motion processing and visuomotor control in a patient with large bilateral lesions of occipitotemporal cortex. J Vis 8:371

Goswami U (2008) Reading. In: Reed J, Warner-Rogers J (eds) Child neuropsychology. Blackwell, Oxford, pp 340–356

Grafman J (2000) Conceptualizing functional neuroplasticity. J Commun Disord 33:345–356

Granrud CE (ed) (1993) Visual perception and cognition in infancy. Erlbaum Assoc, Hillsdale

Granrud CE, Yonas A, Pettersen L (1984) A comparison of monocular and binocular depth perception in 5- and 7-month-old infants. J Exp Child Psychol 38:19–32

Gredebäck G, Johnson S, von Hofsten C (2010) Eye tracking in infancy research. Dev Neuropsychol 35:1–19

Green CR, Mihic AM, Brien DC, Armstrong IT, Nikkel SM, Stade BC, Rasmussen C, Munoz DP, Reynolds JN (2009) Oculomotor control in children with fetal alcohol spectrum using a mobile eye-tracking laboratory. Euro J Neurosci 29:1302–1309

Greenfield DB (1985) Facilitating mentally retarded children's relational learning through novelty-familiarity training. Am J Ment Defic 90:342–348

Grill-Spector K, Malach R (2004) The human visual cortex. Annu Rev Neurosci 27:649–677

Grinter EJ, Maybery MT, Badcock DR (2010) Vision in developmental disorders: is there a dorsal stream deficit? Brain Res Bull 82:147–160

Groenendaal F, van Hof-van Duin J (1990) Partial visual recovery in two fullterm infants after perinatal hypoxia. Neuropediatrics 21:76–78

Groenendaal F, van Hof-van Duin J, Baerts W, Fetter WP (1989) Effects of perinatal hypoxia on visual development during the first year of (corrected) age. Early Hum Dev 20:267–279

Gronqvist H, Brodd KS, Rosander K (2011) Development of smooth pursuit eye movements in very prematurely born infants: 2. The low-risk subgroup. Acta Paediatr 100:e5–e11

Grossberg S, Vladusich T (2010) How do children learn to follow gaze, share joint attention, imitate their teachers, and use tools during social interaction? Neural Netw 23:940–965

Grossmann T (2010) The development of emotion perception in face and voice during infancy. Restor Neurol Neurosci 28:219–236

Grossmann T, Johnson MH (2007) The development of the social brain in the human infancy. Euro J Neurosci 25:909–919

Gupta M, Mulvihill AO, Lascaratos G, Fleck BW, George ND (2012) Nystagmus and reduced visual acuity secondary to drug exposure in utero: long-term follow-up. J Pediatr Ophthalmol Strabismus 49:58–63

Guralnick MJ (1998) Effectiveness of early intervention for vulnerable children: a developmental perspective. Am J Ment Retard 102:319–345

Guralnick MJ (2011) Why early intervention works: a systems perspective. Infants Young Child 24:6–28

Guzzetta A, Mercuri E, Cioni G (2001) Visual disorders in children with brain lesions: 2. visual impairment associated with cerebral palsy. Eur J Paediatr Neurol 5:115–119

Guzzetta A, Frisone MF, Ricci D, Rando T, Guzzetta T (2002) Development of visual attention in West syndrome. Epilepsia 43:757–763

Guzzetta F, Cioni G, Mercuri E, Fazzi E, Biagioni E, Veggiotti P et al (2008) Neurodevelopmental evolution of West syndrome: a 2-year prospective study. Euro J Pediatr Neurol 12:387–397

Guzzetta A, Tinelli F, Del Viva MM, Bancale A, Arrighi R, Pascale RR, Cioni G (2009) Motion perception in preterm children: role of prematurity and brain damage. Neuroreport 20:1339–1343

Guzzetta A, D'Acunto G, Rose S, Tinelli F, Boyd R, Cioni G (2010) Plasticity of the visual system after early brain damage. Dev Med Child Neurol 52:891–900

Gwiazda J, Bauer J, Thorn F, Held R (1997) Development of spatial contrast sensitivity from infancy to adulthood – psychophysical data. Optom Vis Sci 74:785–789

Haber SN, Knutson B (2010) The reward circuit: linking primate autonomy and human imaging. Neuropsychopharmacology 35:4–26

Hainline L (1998) The development of basic visual abilities. In: Slater A (ed) Perceptual development. Visual, auditory, and speech perception in infancy. Psychology Press, Hove, pp 5–50

Haith MM (1980) Rules that babies look by. Hillsdale (NJ) Erlbaum

Hamilton R, McGlone L, MacKinnon JR, Russell HC, Bradnam MS, Mactier H (2010) Ophthalmic, clinical and visual electrophysiological findings in children born to mothers prescribed substitute methadone in pregnancy. Br J Ophthalmol 94:696–700

Hamilton R, Bradnam MS, Dutton GN, Lai Chooi Yan AL, Lavy TE, Livingstone I, Mackay AM, Mackinnon JR (2013) Sensitivity and specificity of the step VEP in suspected functional visual acuity loss. Doc Ophthalmol 126:99–104

Handler SM, Fierson WM (2011) Learning disabilities, dyslexia, and vision. Pediatrics 127:e818–e856

Hansen RM, Fulton AB (1986) Pupillary changes during dark adaptation in human infants. Invest Ophthalmol 27:1726–1729

Hansen RM, Fulton AB (2000) Background adaptation in children with a history of mild retinopathy of prematurity. Invest Ophthalmol Vis Sci 41:320–324

Harbert MJ, Yeh-Na Harbert MJ, Yeh-Nayre LA, O'Halloran HS, Levy ML, Crawford JR (2012) Unrecognized visual field deficits in children with primary central nervous system brain tumors. J Neurooncol 107:545–549

Hargadon DD, Wood J, Twelker JD, Harvey EM, Dobson V (2010) Recognition acuity, grating acuity, contrast sensitivity, and visual fields in 6-year-old children. Arch Ophthalmol 128:70–74

Harris CM, Shawkat F, Russell-Eggitt I, Wilson J, Taylor D (1996) Intermittent horizontal saccade failure ('ocular motor apraxia') in children. Br J Ophthalmol 80:51–158

Hart SJ, Davenport ML, Hooper SR, Belger A (2006) Visuospatial executive function in Turner syndrome: functional MRI and neurocognitive findings. Brain 129:1125–1136

Hartmann EE, Ellis GS Jr, Morgan KS, Love A, May JG (1990) The acuity card procedure: longitudinal assessments. J Pediatr Ophthalmol Strabismus 27:78–184

Hartshorn K, Rovee-Collier C (1997) Infant learning and long-term memory at 6 months: a confirming analysis. Dev Psychobiol 30:71–85

Hartshorn K, Rovee-Collier C, Gerhardstein P, Bhatt RS, Wondoloski TL, Klein P, Gilch J, Wurtzel N, Campos-de-Carvalho M (1998) The ontogeny of long-term memory over the first year-and-a half of life. Dev Psychobiol 32:69–89

Harvey BM, Dumoulin SO (2011) The relationship between cortical magnification factor and population receptive field size in human visual cortex: constancies in cortical architecture. J Neurosci 31:13604–13612

Harvey EM, Dobson V, Luna B (1997) Long-term grating acuity and visual field development in preterm children who experienced brochopulmonary dysplasia. Dev Med Child Neurol 39:167–173

Hayne H (2004) Infant memory development: implications for childhood amnesia. Dev Rev 24:33–73

Hayne H, Boniface J, Barr R (2000) The development of declarative memory in human infants: age-related changes in deferred imitation. Behav Neurosci 114:77–83

Hécaen H, de Ajuriaguerra J (1954) Balint's syndrome (psychic paralysis of fixation) and its minor forms. Brain 77:373–400

Heiervang E, Hugdahl K (2003) Impaired visual attention in children with dyslexia. J Learn Disabil 36:68–73

Held R (1993) Rates of development and underlying mechanisms. In: Granrud CE (ed) Visual perception and cognition in infancy. Erlbaum Assoc, Hillsdale, pp 75–89

Hellgren K, Hellstrom A, Jacobson L, Flodmark O, Wadsby M, Martin L (2007) Visual and cerebral sequelae of very low birth weight in adolescents. Arch Dis Child Fetal Neonatal Ed 92:F259–F264

Hess RF, Zihl J, Pointer S, Schmid C (1990) The contrast sensitivity deficit in cases with cerebral lesions. Clin Vis Sci 5:203–215

Himmelbach M, Erb M, Karnath H-O (2006) Exploring the visual world: the neural substrate of spatial orienting. Neuroimage 32:1747–1759

Hochstein S, Ahissar M (2002) View from the top: hierarchies and reverse hierarchies in the visual system. Neuron 36:791–804

Hodgetts DJ, Simon JW, Sibila TA, Scanlon DM, Vellutino FR (1998) Normal reading despite limited eye movements. J AAPOS 2:182–183

Hoehl S, Reid VM, Parise E, Handl A, Palumbo L, Striano T (2009) Looking at eye gaze processing and its neural correlates in infancy-implications for social development and autism spectrum disorders. Child Dev 80:968–985

Holmes G (1918) Disturbances of visual orientation. Br J Ophthalmol 2:449–468, 506–516

Hong D, Scaletta Kent J, Kesler S (2009) Cognitive profile in Turner syndrome. Dev Disabil Res Rev 15:270–278

Horton JC, Hoyd WF (1991) The representation of the visual field in human striate cortex. Arch Ophthalmol 1091:816–824

Horwood AM, Riddell PM (2008) Gender differences in early accommodation and vergence development. Ophthal Physiol Opt 28:115–126

Houliston MJ, Taguri AH, Dutton GN, Hajivassiliou C, Young DG (1999) Evidence of cognitive visual problems in children with hydrocephalus: a structured clinical history-taking strategy. Dev Med Child Neurol 41:298–306

Hoyt CS (2003) Visual function in the brain-damaged child. Eye 17:369–384

Hoyt CS, Taylor D (2013) Pediatric ophthalmology and strabismus, 4th edn. Elsevier, Edinburgh/London/New York

Huber CH (1962) Homonymous hemianopia after occipital lobectomy. Am J Ophthalmol 54:623–629

Hughes JL, O'Connor PS, Larsen PD, Mumma JV (1985) Congenital vertical ocular motor apraxia. J Clin Neuroophthalmol 5:153–157

Humphreys K, Avidan G, Behrmann M (2007) A detailed investigation of facial expression processing in congenital prosopagnosia as compared to acquired prosopagnosia. Exp Brain Res 176:356–373

Hunnius S (2007) The early development of visual attention and its implications for social and cognitive development. Prog Brain Res 164:187–209

Hunnius S, Bekkering H (2010) The early development of object knowledge: a study of infants' visual anticipations during action observation. Dev Psychol 46:446–454

Hunnius S, Geuze RH, van Geert P (2006) Associations between the developmental trajectories of visual scanning and disengagement of attention in infants. Infant Behav Dev 29:108–125

Hussain Z, Sekuler AB, Bennett PJ (2011) Superior identification of familiar visual patterns a year after learning. Psychol Sci 22:724–730

Huurneman B, Boonstra FN, Cox RF, Cillessen AH, van Rens G (2012) A systematic review on 'foveal crowding' in visually impaired children and perceptual learning as a method to reduce. BMC Ophthalmol 12:27

Huurneman B, Boonstra FN, Cox RF, van Rens G, Cillessen AH (2013) Perceptual learning in children with visual impairment improves near visual acuity. Invest Ophthalmol Vis Sci 54:6208–6216

Huynh SC, Ojaimi E, Robaei D, Rose K, Mitchell P (2005) Accuracy of the Lang II stereotest in screening for binocular disorders in 6-year old children. Am J Ophthalmol 140:1130–1132

Hyvarinen L (2000) Visual evaluation of infants and children. In: Silverstone B, Lang MA, Rosenthal BP, Faye EE (eds) The Lighthouse handbook on vision impairment and vision rehabilitation. Oxford University Press, Oxford, pp 799–820

Hyvarinen L, Jacob N (2011) What and how does this child see? Vistest Ltd., Helsinki

Iliescu BF, Dannemiller JL (2008) Brain-behavior relationships in early visual development. In: Nelson CA, Luciana M (eds) The handbook of developmental cognitive neuroscience, 2nd edn. MIT Press, Cambridge, MA, pp 17–145

Incoccia C, Magnotti L, Iaria G, Piccardi L, Guariglia C (2009) Topographical disorientation in a patient who never developed navigational skills: the (re)bailitation treatment. Neuropsychol Rehabil 19:291–314

Innocenti GM, Kiper DC, Knyazeva MG, Deonna TW (1999) On nature and limits of cortical developmental plasticity after an early lesion, in a child. Restor Neurol Neurosci 15:219–227

Iyer KK, Bradley AP, Wilson SJ (2013) Conducting shorter VEP tests to estimate visual acuity via assessment of SNR. Doc Ophthamol 126:21–28

Jackel B, Wilson M, Hartmann E (2010) A survey of parents of children with cortical or cerebral visual impairment. J Vis Impair Blind 104:613–622

Jacobson L, Dutton GN (2000) Periventricular leukomalacia: an important cause of visual and ocular motility dysfunction in children. Surv Ophthalmol 45:1–13

Jacobson L, Ek E, Fernell E, Flodmark O, Broberger U (1996) Visual impairment in preterm children with periventricular leukomalacia – visual, cognitive and neuropediatric characteristics related to cerebral imaging. Dev Med Child Neurol 38:724–735

Jacobson L, Ygge J, Flodmark O, Ek U (2002) Visual and periventricular characteristics, ocular motility and strabismus in children with periventricular leukomalacia. Strabismus 10: 179–183

Jacobson L, Hård AL, Svensson E, Flodmark O, Hellström A (2003) Optic disc morphology may reveal timing of insult in children with periventricular leucomalacia and/or periventricular haemorrhage. Br J Ophthalmol 87:1345–1349

Jacobson L, Flodmark O, Martin L (2006) Visual field defects in prematurely born patients with white matter damage of immaturity: a multiple-case study. Acta Ophthalmol Scand 84: 357–362

Jacobson L, Hård AL, Horemuzza E, Hammaren H, Hellstrom A (2009) Visual impairment is common in children born before 25 gestational weeks –boys are more vulnerable than girls. Acta Paediatr 98:261–265

Jacobson L, Rydberg A, Eliasson A-C, Kits A, Flodmark O (2010) Visual field function in school-aged children with spastic unilateral cerebral palsy related to different patterns of brain damage. Dev Med Child Neurol 52:e184–e187

Jacobson L, Lennartsson F, Pansell T, Oqvist Seimyr G, Martin L (2012) Mechanisms compensating for visual field restriction in adolescents with damage to the retro-geniculate visual system. Eye (Lond) 26:1437–1445

Jainta S, Kapoula Z (2011) Dyslexic children are confronted with unstable binocular fixation while reading. PLoS One 6:e18694

Jakobson LS, Frisk V, Downie AL (2006) Motion-defined form processing in extremely premature children. Neuropsychologia 44:1777–1786

Jan JE, Freeman RD, Scott EP (1977) Visual impairment in children and adolescents. Grune & Stratton, New York

Jan JE, Farrell K, Wong PK, McCormick AQ (1986) Eye and head movements of visually impaired children. Dev Med Child Neurol 28:285–293

Jan JE, Groenveld M, Sykanda AM (1990) Light-gazing by visually impaired children. Dev Med Child Neurol 32:755–759

Jan JE, Groenveld M, Anderson DP (1993) Photophobia and cortical visual impairment. Dev Med Child Neurol 35:473–477

Janssens A, Uvin K, Van Impe H, Laroche SMF, Van Reempts P, Deboutte D (2009) Psychopathology among preterm infants using the diagnostic classification zero to three. Acta Paediatr 98:1988–1993

Jehee JF, Ling S, Swisher JD, van Bergen RS, Tong F (2012) Perceptual learning selectively refines orientation representations in early visual cortex. J Neurosci 32:16747–16753

John FM, Bromham NR, Woodhouse JM, Candy TR (2004) Spatial vision deficits in infants and children with Down syndrome. Invest Ophthalmol Vis Sci 45:1566–1572

Johnson MH (2001) Functional brain development in humans. Nat Rev Neurosci 2:475–483

Johnson SP (2003) Development of fragmented versus holistic object perception. In: Schwarzer G, Leder H (eds) The development of face processing. Hogrefe & Huber, Cambridge, MA, pp 3–17

Johnson MH, de Haan M (2010) Developmental cognitive neuroscience, 3rd edn. Wiley-Blackwell, Oxford

Johnson MH, Tucker LA (1996) The development and temporal dynamics of spatial orienting in infants. J Exp Child Psychol 63:171–188

Johnson MH, Posner MI, Rothbart MK (1994) Facilitation of saccades toward a covertly attended location in early infancy. Psychol Sci 5:90–93

Johnston CW, Shapiro E (1986) Hemi-inattention resulting from left hemisphere brain damage during infancy. Cortex 22:279–287

Jolles DD, van Buchern MA, Rombouts SA, Crone EA (2012) Practice effects in the developing brain: a pilot study. Dev Cogn Neurosci 2(Suppl 1):S180–S191

Jones L, Rothbart MK, Posner MI (2003) Development of inhibitory control in preschool children. Dev Sci 6:498–504

Jones MW, Branigan HP, Kelly ML (2008) Visual deficits in developmental dyslexia: relationship between non-linguistic visual tasks and their contribution to components of reading. Dyslexia 14:95–115

Jongmans M, Mercuri E, Henderson S, de Vries L, Sonksen P, Dubowitz L (1996) Visual function of prematurely born children with and without perceptual-motor difficulties. Early Hum Dev 45:73–82

Joy P, Brunsdon R (2002) Visual agnosia and prosopagnosia: a prospective case study. Child Neuropsychol 8:1–15

Jurado MB, Rosselli M (2007) The elusive nature of executive functions: a review of our current understanding. Neuropsychol Rev 17:213–233

Kannass KN, Oakes LM, Shaddy DJ (2006) A longitudinal study of the development of attention and distractibility. J Cogn Dev 7:381–409

Kanwisher N (2010) Functional specificity in the human brain: a window into the functional architecture of the mind. Proc Natl Acad Sci 107:11163–11170

Karatekin C (2008) Eye tracking studies of normative and atypical development. In: Nelson CA, Luciana M (eds) The handbook of developmental cognitive neuroscience, 2nd edn. MIT Press, Cambridge, MA, pp 263–299

Katsumi O, Chedid SG, Kronheim JK, Henry RK, Denno S, Hirose T (1995) Correlating preferential looking visual acuity and visual behavior in severely visually handicapped children. Acta Ophthalmol Scand 73:407–413

Katsumi O, Denno S, Arai M, Faria JD, Hirose T (1997) Comparison of preferential looking acuity and pattern reversal visual evoked response acuity in pediatric patients. Graefes Arch Clin Exp Ophthalmol 235:684–690

Katsumi O, Chedid SG, Kronheim JK, Henry RK, Jones CM, Hirose T (1998) Visual ability score – a new method to analyze ability in visually impaired children. Acta Ophthalmol Scand 76:50–55

Kawasaki A, Purvin VA (2002) Photophobia as the presenting visual symptom of chiasmal compression. J Neuroophthalmol 22:3–8

Kaye EM, Herskowitz J (1986) Transient post-traumatic blindness: brief vs. prolonged syndromes in childhood. J Child Neurol 1:206–210

Keane JR (1980) Blindness following tentorial herniation. Ann Neurol 8:186–190

Keating DP, Keniston AH, Manis FR, Bobbitt BL (1980) Development of the search-processing parameter. Child Dev 51:39–44

Kedar S, Zhang X, Lynn MJ, Newman NJ, Biousse V (2006) Pediatric homonymous hemianopia. J AAPOS 10:249–252

Keen R (2011) The development of problem solving in young children: a critical cognitive skill. Annu Rev Psychol 62:1–21

Kellman Ph J (1993) Kinematic foundations of infant visual perception. In: Granrud CE (ed) Visual perception and cognition in infancy. Erlbaum Assoc, Hillsdale, pp 121–173

Kesler SR, Haberecht MF, Menon V, Warsofsky IS, Dyer-Friedman J, Neely EK, Reiss AL (2004) Functional neuroanatomy of spatial orientation processing in Turner syndrome. Cereb Cortex 14:174–180

Khan ZU, Martin-Montanez E, Baxter MG (2011) Visual perception and memory systems: from cortex to medial temporal lobe. Cell Mol Life Sci 68:1737–1754

Khetpal V, Donahue SP (2007) Cortical visual impairment: etiology, associated findings, and prognosis in a tertiary care setting. J AAPOS 11:235–239

Kinnear PR, Sahraie A (2002) New Farnsworth-Munsell 100 hue test norms of normal observers for each eye of age 5–22 and for age decades 30–70. Br J Ophthalmol 86:1408–1411

Kiorpes L, McKee SP (1999) Neural mechanisms underlying amblyopia. Curr Opin Neurobiol 9:480–486

Kivlin JD, Simons KB, Lazoritz S, Ruttum MS (2000) Shaken Baby syndrome. Ophthalmology 107:1246–1254

Klaver P, Marcar V, Martin E (2011) Neurodevelopment of the visual system in typically developing children. Prog Brain Res 189:113–136

Klein JT, Shepard SV, Platt ML (2009) Social attention and the brain. Curr Biol 19:R958–R962

Kleinman JT, Gailloud PH, Jordan LC (2010) Recovery from spatial neglect and hemiplegia in a child despite a large anterior circulation stroke and Wallerian degeneration. J Child Neurol 25:500–503

Klenberg L, Korkman M, Lahti-Nuuttila P (2001) Differential development of attention and executive functions in 3- to 12-year-old Finnish children. Dev Neuropsychol 20:407–428

Kliegel M, Mackinlay R, Jäger T (2008) Complex prospective memory: development across the lifespan and the role of task interruption. Dev Psychol 44:612–617

Knox PJ, Simmers AJ, Gray LS, Cleary M (2012) An exploratory study: prolonged periods of binocular stimulation can provide an effective treatment for childhood amblyopia. Invest Ophthalmol Vis Sci 53:817–824

Koeda T, Inoue M, Takeshita K (1997) Constructional dyspraxia in preterm diplegia: isolation from visual and visual perceptual impairments. Acta Paediatr 86:1068–1073

Kolb B, Teskey GC (2012) Age, experience, injury, and the changing brain. Dev Psychobiol 54:311–325

Kolb B, Mychasiuk R, William P, Gibb R (2011) Brain plasticity and recovery from early cortical injury. Dev Med Child Neurol 53(Suppl 4):4–8

Konen CS, Kastner S (2008) Two hierarchically organised neural systems for object information in human visual cortex. Nat Neurosci 11:224–231

Korkman M, Liikanen A, Fellman V (1996) Neuropsychological consequences of very low birth weight and asphyxia at term: follow-up until school age. J Clin Exp Neuropsychol 18:220–233

Kozeis N, Anogeianaki A, Mitova DT, Anogianakis G, Mitov T, Klisarova A (2007) Visual function and visual perception in cerebral palsied children. Ophthal Physiol Opt 27:44–53

Kravits DJ, Saleem KS, Baker CI, Mishkin M (2011) A neural framework for visuospatial processing. Nat Rev Neurosci 12:217–230

Kronbichler M, Hutzler F, Staffen W, Mair A, Ladurner G, Wimmer H (2006) Evidence for a dysfunction of left posterior reading area in German dyslexic readers. Neuropsychologia 44:1822–1832

Kronbichler M, Klackl J, Richlan F, Schurz M, Staffen W, Ladurner G, Wimmer H (2009) On the functional neuroanatomy of visual word processing: effects of case and letter deviance. J Cogn Neurosci 21:222–229

Kuba M, Liláková D, Hejcmanová D, Kremlácek J, Langrová J, Kubová Z (2008) Ophthalmological examination and VEPs in preterm children with perinatal CNS involvement. Doc Ophthalmol 117:137–145

Kvarnstrom G, Jakobsson P (2005) Is vision screening in 3-year-old children feasible? Comparison between the Lea Symbol chart and the HVOT (LM) chart. Acta Ophthalmol Scand 83: 76–80

Lambert SR, Hoyt CS, Jan JE, Barkovich J, Flodmark O (1987) Visual recovery from hypoxic cortical blindness during childhood. Arch Ophthalmol 105:1371–1377

Lambert SR, Kriss A, Taylor D (1989) Delayed visual maturation. A longitudinal clinical and electrophysiological assessment. Ophthalmology 96:524–528

Landis T, Regard M, Bliestle A, Kleihues P (1988) Prosopagnosia and agnosia for noncanonical views. An autopsied case. Brain 111:1287–1297

Landry SH, Smith KE, Swank PR (2006) Responsive parenting: establishing early foundations for social, communication, and independent problem-solving skills. Dev Psychol 42:627–642

Lanzi G, Fazzi E, Uggetti C, Cavallini A, Danova S, Egitto MG et al (1998) Cerebral visual impairment in periventricular leukomalacia. Neuropediatrics 29:145–150

Larson RW, Rusk N (2011) Intrinsic motivation and positive development. Adv Child Dev Behav 41:89–130

Larsson E, Rydberg A, Holmstrom G (2006) Contrast sensitivity in 10 year old preterm and full term children: a population based study. Br J Ophthalmol 90:87–90

Lassus-Sangousse D, N'guyen-Morel MA, Valdois S (2008) Sequential or simultaneous visual processing deficit in developmental dyslexia? Vision Res 48:978–988

Laurent-Vannier A, Pradat-Diehl P, Chevignard M, Abada G, De Agostini M (2003) Spatial and motor neglect in children. Neurology 60:202–207

Laurent-Vannier A, Chevignard M, Pradat-Diehl P, Abada G, De Agostini M (2006) Assessment of unilateral spatial neglect in children using the Teddy Bear Cancellation test. Dev Med Child Neurol 48:120–125

Lê S, Cardebat D, Boulanouar K, Hénaff M-A, Michel F, Milner D et al (2002) Seeing, since childhood, without ventral stream: a behavioural study. Brain 125:58–74

Leat SJ (1996) Reduced accommodation in children with cerebral palsy. Ophthal Physiol Opt 16:385–390

Leat SJ, Wegmann D (2004) Clinical testing of contrast sensitivity in children: age-related norms and validity. Optom Vis Sci 81:245–254

Leaverton DR, Rupp JW, Poff MG (1977) Brief therapy for monocular hysterical blindness in childhood. Child Psychiatry Hum Dev 7:254–263

Lee Y, Duchaine B, Wilson HR, Nakayama K (2009) Three cases of developmental prosopagnosia from one family: detailed neuropsychological and psychophysical investigation of face processing. Cortex 46:949–964

Leigh RJ, Zee DS (2006) The neurology of eye movements, 4th edn. F.A. Davis Company, Philadelphia

Lenassi E, Likar K, Stirn-Kranjc B, Brecelj J (2008) VEP maturation and visual acuity in infants and preschool children. Doc Ophthalmol 117:111–120

Leppanen JM, Nelson CA (2009) Tuning the developing brain to social signals of emotions. Nat Rev Neurosci 10:37–47

Lerner Y, Hendler T, Malach R, Harel M, Leiba H, Stolovitch C et al (2006) Selective fovea-related deprived activation in retinotopic and high-order visual cortex of human amblyopes. Neuroimage 33:169–179

Levi DM, Li RW (2009) Perceptual learning as a potential treatment for amblyopia: a mini-review. Vision Res 49:2535–2549

Lewis TL, Maurer D (2009) Effects of early pattern deprivation on visual development. Optom Vis Sci 86:640–646

Lewis TL, Maurer D, Brent HP (1995) Development of grating acuity in children treated for unilateral or bilateral congenital cataract. Invest Ophthalmol Vis Sci 36:2080–2095

Lezak MD, Howieson DB, Bigler ED, Tranel D (2012) Neuropsychological assessment, 5th edn. Oxford University Press, Oxford

Li SC (2003) Biocultural orchestration of developmental plasticity across levels: the interplay of biology and culture in shaping the mind and behavior across the life span. Psychol Bull 129:171–194

Li SC, Brehmer Y, Shing YL, Werkle-Bergner M, Lindenberger U (2006) Neuromodulation of associative and organizational plasticity across the life span: empirical evidence and neurocomputational models. Neurosci Biobehav Rev 30:775–790

Libertus K, Needham A (2010) Teach to reach: the effects of active vs. passive reaching experiences on action and perception. Vision Res 50:2750–2757

Lim M, Soul JS, Hansen RM, Mayer DL, Moskowitz A, Fulton AB (2005) Development of visual acuity in children with cerebral visual impairment. Arch Ophthalmol 123:1215–1220

Ling BY, Stephen J (2008) Color vision in children and the Lanthony New Color Test. Vis Neurosci 25:441–444

Lions C, Bui-Quoc E, Seassau M, Bucci MP (2013) Binocular coordination of saccades during reading in strabismic children. Invest Ophthalmol Vis Sci 54:620–628

Lissauer H (1890) Ein Fall von Seelenblindheit nebst einem Beitrag zur Theorie derselben. Arch Psychiatr Nervenkr 21:222–270

Liszkowski U, Carpenter M, Henning A, Striano T, Tomasello M (2004) Twelve-month-olds point to share attention and interest. Dev Sci 7:297–307

Lithander J (1997) Visual development in healthy eyes from 24 months to four years of age. Acta Ophthalmol Scand 75:275–276

Little S, Dutton GN (2014) Children with complex needs can engage when enclosed by a 'tent': is this due to Balint's syndrome? B J Vis Impair (in press)

Little JA, Woodhouse JM, Lauritzen JS, Saunders KJ (2009) Vernier acuity in Down syndrome. Invest Ophthalmol Vis Sci 50:567–572

Liu GT, Volpe NJ, Galetta SL (2001) Neuro-ophthalmology. Diagnosis and management. W.B. Saunders Company, Philadelphia

Lorusso ML, Facoetti A, Paganoni P, Pezzani M, Molteni M (2006) Effects of visual hemisphere-specific stimulation versus reading-focused training in dyslexic children. Neuropsychol Rehabil 16:194–212

Lorusso ML, Facoetti A, Bakker DJ (2011) Neuropsychological treatment of dyslexia: does type of treatment matter? J Learn Disabil 44:136–149

Lueck AH (2004) Functional vision. A practitioner's guide to evaluation and intervention. AFB Press, New York

Lueck AH (2006) Issues in intervention for children with visual impairment or visual dysfunction due to brain injury. In: Dennison E, Lueck AH (eds) Proceedings of the summit on cerebral/cortical visual impairment: educational, family, and medical perspectives, April 30, 2005. AFB Press, New York, pp 121–130

Lueck AH (2010) Cortical or cerebral visual impairment in children: a brief overview. J Vis Impair Blind 104:585–592

Lundh BL (1989) Two years clinical experience with the preferential looking technique for visual acuity determination in infants and young children. Acta Ophthalmol 64:674–680

Luria AR (1959) Disorders of "simultaneous perception" in a case of bilateral occipito-parietal brain injury. Brain 82:437–449

MacIntyre-Béon C, Mitchell K, Gallagher I, Cockburn D, Dutton GD, Bowman R (2010) My voice heard: the journey of a young man with a cerebral visual impairment. J Vis Impair Blind 106:166–176

Macintyre-Béon C, Young D, Calvert J, Ibrahim H, Dutton GN, Bowman R (2012) Reliability of a question inventory for structured history taking in children with cerebral visual impairment. Eye (Lond) 26:1393

Macintyre-Béon C, Young D, Dutton GN, Mitchell K, Simpson J, Loffler G et al (2013) Cerebral visual dysfunction in prematurely born children attending mainstream school. Doc Ophthalmol 127:89–102

MacKay TL, Jakobson LS, Ellemberg D, Lewis TL, Maurer D, Casiro O (2005) Deficits in the processing of local and global motion in very low birthweight children. Neuropsychologia 43:1738–1748

Mackay AM, Bradnam MS, Hamilton R, Elliot AT, Dutton GN (2008) Real-time rapid acuity assessment using VEPs: development and validation of the step VEP technique. Invest Ophthalmol Vis Sci 49:438–441

Mackeben M, Trautzettl-Klosinski S, Reinhard J, Durrwachter U, Adler M, Klosinski G (2004) Eye movement control during single-word reading in dyslexics. J Vis 4:388–402

Mackie RT, McCulloch DL, Saunders KJ, Ballantyne J, Day RE, Bradnam MS et al (1995) Comparison of visual assessment tests in multiply handicapped children. Eye (Lond) 9:136–141

Maisog JM, Einbinder ER, Flowers DL, Turkeltaub PE, Eden EF (2008) Meta-analysis of functional neuroimaging studies of dyslexia. Ann N Y Acad Sci 1145:237–259

Malkowicz EM, Myers G, Leisman G (2006) Rehabilitation of cortical visual impairment in children. Int J Neurosci 116:1015–1033

Martelli M, Di Filippo G, Spinelli D, Zoccolotti P (2009) Crowding, reading, and developmental dyslexia. J Vis 9:1–18

Martin L, Aring E, Landgren M, Hellstrom A, Andersson Gronlund M (2008) Visual fields in children with attention-deficit/hyperactivity disorder before and after treatment with stimulants. Acta Ophthalmol 86:259–265

Martinez-Conde S, Macknik SL, Hubel DH (2004) The role of fixational eye movements in visual perception. Nat Rev Neurosci 5:229–239

Mash C, Dobson V (2005) Intraobserver reliability of the Teller Card procedure in infants with perinatal complications. Optom Vis Sci 82:817–822

Mather G (2006) Foundations of perception. Psychology Press, Hove/New York

Matsuba CA, Jan JE (2006) Long-term outcome of children with cortical visual impairment. Dev Med Child Neurol 48:508–512

Maurer D, Lewis TL (2001a) Visual acuity: the role of visual input in inducing postnatal change. Clin Neurosci Res 1:239–247

Maurer D, Lewis TL (2001b) Visual acuity and spatial contrast sensitivity: normal development and underlying mechanisms. In: Nelson CA, Luciana M (eds) The handbook of developmental cognitive neuroscience. MIT Press, Cambridge, MA, pp 237–251

Maurer D, Lewis TL, Mondloch CJ (2005) Missing sights: consequences for visual cognitive development. Trends Cogn Sci 9:144–151

Maurer D, Ellemberg D, Lewis TL (2006) Repeated measurements of contrast sensitivity reveals limits to visual plasticity after early binocular deprivation in humans. Neuropsychologia 44:2104–2112

Maurer D, Lewis TL, Mondloch CJ (2008) Plasticity of the visual system. In: Nelson CA, Luciana M (eds) The handbook of developmental cognitive neuroscience, 2nd edn. MIT Press, Cambridge, MA, pp 415–437

Max JE, Robin DA, Lindgren SD, Smith WL Jr, Sato Y, Mattheis PJ et al (1998) Traumatic brain injury in children and adolescents: psychiatric disorders at one year. J Neuropsychiatry Child Neurosci 10:290–297

May A (2011) Experience-dependent structural plasticity in the adult human brain. Trends Cogn Sci 15:475–482

Maylor EA, Logie RH (2010) A large-scale comparison of prospective and retrospective memory development from childhood to middle age. Q J Exp Psychol 63:442–451

McClelland JF, Parkes J, Hill N, Jackson AJ, Saunders KJ (2006) Accommodative dysfunction in children with cerebral palsy: a population-based study. Invest Ophthalmol Vis Sci 47: 1824–1830

McCloskey M (2004) Spatial representations and multiple-visual-systems hypotheses: evidence from a developmental deficit in visual location and orientation processing. Cortex 40:677–694

McCulloch DL, Mackie RT, Dutton GN, Bradnam MS, Day RE, McDaid GJ, Phillips S, Napier A, Herbert AM, Saunders KJ, Sheperd AJ (2007) A visual skills inventory for children with neurological impairments. Dev Med Child Neurol 49:757–763

McGlone L, Hamilton R, McCulloch DL, Mackinnon JR, Bradnam M, Mactier H (2013) Visual outcome in infants born to drug-misusing mothers prescribed methadone in pregnancy. Br J Ophthalmol 98:238–245

McGraw PV, Winn B, Gray LS, Elliott DB (2000) Improving the reliability of visual acuity measures in young children. Ophthal Physiol Opt 20:173–184

McKillop E, Dutton GN (2008) Impairment of vision due to damage to the brain: a practical approach. Br Ir Orthop J 5:8–14

McKillop E, Bennett D, McDaid G, Holland B, Smith G, Spowart K et al (2006) Problems experienced by children with cognitive visual dysfunction due to cerebral visual impairment – and the approaches which parents have adopted to deal with these problems. Br J Vis Impair 24:121–127

McKone E, Crookes K, Kanwisher N (2009) The cognitive and neural development of face recognition in humans. In: Gazzaniga MS (ed) The cognitive neurosciences, 4th edn. MIT Press, Cambridge, MA, pp 467–482

Medland C, Walter H, Woodhouse JM (2010) Eye movements and poor reading: does the Developmental Eye Movement test measure cause or effect? Ophthal Physiol Opt 30:740–747

Meerwaldt JD, van Dongen HR (1988) Disturbances of spatial perception in children. Behav Brain Res 31:131–134

Mellor DH, Fielder AR (1980) Dissociated visual development: electrodiagnostic studies in infants who are 'slow to see'. Dev Med Child Neurol 22:327–335

Menghini D, Finzi A, Benassi M, Bolzani R, Facoetti A, Giovagnoli S, Ruffino M, Vicari S (2010) Different underlying neurocognitive deficits in developmental dyslexia: a comparative study. Neuropsychologia 48:863–872

Mercer ME, Courage ML, Adams RJ (1991) Contrast/color card procedure: a new test of young infants' color vision. Optom Vis Sci 68:522–532

Mercuri E, Atkinson J, Braddick O, Anker S, Cowan F, Rutherford M et al (1997) Visual function in full-term infants with hypoxic-ischemic encephalopathy. Neuropediatrics 28:155–161

Mercuri E, Haataja L, Guzzetta A, Anber S, Cowan F, Rutherford M et al (1999) Visual function in term infants with hypoxic-ischaemic insults: correlation with neurodevelopment at 2 years of age. Arch Dis Child Fetal Neonatal Ed 80:F99–F104

Mervis CA, Boyle CA, Yeargin-Allsopp M (2002) Prevelance and selected characteristics of childhood vision impairment. Dev Med Child Neurol 44:538–541

Mezey LE, Harris CM, Shawkat FS, Timms C, Kriss A, West P et al (1998) Saccadic strategies in children with hemianopia. Dev Med Child Neurol 40:626–630

Mian JF, Mondloch CJ (2012) Recognizing identity in the face of change: the development of an expression-independent representation of facial identity. J Vis 12(17):1–11

Miller LJ, Mittenberg S, Carey VM, McMorrow MA, Kushner TE, Weinstein JM (1999) Astereopsis caused by traumatic brain injury. Arch Clin Neuropsychol 14:537–543

Milner AD, Goodale MA (2006) The visual brain in action, 2nd edn. Oxford University Press, Oxford

Milner AD, Goodale MA (2008) Two visual systems re-viewed. Neuropsychologia 46:774–785

Milner AD, MacIntosh RD (2005) The neurological basis of visual neglect. Curr Opin Neurol 18:748–753

Mirabella G, Westall CA, Asztalos E, Perlman K, Koren G, Rovet J (2005) Development of contrast sensitivity in infants with prenatal and neonatal thyroid hormone insufficiencies. Pediatr Res 57:902–907

Miranda S (1970) Visual abilities and patterns preferences of premature infants and full-term neonates. J Exp Child Psychol 10:189–205

Mondloch CJ, Geldart S, Maurer D, Le Grand R (2003) Developmental changes in face processing skills. J Exp Child Psychol 86:67–84

Moore Q, Al-Zubidi N, Yalamanchili S, Lee AG (2012) Non-organic visual loss in children. Int Ophthalmol Clin 52:107–123

Moreaud O (2003) Balint syndrome. Arch Neurol 60:1329–1331

Morrone MC, Burr DC, Fiorentini A (1990) Development of contrast sensitivity and acuity of the infant colour system. Proc Royal Soc Lond B 242:134–139

Morrone MC, Gazzetta A, Tinelli F, Tosetti M, Del Viva M, Montanaro D, Burr D, Cioni C (2008) Inversion of perceived direction of motion caused by spatial undersampling in two children with periventricular leukomalacia. J Cogn Neurosci 20:1094–1106

Muckli L, Naumer MJ, Singer W (2009) Bilateral visual field maps in a patient with only one hemisphere. Proc Natl Acad Sci U S A 106:13034–13039

Mueller ST, Weidemann CT (2012) Alphabetic letter identification: effects of perceivability, similarity, and bias. Acta Psychol (Amst) 139:19–37

Müller D, Kandzia C, Roider J (2009) Computer-animated children's picture for assessing visual acuity. Ophthalmologe 106:328–333

Mulvihill AO, Cackett PD, George ND, Fleck BW (2007) Nystagmus secondary to drug exposure in utero. Br J Ophthalmol 91:613–615

Mundy P, Jarrold W (2010) Infant joint attention, neural networks and social cognition. Neural Netw 23:985–997

Murphy KM, Beston BR, Boley PM, Jones DG (2005) Development of human visual cortex: a balance between inhibitory and excitatory plasticity mechanisms. Dev Psychobiol 46:209–221

Murray K, Lillikas L, Weber R, Moore S, Irving E (2007) Development of head movements propensity in 4–15 year old children in response to visual step stimuli. Exp Brain Res 177:15–20

Murray IC, Fleck BW, Brash HM, Macrae ME, Tan LL, Minns RA (2009) Feasibility of saccadic vector optokinetic perimetry: a method of automated static perimetry for children using eye tracking. Ophthalmology 116:2017–2026

Murray I, Perperidis A, Brash H, Cameron L, McTrusty A, Fleck B, Minns R (2013) Saccadic Vector Optokinetic Perimetry (SVOP): a novel technique for automated static perimetry in children using eye tracking. Conf Proc IEEE Eng Med Biol Soc 978-1-4577-2160-7/13;3186–3189. http://www.i2eyediagnostics.com/maintenance.html

Nackaerts E, Wagemans J, Helsen W, Swinnen SP, Wenderoth N, Alaerts K (2012) Recognizing biological motion and emotions from point-light displays in autism spectrum disorder. PLoS One 7:e44473

Nagai C, Inui T, Iwata M (2011) Fading-figure tracing in Williams syndrome. Brain Cogn 75:10–17

Nardini M, Atkinson J, Braddick O, Burgess N (2008) Developmental trajectories for spatial frames of reference in Williams syndrome. Dev Sci 11:583–595

Nava E, Roder B (2011) Adaptation and maladaptation insights from brain plasticity. Prog Brain Res 191:177–194

Nelson CA (1995) The ontogeny of human memory: a cognitive neuroscience perspective. Dev Psychol 31:723–738

Netelenbos JB, Savelsbergh GJP (2003) Children's search for targets located within and beyond the field of view: effects of deafness and age. Perception 32:485–497

Netelenbos JB, Van Rooij L (2004) Visual search in school-aged children with unilateral brain lesions. Dev Med Child Neurol 46:334–349

Nielsen LS, Skov L, Jensen H (2007a) Visual dysfunctions and ocular disorders in children with developmental delay. I. Prevalence, diagnoses and aetiology of visual impairment. Acta Ophthalmol Scand 85:149–156

Nielsen LS, Nielsen SK, Skov L, Jensen H (2007b) Contrast sensitivity – an unnoticed factor of visual perception in children with developmental delay: normal data of the Cambridge Low Contrast Gratings test in children. J Child Neurol 22:151–155

Nijboer TCW, van Zaandvort MJE, de Haan EHF (2007) A familial factor in the development of colour agnosia. Neuropsychologia 45:1961–1965

Nithianantharajah J, Hannan AJ (2006) Enriched environments, experience-dependent plasticity and disorders of the nervous system. Nat Rev Neurosci 7:697–709

Novak C (2000) Sehbehindertengerechter Arbeitsplatz – Kommunikation im Internet mit Farben. (Workplace accessible for low vision handicapped – communication in the Internet with colours. In German). Unpublished master's thesis, Advanced Technical College, Hagenberg

O'Connor AR, Stephenson TJ, Johnson A, Tobin MJ, Ratib S, Moseley M, Fielder AR (2004) Visual function in low birthweight children. Br J Ophthalmol 88:1149–1153

O'Reilly M, Vollmer B, Vargha-Kadem F, Neville B, Connelly A, Wyatt J, Timms C, de Haan M (2010) Ophthalmological, cognitive electrophysiological and MRI assessment of visual processing in preterm children without major neuromotor impairment. Dev Sci 13:692–705

Ohlsson J, Villareal G, Abrahamsson M, Cavazos H, Sjostrom A, Sjostrand J (2001) Screening merits of the Lang II, Frisby, Randot, Titmus, and TNO stereo tests. J AAPOS 5:316–322

Ortibus E, Lagae L, Casteels I, Demaerel P, Stiers P (2009) Assessment of cerebral visual impairment with the L94 visual perceptual battery: clinical value and correlation with MRI findings. Dev Med Child Neurol 51:209–217

Ortibus E, Laenen A, Verhoeven J, De Cock P, Casteels I, Schoolmeesters B, Buyck A, Lagae L (2011) Screening for cerebral visual impairment: value of a CVI questionnaire. Neuropediatrics 42:138–147

Osterrieth P (1946) Le test de copie d'une figure complexe. Les Arch Psycho 31:206–356

Ostrovsky Y, Amaldam A, Sinha P (2006) Vision following extended congenital blindness. Psychol Sci 17:1009–1014

Ozonoff S, Macari S, Young GS, Goldring S, Thompson M, Rogers SJ (2008) Atypical visual exploration at 12 months of age is associated with autism in a prospective sample. Autism 12:457–472

Palermo R, Willis MR, Rivolta D, McKone E, Wilson CE, Calder AJ (2011) Impaired holistic processing of facial expression and facial identity in congenital prosopagnosia. Neuropsychologia 49:1226–1235

Palomares M, Landau B, Egeth H (2008) Visuospatial interpolation in typically developing children and in people with Williams syndrome. Vision Res 48:439–450

Pantev C, Ross B, Fujioka T, Trainor LJ, Schulte M, Schulz M (2003) Music and learning-induced cortical plasticity. Ann N Y Acad Sci 999:438–450

Pascalis O, Slater A (eds) (2003) The development of face processing in infancy and early childhood: current perspectives. Nova Science, New York

Pasqualotto A, Proulx MJ (2012) The role of visual experience for the neural basis of spatial cognition. Neurosci Biobehav Rev 36:1179–1187

Pavlova M, Staudt M, Sokolov A, Birbaumer N, Krägeloh-Mann I (2003) Perception and production of biological movement in patients with early periventricular brain lesions. Brain 126:692–701

Pavlova M, Sokolov A, Krägeloh-Mann I (2007) Visual navigation in adolescents with early periventricular lesions: knowing where, but not getting there. Cereb Cortex 17:363–369

Pel JJ, Manders JC, van der Steen J (2010) Assessment of visual orienting behaviour in young children using remote eye tracking: methodology and reliability. J Neurosci Methods 189:252–256

Pel J, Does LV, Boot F, Faber TD, Steen-Kant SV, Willemsen S, Steen HV (2011) Effects of visual processing and congenital nystagmus on visually guided ocular motor behavior. Dev Med Child Neurol 53:344–349

Pereira AF, James KH, Jones SS, Smith LB (2010) Early biases and development changes in self-generated object views. J Vis 10:22

Petersen SE, Posner MI (2012) The attention system of the human brain: 20 years after. Annu Rev Neurosci 35:73–89

Peterson RL, Pennington BF (2012) Developmental dyslexia. Lancet 379:1997–2007

Phillipou A, Douglas J, Krieser D, Ayton L, Abel L (2014) Changes in saccadic eye movement and memory function after mild closed head injury in children. Dev Med Child Neurol 56:337–345

Picard L, Reffuveille I, Eustache F, Piolino P (2009) Development of autonoetic autobiographical memory in school-age children: genuine age effect or development of basic cognitive abilities? Conscious Cogn 18:864–876

Pierrot-Deseilligny C, Rivaud S, Gaymard B, Muri R, Vermersch AI (1995) Cortical control of saccades. Ann Neurol 37:557–567

Pike MG, Holmstrom G, de Vries LS, Pennock JM, Drew KJ, Sonksen PM et al (1994) Patterns of visual impairment associated with lesions of the preterm infant brain. Dev Med Child Neurol 36:849–862

Poggi G, Calori G, Mancarella G, Colombo E, Profice P, Martinelli F et al (2000) Visual disorders after traumatic brain injury in developmental age. Brain Inj 14:833–845

Pola JR (2006) Development of eye movements in infants. In: Duckman RH (ed) Visual development, diagnosis, and treatment of the pediatric patient. Lippincott Williams & Wilkins, Philadelphia, pp 89–109

Polat U, Ma-Naim T, Spierer A (2009) Treatment of children with amblyopia by perceptual learning. Vision Res 49:2599–2603

Pollen DA (2011) On the emergence of primary visual perception. Cereb Cortex 21:1941–1953

Ponsonby AL, Williamson E, Smith K, Bridge D, Carmichael A, Jacobs A et al (2009) Children with low literacy and poor stereoacuity: an evaluation of complex interventions in a community-based randomized trial. Ophthalmic Epidemiol 16:311–321

Porro G, Wittebol-Post D, de Graaf M, van Nieuwenhuizen O, Schenk-Rootlieb AJF, Treffers WF (1998) Development of visual function in hemihydranencephaly. Dev Med Child Neurol 40:563–567

Porro G, van der Linden D, van Nieuwenhuizen O, Wittebol-Post D (2005) Role of visual dysfunction in postural control in children with cerebral palsy. Neural Plast 12:205–210

Porter MA, Colheart M (2006) Global and local processing in Williams syndrome, autism, and Down syndrome: perception, attention, and construction. Dev Neuropsychol 30:771–789

Porton-Deterne IF, Bloch H, Lacert P (2000) Ocular motility and visuo-spatial attention in children with periventricular leukomalacia. Brain Cogn 43:362–364

Posner MI, Petersen SE (1990) The attention system of the human brain. Annu Rev Neurosci 13:25–42

Powers MK (2009) Paper tools for assessing visual function. Optom Vis Sci 86:613–618

Prado C, Dubois M, Valdois S (2007) The eye movements of dyslexic children during reading and visual search: impact of the visual attention span. Vision Res 47:2521–2530

Pula J (2012) Functional visual loss. Curr Opin Opthalmol 23:460–465

Quadrato G, Di Giovanni S (2013) Waking up the sleepers: shared transcriptional pathways in axonal regeneration and neurogenesis. Cell Mol Life Sci 70:993–1007

Quaid P, Simpson T (2013) Association between reading speed, cycloplegic refractive error, and oculomotor function in reading disabled children versus controls. Graefes Arch Clin Exp Ophthalmol 251:169–187

Quin W, Liu Y, Jiang T, Yu C (2013) The development of visual areas depends differentially on visual experience. PLoS One 8:e53784

Quinn PC (1998) Object and spatial categorisation in young infants: "what" and "where" in early visual perception. In: Slater A (ed) Perceptual development. Visual, auditory, and speech perception in infancy. Psychology Press, Hove, pp 131–165

Quinn PC (2003) Concepts are not just for objects. Categorization of spatial relation information by infants. In: Rakinson D, Oakes LM (eds) Early category and concept development. Oxford University Press, New York, pp 50–75

Quinn PC, Bhatt RS (2001) Object recognition and object segregation in infancy: historical perspective, theoretical significance, "kinds" of knowledge, and relation to object categorization. J Exp Child Psychol 78:25–34

Quinn PC, Bhatt RS (2009) Perceptual organization in infancy: bottom-up and top-down influences. Optom Vis Sci 86:589–594

Ragge NK, Barkovich AJ, Hoyt WF, Lambert SR (1991) Isolated congenital hemianopia caused by prenatal injury to the optic radiation. Arch Neurol 48:1088–1091

Rainer G, Logothetis N (2003) Vision, behavior, and the single neuron. In: Fahle M, Greenlee M (eds) The neuropsychology of vision. Oxford University Press, Oxford, pp 3–22

Rakinson D, Oakes LM (eds) (2003) Early category and concept development. Oxford University Press, New York

Ramenghi LA, Ricci D, Mercuri E, Groppo M, De Carli A, Ometto A et al (2010) Visual performance and brain structures in the developing brain of pre-term infants. Early Hum Dev 86(Suppl 1):73–75

Ramon M, Rossion B (2010) Impaired processing of relative distances between features and of the eye region in acquired prosopagnosia – two sides of the same holistic coin? Cortex 46:374–389

Rapport LJ, Millis SR, Bonello PJ (1998) Validation of the Warrington theory of visual processing and the Visual Object and Space Perception Battery. J Clin Exp Neuropsychol 20:211–220

Rauschecker AM, Bowen RF, Perry LM, Kevan AM, Dougherty RF, Wandell BA (2011) Visual feature-tolerance in the reading network. Neuron 71:941–953

Rauschecker AM, Bowen RF, Parvizi J, Wandell BA (2012) Position sensitivity in the visual word form area. Proc Natl Acad Sci U S A 109:E1568–E1577

Rayner K (2009) Eye movements and attention in reading, scene perception, and visual search. Q J Exp Psychol 62:1457–14506

Rayner K, Foorman BR, Perfetti CA, Pesetsky D, Seidenberg MS (2001) How psychological science informs the teaching of reading. Psychol Sci 2:31–74

Reese E (2002) Social factors in the development of autobiographical memory: the state of the art. Soc Dev 11:124–142

Regal DM, Ashmead DH, Salapatek P (1983) The co-ordination of eye and head movements during early infancy: a selective review. Behav Brain Res 10:125–132

Reinis S, Goldman JM (1980) The development of the brain: biological and functional perspectives. Charles C. Thomas, Springfield

Ribeiro MJ, Violante IR, Bernardino I, Ramos F, Saraiva J, Reviriego P et al (2012) Abnormal achromatic and chromatic contrast sensitivity in neurofibromatosis type 1. Invest Ophthalmol Vis Sci 53:287–293

Riby DM, Back E (2010) Can individuals with Williams syndrome interpret mental stats from moving faces? Neuropsychologia 48:1914–1922

Ricci D, Anker S, Cowan F, Pane M, Gallini F, Luciano R et al (2006) Thalamic atrophy in infants with PVL and cerebral visual impairment. Early Hum Dev 82:591–595

Richards JE (2008) Attention in young infants: a developmental psychophysiological perspective. In: Nelson CA, Luciana M (eds) The handbook of developmental cognitive neuroscience, 2nd edn. MIT Press, Cambridge, MA, pp 479–497

Richards JE, Hunter SK (1998) Attention and eye movement control in young infants: neural control and development. In: Richards JE (ed) Cognitive neuroscience of attention. A developmental perspective. Erlbaum Assoc, London, pp 131–162

Ridder WH (2004) Methods of visual acuity determination with the spatial frequency sweep visual evoked potential. Doc Ophthalmol 109:239–247

Riva D, Cazzaniga L (1986) Late effects of unilateral brain lesions sustained before and after age one. Neuropsychologia 24:423–428

Rizzo M, Vecera SP (2002) Psychoanatomical substrates of Bálint's syndrome. J Neurol Neurosurg Psychiatry 72:162–178

Rizzolatti G, Sinigaglia C (2010) The functional role of the parieto-frontal mirror circuit: interpretations and misinterpretations. Nat Rev Neurosci 11:264–274

Robertson SS, Bacher LF, Huntington NL (2001) The integration of body movement and attention in young infants. Psychol Sci 12:523–526

Roman-Lantzy C (2007) Cortical visual impairment: an approach to assessment and intervention. AFB Press, New York

Roman C, Baker-Nobles L, Dutton GN, Luiselli TE, Flener BS, Jan JE, Lantzy A, Matsuba C, Mayer DL, Newcomb S, Nielsen AS (2010) Statement on cortical visual impairment. J Vis Impair Blind 104:69–72

Romine CB, Reynolds C (2005) A model of the development of frontal lobe functioning: findings from a meta-analysis. Appl Neuropsychol 12:190–201

Rosander K (2007) Visual tracking and its relationship to cortical development. Prog Brain Res 164:105–122

Rose SA, Feldman JF, Jankowski JJ (2001) Attention and recognition memory in the 1st year of life: a longitudinal study of preterm and full-term infants. Dev Psychol 37:135–151

Rosenbaum P, Paneth N, Leviton A et al (2007) A report: the definition and classification of cerebral palsy. Dev Med Child Neurol Suppl 109:8–14

Rosenfield M (2006) Development of accommodation in human infants. In: Duckman RH (ed) Visual development, diagnosis, and treatment of the pediatric patient. Lippincott Williams & Wilkins, Philadelphia, pp 110–123

Roucoux A, Culee C, Roucoux M (1983) Development of fixation and pursuit eye movements in human infants. Behav Brain Res 10:133–139

Rovet J, Simic N (2008) The role of transient hypothyroxinemia of prematurity n development of visual abilities. Semin Perinatol 32:431–437

Rubinstein AJ, Kalakanis L, Langlois JH (1999) Infant preferences for attractive faces: a cognitive explanation. Dev Psychol 35:848–855

Rudanko SL, Fellman V, Laatikainen L (2003) Visual impairment in children born prematurely from 1972 through 1989. Ophthalmology 110:1639–1645

Ruddock GA, Harding GF (1994) Visual electrophysiology to achromatic and chromatic stimuli in premature and full term infants. Int J Psychophysiol 16:209–218

Rudolph D, Sterker I, Graefe G, Till H, Ulrich A, Geyer C (2010) Visual field constriction in children with shunt-treated hydrocephalus. J Neurosurg Pediatr 6:481–485

Ruff HA, Cappozoli MC (2003) Development of attention and distractibility in the first 4 years of life. Dev Psychol 39:877–890

Rushton WAH (1972) Light and dark adaptation. Invest Ophthalmol 11:503–517

Ruskin EM, Kasari C, Mundy P, Sigman M (1994) Attention to people and toys during social and object mastery in children with Down syndrome. Am J Ment Retard 99:103–111

Rutsche A, Baumann A, Jiang X, Mojon DS (2006) Development of visual pursuit in the first 6 years of life. Graefes Arch Clin Exp Ophthalmol 244:1406–1411

Ryan RM, Kuhl J, Deci EL (1997) Nature and autonomy – an organizational view of social and neurobiological aspects of self-regulation in behavior and development. Dev Psychopathol 9:701–728

Rydberg A, Ericson B (1998) Assessing visual function in children younger than 1 1/2 years with normal and subnormal vision: evaluation of methods. J Pediatr Ophthalmol Strabismus 35:312–319

Rydberg A, Han Y (1999) Assessment of contrast sensitivity in children aged 3 years 3 months – 6 years with normal vision, visual impairment due to ocular disease and strabismic amblyopia. Strabismus 7:79–95

Rydberg A, Ericson B, Lennerstrand G, Jacobson L, Lindstedt E (1999) Assessment of visual acuity in children aged 1½–6 years, with normal and subnormal vision. Strabismus 7:1–24

Sadato N, Pascual-Leone A, Grafman J, Deiber MP, Ibanez V, Hallett M (1998) Neural networks for Braille reading by the blind. Brain 121:1213–1229

Saeed M, Henderson G, Dutton GN (2007) Hyoscine skin patches for drooling dilate pupils and impair accommodation: spectacle correction for photophobia and blurred vision may be warranted. Dev Med Child Neurol 49:426–428

Sai FZ (2005) The role of the mother's voice in developing mother's face preference: evidence for intermodal perception at birth. Infant Child Dev 14:29–50

Saidkasimova S, Bennet DM, Butler S, Dutton GN (2007) Cognitive visual impairment with good visual acuity in children with posterior periventricular white matter injury: a series of 7 cases. J AAPOS 11:426–430

Salati R, Borgatti R, Giammari G, Jacobson L (2002) Oculomotor dysfunction in cerebral visual impairment following perinatal hypoxia. Dev Med Child Neurol 44:542–550

Sanes DH, Reh TA, Harris WA (2006) Development of the nervous system, 2nd edn. Elsevier Inc., Amsterdam

Sanocki T, Dyson MC (2012) Letter processing and font information during reading: beyond distinctiveness, where vision meets design. Atten Percept Psychophys 74:132–145

Saunders KJ, McClelland JF, Richardson PM, Stevenson M (2008) Clinical judgment of near pupil responses provides a useful indicator of focusing ability in children with cerebral palsy. Dev Med Child Neurol 50:33–37

Saunders KJ, Little JA, McClelland JF, Jackson AJ (2010) Profile of refractive errors in cerebral palsy: impact of severity of motor impairment (GMFCS) and CP subtype on refractive outcome. Invest Ophthalmol Vis Sci 51:2885–2890

Scerif G, Cornish K, Wilding J, Driver J, Karmiloff-Smith A (2004) Visual search in typically developing toddlers and toddlers with Fragile X or Williams syndrome. Dev Sci 7: 116–130

Schenk T (2006) An allocentric rather than perceptual deficit in patient DF. Nat Neurosci 9:1369–1370

Schenk T, McIntosh RD (2010) Do we have independent visual streams for perception and action? Cogn Neurosci 1:52–62

Schenk-Rootlieb AJF, van Nieuwenhuizen O, van Waes PFGM, van der Graaf Y (1994) Cerebral visual impairment in cerebral palsy: relation to structural abnormalities of the cerebrum. Neuropediatrics 25:68–72

Schlaggar BL, Church JA (2009) Functional neuroimaging insights into the development of skilled reading. Curr Dir Psychol Sci 18:21–26

Schlaggar BL, McCandliss BD (2007) Development of neural systems for reading. Annu Rev Neurosci 30:475–503

Schmalzl L, Palermo R, Green M, Brunsdon R, Coltheart M (2008) Training of familiar face recognition and visual scan paths for faces in a child with congenital prosopagnosia. Cogn Neuropsychol 25:704–729

Schmidt PP (1994) Visual acuity measurement in exceptional children. J Am Optom Assoc 65:627–633

Schmitt KU, Moser MH, Lanz C, Walz F, Schwarz U (2007) Comparing eye movements recorded by search coil and infrared eye tracking. J Clin Monit Comput 21:49–53

Schmuckler MA (2001) What is ecological validity? A dimensional analysis. Infancy 2:419–436

Schoenfeld MA, Hassa T, Hopf JM, Eulitz C, Schmidt R (2011) Neural correlates of hysterical blindness. Cereb Cortex 21:2394–2398

Schor CM (1985) Development of stereopsis depends upon contrast sensitivity and spatial tuning. J Am Optom Assoc 56:628–635

Schroeder CE, Tenke CE, Arezzo JC, Vaughan HG (1989) Timing and distribution of flash-evoked activity in the lateral geniculate nucleus of the alert monkey. Brain Res 477:183–195

Schwartz TL, Dobson V, Sandstrom DJ, van Hof-van Duin J (1987) Kinetic perimetry assessment of binocular visual field shape in size in young infants. Vision Res 27:2163–2175

Schwenck C, Bjorklund DF, Schneider W (2009) Developmental and individual differences in young children's use and maintenance of a selective memory strategy. Dev Psychol 45:1034–1050

Senbil N, Aydin OF, Orer H, Gürer YK (2004) Subacute sclerosing panencephalitis: a cause of acute vision loss. Pediatr Neurol 31:214–217

Senju A, Johnson MH (2009) The eye contact effect: mechanisms and development. Trends Cogn Sci 13:127–134

Serino A, Cecere R, Dundon N, Bertini C, Sanchez-Castaneda C, Làdavas E (2014) When apperceptive agnosia is explained by a deficit of primary visual processing. Cortex 52: 12–27

Serna RW, Dube WV, McIlvane WJ (1997) Assessing same/different judgements in individuals with severe intellectual disabilities: a status report. Res Dev Disabil 18:343–368

Sewards TV (2011) Neural structures and mechanisms involved in scene recognition: a review and interpretation. Neuropsychologia 49:277–298

Sexton CC, Gelhorn HL, Bell JA, Classi PM (2012) The co-occurrence of reading disorder and ADHD: epidemiology, treatment, psychosocial impact, and economic burden. J Learn Disabil 45:538–564

Sharpe JA, Lo AW, Rabinovitch HE (1979) Control of saccadic and smooth pursuit systems after hemidecortication. Brain 102:387–403

Shaywitz SE, Shaywitz BA (2008) Paying attention to reading: the neurobiology of reading and dyslexia. Dev Psychopathol 20(Special Issue S1):1329–1349

Shute RH, Westall CA (2000) Use of Mollon-Reffin Minimalist color vision test with young children. J AAPOS 4:366–372

Sidman M, Stoddard LT (1967) The effectiveness of fading in programming a simultaneous form discrimination for retarded children. J Exp Anal Behav 10:3–15

Siegler RS, DeLaoche JS, Eisenberg N (2011) How children develop, 3rd edn. Worth Publishers, New York

Sigmundsson H, Hansen PC, Talcott JB (2003) Do "clumsy" children have visual deficits. Behav Brain Res 139:123–129

Simion F, Leo I, Turati C, Valenza E, Dalla Barba B (2007) How face specialisation emerges in the first months of life. Prog Brain Res 164:169–185

Sinclair M, Taylor E (2008) The neuropsychology of attention development. In: Reed J, Warner-Rogers J (eds) Child neuropsychology. Blackwell, Oxford, pp 235–263

Singh-Curry V, Husain M (2009) The functional role of the inferior parietal lobe in the dorsal and ventral stream dichotomy. Neuropsychologia 47:1434–1448

Sinigaglia C (2013) What type of action understanding is subserved by mirror neurons? Neurosci Lett 540:59–61

Sireteanu R (2000) The binocular visual system in amblyopia. Strabismus 8:39–51

Sireteanu R, Encke I, Bachert I (2003) Infants' preference for texture-defined targets of different saliency: evidence for local processing. In: Schwarzer G, Leder L (eds) The development of face processing. Hogrefe & Huber, Cambridge, MA, pp 19–34

Sireteanu R, Goebel C, Goertz R, Wandert T (2006) Do children with developmental dyslexia show a selective visual attention deficit? Strabismus 14:85–93

Sireteanu R, Goebel C, Goertz R, Werner I, Nalewajko M, Thiel A (2008) Impaired visual search in children with developmental dyslexia. Ann N Y Acad Sci 1145:199–211

Skoczenski AM, Good WV (2004) Vernier acuity is selectively affected in infants and children with cortical visual impairment. Dev Med Child Neurol 46:526–532

Slater A (ed) (1998a) Perceptual development. Psychology Press, Hove

Slater A (1998b) The competent infant: innate organisation and early learning in infant visual perception. In: Slater A (ed) Perceptual development. Visual, auditory, and speech perception in infancy. Psychology Press, Hove, pp 105–130

Slater A, Mattock A, Brown E (1990) Size constancy at birth: newborn infants' responses to retinal and real size. J Exp Child Psychol 49:314–322

Smith AD, Gilchrist ID, Hood BM (2005) Children's search behaviour in large-scale space: developmental components of exploration. Perception 34:1221–1229

Smith-Spark JH, Fisk JE (2007) Working memory in developmental dyslexia. Memory 15:34–56

Solan HA, Larson S, Shelley-Tremblay J, Ficarra A, Silverman M (2001) Role of visual attention in cognitive control of oculomotor readiness in students with reading disabilities. J Learn Disabil 34:107–118

Song Y, Tian M, Liu J (2012) Top-down processing of symbolic meanings modulates the visual word form area. J Neurosci 32:12277–12283

Soul J, Matsuba C (2010) Common aetiologies of cerebral visual impairment. In: Dutton GN, Bax M (eds) Visual impairment in children due to damage to the brain. MacKeith Press, London, pp 20–26

Sourander A, Ronning J, Brunstein-Klomek A, Gyllenberg D, Kumpulainen K, Niemela S et al (2009) Childhood bullying behavior and later psychiatric hospital and psychopharmacological treatment: Findings from the Finnish 1981 Birth Cohort Study. Archives of General Psychiatry 66:1005–12

Spreen O, Risser AH, Edgell D (1995) Developmental neuropsychology. Oxford University Press, New York/Oxford

Squire LR, Wixted JT (2011) The cognitive neuroscience of human memory since H.M. Annu Rev Neurosci 34:259–288

Stevens DJ, Hertle RW (2003) Relationships between visual acuity and anomalous head posture in patients with congenital nystagmus. J Paediatr Ophthalmol Strabismus 40:259–264

Stewart RE, Woodhouse JM, Cregg M, Pakeman VH (2007) Association between accommodative accuracy, hypermetropia, and strabismus in children with Down's syndrome. Optom Vis Sci 844:149–155

Stiers P, Vandenbussche E (2004) The dissociation of perception and cognition in children with early brain damage. Brain Dev 26:81–92

Stiers P, De Cock P, Vandenbussche E (1998) Impaired visual perceptual performance on an Object Recognition Task. Neuropediatrics 29:80–88

Stiers P, Vanderkelen R, Vanneste G, Coene S, De Rammelaere M, Vandenbussche E (2002) Visual-perceptual impairment in a random sample of children with cerebral palsy. Dev Med Child Neurol 44:370–382

Stiers P, Vanderkelen R, Vandenbussche E (2004) Optotype and grating visual acuity in patients with ocular and cerebral visual impairment. Invest Ophthalmol Vis Sci 45:4333–4339

Stiles J, Paul B, Ark W (2008) The development of visuospatial processing. In: Nelson CA, Luciana M (eds) The handbook of developmental cognitive neuroscience, 2nd edn. MIT Press, Cambridge, MA, pp 521–540

Strand-Brodd K, Ewald U, Gronqvist H, Holmstrom G, Stromberg G, Gronqvist E et al (2011) Development of smooth pursuit eye movements in very preterm infants: 1. General aspects. Acta Paediatr 100:983–991

Strand-Brodd K, Gronqvist H, Holmstrom G, Gronqvist E, Rosander K, Ewald U (2012) Development of smooth pursuit eye movements in very preterm infants: 3. Association with perinatal risk factors. Acta Paediatr 101:164–171

Straßburg HM, Dacheneder W, Kreß W (1997) Entwicklungsstörungen bei Kindern. Grundlagen der interdisziplinären Betreuung. English edition: Developmental disorders in children. Principles of interdisciplinary care. Lübeck: Gustav Fischer Verlag

Stuss DT, Alexander MP (2007) Is there a dysexecutive syndrome? Philos Trans R Soc Lond B Biol Sci 362:901–915

Suchan J, Rorden C, Karnath HO (2012) Neglect severity after left and right brain damage. Neuropsychologia 50:1136–1141

Summers CG, MacDonald JT (1990) Vision despite tomographic absence of the occipital cortex. Surv Ophthalmol 35:188–190

Sun J, Mohay H, O'Callaghan M (2009) A comparison of executive function in very preterm and term infants at 8 months corrected age. Early Hum Dev 85:225–230

Susilo T, Duchaine B (2013) Advances in developmental prosopagnosia research. Curr Opin Neurobiol 23:423–429

Szwed M, Dehaene S, Kleinschmidt A, Eger E, Valabregue R, Amadon A, Cohen L (2011) Specialization for written words over objects in the visual cortex. Neuroimage 56: 330–344

Tadic V, Pring L, Dale N (2009) Attentional processes in young children with congenital visual impairment. Br J Dev Psychol 27:311–330

Tallal P, Miller SL, Bedi G, Byma G, Wang X, Nagarajan SS, Schreiner C, Jenkins WM, Merzenich MM (1996) Language comprehension in language-learning impaired children improved with acoustically modified speech. Science 271(5245):81–84

Tam EW, Widjaja E, Blaser SI, MacGregor DL, Satodia P, Moore AM (2008) Occipital lobe injury and cortical visual outcomes after neonatal hypoglycemia. Pediatrics 122:507–512

Tasker SL, Schmidt L (2008) The "dual usage problem" in the explanations of "joint attention" and children's socioemotional development: a reconceptualization. Dev Rev 28:263–288

Taylor MJ, Khan SC (2000) Top-down modulation of early selective attention processes in children. Int J Psychophysiol 37:135–147

Taylor MJ, McCulloch DL (1992) Visual evoked potentials in infants and children. J Clin Neurophysiol 9:357–372

Teller DY, Lindsey DT (1993) Motion nulling techniques and infant color vision. In: Granrud CE (ed) Visual perception and cognition in infancy. Erlbaum Assoc, Hillsdale, pp 47–73

Teller DY, McDonald MA, Preston K, Sebris SL, Dobson V (1986) Assessment of visual acuity in infants and children: the acuity card procedure. Dev Med Child Neurol 28:779–789

Thaler L, Arnott SR, Goodale MA (2011) Neural correlates of natural human echolocation in early and late blind echolocation experts. PLoS One 6:e20162. doi:10.1371/journal.pone.0020162

Thomas C, Kveraga K, Huberle E, Karnath HO, Bar M (2012) Enabling global processing in simultanagnosia by psychophysical biasing of visual pathways. Brain 135:1578–1585

Tian N, Copenhagen DR (2003) Visual stimulation is required for refinement of ON and OFF pathways in postnatal retina. Neuron 39:85–96

Tinelli F, Pei F, Guzzetta A, Bancale A, Mazzotti S, Baldassi S, Cioni G (2008) The assessment of visual acuity in children with periventricular damage: a comparison of behavioral and electrophysiological techniques. Vision Res 48:1233–1241

Ting DS, Pollock A, Dutton GN, Doubal FN, Ting DS, Thompson M, Dhillon B (2011) Visual neglect following stroke: current concepts and future focus. Surv Ophthalmol 56:114–134

Toldo I, Pinello L, Suppiej A, Ermani M, Cermakova I, Zanin E, Sartori S, Battistella PA (2010) Nonorganic (psychogenic) visual loss in children: a retrospective series. J Neuroophthalmol 30:26–30

Tomac S, Altay Y (2000) Near stereoacuity: development in preschool children; normative values and screening for binocular vision abnormalities; a study of 115 children. Binocul Vis Strabismus Q 15:221–228

Tommiska V, Heinonen K, Kero P, Pokela ML, Tammela O, Jarvenpaa AL et al (2003) A national two year follow up study of extremely low birthweight infants born in 1996–1997. Arch Dis Child Fetal Neonatal Ed 88:F29–F35

Tondel GM, Candy TR (2008) Accommodation and vergence latencies in human infants. Vision Res 48:564–576

Tootell RBH, Dale AM, Sereno MI, Malach R (1996) New images from human visual cortex. Trends Neurosci 19:481–489

Topor IL, Erin JN (2000) Educational assessment of vision function in infants and children. In: Silverstone B, Lang MA, Rosenthal BP, Faye EE (eds) The Lighthouse handbook on vision impairment and vision rehabilitation. Oxford University Press, Oxford, pp 821–832

Torgrud LJ, Holborn SW (1989) Effectiveness and persistence of precurrent mediating behavior in delaying matching to sample and oddity matching with children. J Exp Anal Behav 52:181–191

Trauner D (2003) Hemispatial neglect in young children with early unilateral brain damage. Dev Med Child Neurol 45:160–166

Tree JJ, Wilkie J (2010) Face and object imagery in congenital prosopagnosia: a case series. Cortex 46:1189–1198

Treue S (2003) Visual attention: the where, what, how and why of saliency. Curr Opin Neurobiol 13:428–432

Turati C, Bulf H, Simion F (2008) Newborns' face recognition over changes in viewpoint. Cognition 106:1300–1321

Turnbull OH, Carey DP, McCarthy RA (1997) The neuropsychology of object constancy. J Int Neuropsychol Soc 3:288–298

Ungerleider LG, Mishkin M (1982) Two cortical systems. In: Ingle DJ, Mansfield JW, Goodale MA (eds) Advances in the analysis of visual behaviour. MIT Press, Cambridge, MA, pp. 549–596

Valdois S, Bosse ML, Tainturier MJ (2004) The cognitive deficits responsible for developmental dyslexia: review of evidence for a selective visual attentional disorder. Dyslexia 10:339–363

van Braeckel K, Butcher PR, Geuze RH, van Duijn MAJ, Bos AF, Bouma A (2010) Difference rather than delay in development of elementary visuomotor processes in children born preterm without cerebral palsy: a quasi-longitudinal study. Neuropsychology 24:90–100

Van den Hout BM, Eken P, Van der Linden D, Wittebol-Post D, Aleman S, Jennekens-Schinkel A et al (1998) Visual, cognitive, and neurodevelopmental outcome at 5½ years in children with perinatal haemorrhagic-ischaemic brain lesions. Dev Med Child Neurol 40:820–828

Van der Aa NE, Dudink J, Benders MJNL, Govarert P, van Straaten HLM, Porro GL et al (2013) Neonatal posterior cerebral artery stroke: clinical presentation, MRI findings, and outcome. Dev Med Child Neurol 55:283–290

Van der Geest JN, Lagers-van Haselen GC, van Hagen JM, Brenner E, Govaerts LC, de Coo IF et al (2005) Visual depth perception in Williams-Beuren syndrome. Exp Brain Res 166:200–209

Van der Mark S, Bucher K, Maurer U, Schulz E, Brem S, Buckelmüller J et al (2009) Children with dyslexia lack multiple specializations along the visual word-form (VWF) system. Neuroimage 47:1940–1949

Van der Mark S, Klaver P, Bucher K, Maurer U, Schulz E, Brem S et al (2011) The left occipitotemporal system in reading: disruption of focal fMRI connectivity to left inferior frontal and inferior parietal language areas in children with dyslexia. Neuroimage 54:2426–2436

Van Genderen M, Riemslag F, Jorritsma F, Hoeben F, Meire F, Stilma J (2006) The key role of electrophysiology in the diagnosis of visually impaired children. Acta Ophthalmol Scand 84:799–806

van Genderen M, Dekker M, Pilon F, Bals I (2012) Diagnosing cerebral visual impairment in children with good visual acuity. Strabismus 20:78–83

Van Hecke Vaughan A, Mundy P, Block JJ, Delgado CE, Parlade MV, Pomares YB et al (2012) Infant responding to joint attention, executive processes, and self-regulation in preschool children. Infant Behav Dev 35:303–311

Van Hof-van Duin J, Mohn G (1984) Visual defects in children after cerebral hypoxia. Behav Brain Res 14:147–155

Van Hof-van Duin J, Cioni G, Bertuccelli B, Fazzi B, Romano C, Boldrini A (1998) Visual outcome at 5 years of newborn infants at risk of cerebral visual impairment. Dev Med Child Neurol 40:302–309

Van Nieuwenhuizen O, Willemse J (1984) CT-Scanning in children with cerebral disturbance and its possible relation to hypoxia and ischaemia. Behav Brain Res 14:143–145

Van Praag H, Kempermann G, Gage FH (2000) Neural consequences of environmental enrichment. Nat Rev Neurosci 1:191–198

Van Zaandvort MJE, Nijboer TCW, de Haan EHF (2007) Developmental colour agnosia. Cortex 43:750–757

Van Zomeren AH, Brouwer WH (1994) Clinical neuropsychology of attention. Oxford University Press, New York

Venkateswaran S, Shevell MI (2008) Comorbidities and clinical determinants of outcome in children with spastic quadriplegic cerebral palsy. Dev Med Child Neurol 50:216–222

Vidyasagar TR, Pammer K (2010) Dyslexia: a deficit in visuo-spatial attention, not in phonological processing. Trends Cogn Sci 14:57–63

Voeller KKS, Heilman KM (1988) Attention deficit disorder in children: a neglect syndrome? Neurology 389:806–808

Volpe JJ (2009a) The encephalopathy of prematurity – brain injury and impaired brain development inextricably intertwined. Semin Pediatr Neurol 16:167–178

Volpe JJ (2009b) Brain injury in premature infants: a complex amalgam of destructive and developmental disturbances. Lancet Neurol 8:110–124

Vuilleumier P (2005) Hysterical conversion and brain function. Prog Brain Res 150:309–329

Waber SP, Holmes JM (1985) Assessing children's copy productions of the Rey-Osterrieth Complex Figure. J Clin Exp Neuropsychol 7:264–280

Wan CY, Wood AG, Reutens DC, Wilson SJ (2010) Early but not late-blindness leads to enhanced auditory perception. Neuropsychologia 48:344–348

Wandell BA (2011) The neurobiological basis of seeing words. Ann N Y Acad Sci 1224:63–80

Wandell BA, Dumoulin SO, Brewer AA (2007) Visual field maps in human cortex. Neuron 56:366–383

Watson T, Orel-Bixler D, Haegerstrom-Portnoy G (2007) Longitudinal quantitative assessment of vision function in children with cortical visual impairment. Optom Vis Sci 84:471–480

Watson T, Orel-Bixler D, Haegerstrom-Portnoy G (2009) VEP vernier, VEP grating, and behavioral grating acuity in patients with cortical visual impairment. Optom Vis Sci 86:774–780

Watson T, Orel-Bixler D, Haegerstrom-Portnoy G (2010) Early visual-evoked potential acuity and future behavioral acuity in cortical visual impairment. Optom Vis Sci 87:80–86

Wattam-Bell J (1992) The development of maximum displacement limits for discrimination of motion direction in infancy. Vision Res 32:621–630

Wattam-Bell J (1996a) Visual motion processing in one-month-old infants: preferential looking experiments. Vision Res 36:1671–1677

Wattam-Bell J (1996b) Visual motion processing in one-month-old infants: habituation experiments. Vision Res 36:1679–1685

Weber P, Pache M, Lutschg J, Kaiser HJ (2004) Visual object and space perception battery: normal values for children from 8 to 12. Klin Monbl Augenheilkd 221:583–587

Weinstein JM, Gilmore RO, Shaikh SM, Kunselman AR, Trescher WV, Tashima LM et al (2012) Defective motion processing in children with cerebral visual impairment due to periventricular white matter damage. Dev Med Child Neurol 54:1–8

Weir CR, Cleary M, Parks S, Dutton GN (2000) Spatial localization in esotropia: does extraretinal eye position information change? Invest Ophthalmol Vis Sci 41:3782–3786

Weiskrantz L (2004) Roots of blindsight. Prog Brain Res 144:229–241

Weiss AH, Kelly JP, Phillips JO (2001) The infant who is visually unresponsive on a cortical basis. Ophthalmology 108:2076–2087

Werth R (2006) Visual functions without the occipital lobe or after cerebral hemispherectomy in infancy. Euro J Neurosci 24:2932–2944

Werth R (2007) Residual visual function after loss of both cerebral hemispheres in infancy. Invest Ophthalmol Vis Sci 48:3098–3106

Werth R (2008) Cerebral blindness and plasticity of the visual system in children. A review of visual capacities in patients with occipital lesions, hemispherectomy or hydranencephaly. Restor Neurol Neurosci 26:377–389

Werth R, Moehrenschlager M (1999) The development of visual functions on cerebrally blind children during a systematic visual field training. Restor Neurol Neurosci 15:229–241

Werth R, Seelos K (2005) Restitution of visual functions in cerebrally blind children. Neuropsychologia 43:2011–2023

White CP, Jan JE (1992) Visual hallucinations after acute visual loss in a young child. Dev Med Child Neurol 34:259–261

White SJ, Staub A (2012) The distribution of fixation durations during reading: effects of stimulus quality. J Exp Psychol Hum Percept Perform 38:603–617

Wijnroks L (1998) Early maternal stimulation and the development of cognitive competence and attention of preterm infants. Early Dev Parent 7:19–30

Williams LM, Hermens DF, Palmer D, Kohn M, Clarke S, Keage H et al (2008) Misinterpreting emotional expressions in attention-deficit/hyperactivity disorder: evidence for a neural marker and stimulant effects. Biol Psychiatry 63:917–926

Williams C, Northstone K, Sabates R, Feinstein L, Emond A, Dutton GN (2011) Visual perceptual difficulties and under-achievement at school in a large community-based sample of children. PLoS One 6(3):e14772

Williams C, Northstone K, Borwick C, Gainsborough M, Roe J, Howard S et al (2014) How to help children with neurodevelopmental and visual problems: a scoping review. Br J Ophthalmol 98:6–12

Wilson CE, Palermo R, Schmalzl L, Brock J (2010) Specificity of impaired facial identity recognition in children with suspected developmental prosopagnosia. Cogn Neuropsychol 27:30–45

Wilson CE, Palermo R, Brock J (2012) Visual scan path and recognition of facial identity in autism spectrum disorder and typical development. PLoS One 7:e37681

Wittenberg GF, Werhahn KJ, Wassermann EM, Herscovitch P, Cohen LG (2004) Functional connectivity between somatosensory and visual cortical areas in early blind humans. Euro J Neurosci 20:1923–1927

Wong AM, Sharpe JA (1999) Representation of the visual field in the human occipital cortex: a magnetic resonance imaging and perimetric correlation. Arch Ophthalmol 117:208–217

Wygnanksi-Jaffe T, Panton CM, Buncic JR, Westall CA (2009) Paradoxical robust visual evoked potentials in young patients with cortical blindness. Doc Ophthalmol 119:101–107

Xerri C, Merzenich MM, Jenkins W, Santucci S (1999) Representational plasticity in cortical area 3b paralleling tactual-motor skill acquisition in adult monkeys. Cereb Cortex 9:264–276

Yantis S (2013) Sensation and perception. Worth Publishers, New York

Ying GS, Maguire MG, Cyert LA, Ciner E, Quinn GE, Kulp MT, Vision In Preschoolers (VIP) Study Group et al (2014) Prevalence of vision disorders by racial and ethnic group among children participating in head start. Ophthalmology 121:630–636

Yokochi K (1991) Paroxysmal ocular downward deviation in neurologically impaired infants. Pediatr Neurol 7:426–428

Zeki S (1993) A vision of the brain. Blackwell Scientific, Oxford

Zemach IK, Teller DY (2007) Infant color vision: infants' spontaneous preferences are well behaved. Vision Res 47:1362–1367

Zemach IK, Chang S, Teller DY (2007) Infant color vision: prediction of infants' spontaneous color preferences. Vision Res 47:1368–1381

Zihl J (2011) Rehabilitation of cerebral visual disorders, 2nd edn. Psychology Press, Hove

Zihl J (2014) Perceptual disorders. In: Ochsner K, Kosslyn SM (eds) The Oxford handbook of cognitive neuroscience. Oxford University Press, Oxford, pp 193–211

Zihl J, Hebel N (1997) Oculomotor scanning patterns in patients with unilateral posterior parietal or frontal lobe damage. Neuropsychologia 33:287–303

Zihl J, von Cramon D, Mai N (1983) Selective disturbance of movement vision after bilateral brain damage. Brain 106:313–340

Zihl J, Fink T, Pargent F, Ziegler M, Bühner M (2014) Cognitive reserve in young and old subjects: differences and similarities in a testing-the-limits paradigm with DSST. PLoS One 9(1):e84590. doi:10.1371/journal.pone.0084590

Index

J. Zihl, G. Dutton, *Cerebral Visual Impairment in Children: Visuoperceptive and Visuocognitive Disorders*, DOI 10.1007/978-3-7091-1815-3

Printed in the United States
By Bookmasters